HEARING LOSS

JOSEPH SATALOFF, M.D., D.SC. (MED.)

Visiting Professor of Otology and Co-director of Industrial Deafness and Otolaryngology Courses, Colby College; Professor of Otology, The Jefferson Medical College of Philadelphia; Consultant in Audiology, Veterans Administration; Associate Editor, A.M.A. Archives of Otolaryngology; Chief of Otology, St. Joseph's Hospital of Philadelphia

HEARING LOSS

J. B. LIPPINCOTT COMPANY

PHILADELPHIA AND TORONTO

Distributed in Great Britain by
Pitman Medical Publishing Co., Limited, London

Library of Congress Catalog Card Number 66-11670

Printed in the United States of America

Dedicated to
FREDERICK THAYER HILL, M.D.,
and
FRED HARBERT, M.D.,
Friends

Preface

The principal purpose of this book is to present in practical but comprehensive form the principles and procedures for determining the causes of hearing loss, including the otologic history, otologic examination and hearing tests. Although most of this information has appeared at some time in isolated form in medical journals or has been touched upon briefly in books on otology and audiology, to the author's knowledge it has not been reviewed systematically in a single volume.

This book has been written with special awareness of the need of busy general practitioners, industrial physicians, internists, pediatricians and others whose practices intersect only incidentally with problems of hearing loss and deafness to have available a handy reference volume that would enable them to be of greater service to their patients.

In addition, medical students, audiologists and other paramedical personnel who lack the time to search through the literature for essential background information may find in this book ready answers to problems that arise in their daily work.

Unavoidably, much of what appears here must seem elementary to specialists in otolaryngology. Nevertheless, it is hoped that they may find this book useful because it seeks to establish a long-needed bridge between otolaryngology and medicine as a whole, and because it fosters greater awareness on the part of nonspecialists of the vital importance of the early recognition and diagnosis of hearing loss so that the patient may have the best opportunity for treatment or rehabilitation.

Many users of this book may be mainly interested in refreshing their recollection of correct technics for testing hearing with a tuning fork and other tests and procedures that can be carried out with simple office equipment. Others may be willing to invest about $300 in an audiometer because of the more accurate and quantitative measurements possible with this device. Regardless of how the physician resolves this question, he should be familiar with the uses of this instrument and know how to interpret an audiogram when an otolaryngologist or a hearing clinic sends him such a chart on a patient whom he has referred.

Therefore, while full consideration is given to the great usefulness and scope of simple tests with a 500-cycle tuning fork, the limitations of such tests are realistically pointed out, and the reader is given systematic instruction in the interpretation of audiometric findings, not only in the more common, uncomplicated cases but also in the more complex situations with which the physician should have some degree of familiarity.

Treatment of disorders of the ear, nose and throat receives only incidental mention in this book, since this subject is rather frequently discussed in medical journals. Nevertheless, forceful references will be made to common errors and misconceptions in treatment that have an unhappy tendency to survive the passage of time.

Since it is hoped that many physicians will use this volume as a general reference work, an effort has been made to include practically all known causes of hearing impairment. Both typical and atypical clinical case reports are presented, with emphasis on the criteria used to establish the diagnosis. All case reports are from the author's personal practice or from that of one of his colleagues, as specified.

Industrial physicians will find this book helpful in deciding whether hearing loss among personnel is related to industrial noise, head injury or nonoccupational causes.

Almost any physician may be the first port of call in cases of hearing loss. This book should help any physician to answer the hard-of-hearing patient's most urgent question, "Can anything be done to restore my hearing, doctor?"

Although this book is based on the author's experience in clinical practice and at the hearing center of the U. S. Naval Hospital in Philadelphia, many colleagues indirectly have contributed to its writing. I particularly express my deep appreciation to Philip H. Van Itallie, whose editorial judgment has helped me achieve the desired clarity and organization of my manuscript. The real motivating force for the actual completion of this book came from two close friends, Dr. E. A. Irvin, Medical Director of the Ford Motor Company, and Floyd Frazier, Executive Director of the National Association of Mutual Casualty Companies. Both men emphasized the vital need among industrial physicians and general practitioners for a book of this type. I am also indebted to Drs. John Zapp and George Shambaugh, special friends, for their kind encouragement and friendship.

To the faculty and students of Colby College, Waterville, Maine, and to the college administration I also express my thanks for the many summers of delight spent in exchanging otologic information during the courses in Occupational Deafness and Otolaryngology. To my good friends, Dr. Ted Hill and Dr. Fred Harbert, I feel a special debt of gratitude. Their friendship and that of the late Dr. George M. Coates played a major role in the modest success I have achieved in my chosen profession.

A special word of thanks for tirelessly typing and retyping this manuscript goes to Mary Jane Grooms and Jean Mason, and many thanks also are due to Larry Vassallo, who carefully reread this manuscript and made many useful suggestions.

I should like to pay a warm tribute to the Felician Sisters of St. Joseph's Hospital for their unselfish devotion to the care of patients. Their dedicated example has been an inspiration in my practice of otology.

JOSEPH SATALOFF

Contents

xi

Chapter 1

Hearing Loss and the Physician

When hard-of-hearing patients are set adrift without a physician's responsible guidance, they may go directly to hearing aid dealers without a diagnosis or even a medical examination. Though many "hearing centers" are conducted in an ethical manner, there are countless instances in which a patient whose deafness could have been cured ends instead with a hearing aid. Others are sold hearing aids that they cannot use satisfactorily, because they are high-pressured into making a choice from an inadequate selection of instruments; when they become dissatisfied, they are told they have to stick with their bargain.

On the other hand, in fairness to hearing aid dealers, it must be admitted that in many types of hearing loss, a hearing aid provides the only possible way in which a patient can be helped to hear, and this help is by no means perfect. It is necessary for the patient to realize that no hearing aid can overcome the distortion produced by sensorineural deafness. Yet it is painful for a patient to accept these disagreeable facts. It takes time to learn to use a hearing aid, and the patient must be willing to live within his limitations. It takes time, effort and patience to get these ideas across, and often the patient's only chance to receive a clear explanation of his hearing trouble—what he has to look forward to, and what can be done about it— is to go to a physician who can give him the facts and advise him properly.

The patient's personality and financial need to hear also enter into the way he adapts to his handicap, including his willingness to wear a hearing aid and perhaps to take up speech reading. A person who must make a living will put up with these discomforts more readily than an old person who is willing to retire into the comfortable silence of a restricted existence.

A Challenging Problem and Its Effect on Personality. Deafness is one of the most challenging problems confronting medicine, not only because of its high incidence but especially because no physical disability can

1

affect personality so adversely as a hearing loss—and the loss need not even be severe. On the contrary, a mild hearing loss, particularly one caused by otosclerosis, may at times produce more psychological disturbance than a severe hearing deficit. It is this effect of hearing loss on the patient's emotions rather than the actual deafness that persuades the patient to seek the help of a physician. The hearing loss itself bothers the people around him, but it may not disturb the patient greatly. It is a rather strange symptom, for it is not accompanied by pain, discomfort, itch or fear, as is true of cancer and other diseases that impel patients to seek medical aid. Hearing loss is a symptom, not a disease.

Consider for a moment what motivates a patient to visit a doctor and complain of hearing trouble. More than likely it is the embarrassing situations that arise with increasing frequency in his everday living. He may fail to hear or to understand his employer when he is given directions, especially when there is much noise around him. Or a secretary may fail to take dictation correctly, and the resulting mistakes cause a great deal of tension in the office. Or a young lady may have been trying to hide from herself and her friends that she has a hearing loss, but when she goes out on a date, she repeatedly may give the wrong answers, especially when it is dark in the car, and she is unable to read the face of her companion. A husband may sit and read his newspaper and fail to understand what his wife is saying while she is washing dishes in the kitchen; this situation may lead to constant friction between husband and wife, with complete lack of communication, and eventually it may grow into marital strife.

These situations are typical of the embarrassing circumstances that produce feelings of inadequacy and insecurity. Yet the patient is unable forthrightly to face the problem that eventually leads him to seek the help of a physician. Furthermore, even when he does come to a physician to complain of deafness, he rarely comes of his own free will. He usually is nagged into coming by his spouse, friends or boss, who have been trying for years to get him to do something about his hearing difficulty.

Not infrequently, when a husband and a wife walk into the otologist's office, the dialogue follows a familiar pattern. The physician asks the man what his difficulty is, and before he has a chance to answer, his wife blurts out that he is deaf, and he doesn't pay attention to her. The husband generally looks meek and bewildered, as if he is not sure what is going on, but he certainly doesn't want to assume the blame for all of his difficulty. It soon becomes apparent that bickering and strife are the keynote of the troubles brought on by his hearing difficulty.

Early Stages of a Hearing Loss. Unfortunately, patients do not really notice any hearing loss until their hearing level has deteriorated rather markedly. In the early stages of a measurable hearing loss, one that can be detected with good hearing tests, there are actually no symptoms except perhaps in the higher frequencies, and the patient may say that he cannot hear his watch tick in one ear as well as he can in the other. If he is of this observant turn of mind, he may seek help for not being able to hear his watch tick.

Every Patient Can Be Helped. The serious effect on the emotions caused by deficient hearing is the major reason for the categorical statement that every patient with a hearing loss who visits his physician can be helped in some way. Not always may it be possible to restore hearing to normal or to improve it to a nonhandicapping level, but it is possible always to mitigate the psychological impact of a hearing loss on the patient. He can be taught to hear better with the hearing he has left, his pessimistic and antagonistic attitude toward his problem can be corrected, and in many ways he can be instructed to communicate better.

Referral of Patients by Various Specialists. Interestingly enough, many patients are referred to an otolaryngologist, not by the general practitioner, internist, or pediatrician, but by a surprising variety of other physicians, such as obstetricians, dermatologists, psychiatrists and even proctologists. Patients seem to have a strange inclination to reveal their hearing loss symptoms under the most unusual circumstances. For example, astute obstetricians have referred to me many patients who had complained of buzzing in their ears during the last month of pregnancy or shortly post-partum. The usual finding in these cases is otosclerosis, which accounts for the buzzing tinnitus. Obstetricians should be alert to a family history of hearing loss, because this is associated with otosclerosis, a condition often aggravated by pregnancy or possibly presenting initially after delivery.

Hearing loss is reported commonly in dermatologists' offices by patients whose ear canals repeatedly collect debris from an exfoliative dermatitis. Unless the debris is removed carefully, the canal walls can be injured and the dermatitis aggravated. Psychiatrists should be cognizant of the relationship of hearing loss to emotional disturbances. Hard-of-hearing patients often have been under a psychiatrist's care for a long time before being referred to an otologist for a hearing evaluation. Many psychological and emotional disturbances can be corrected or mitigated by early attention to the patient's hearing. Some deaf but otherwise normal children lamentably have been found in mental institutions.

Although it may appear to be morbidly humorous, it is an actual fact that some patients are most disturbed by their hearing loss when they fail to hear the little sounds that eventually may cause them serious embarrassment, such sounds as the passing of urine or flatus. Several patients have been referred to me by proctologists and urologists for complaints that the patients never had discussed with their general practitioners.

The Value of Understanding and Making Hearing Tests. Detecting hearing loss is often such a simple procedure that physicians of every specialty should have some understanding of hearing tests and be able to make them in their offices whenever the need arises. In most instances a simple test can be done with a 500-cycle tuning fork. However, this instrument will not be of great help in the detection of very minimal high frequency losses above 1,000 and 2,000 cycles and in other very mild hearing losses, but it can prove to be invaluable and very reliable in discovering instances of handicapping hearing impairment.

Although it is usually possible with a 500-cycle tuning fork to determine whether a hearing loss is due to damage to the middle ear or to the sensorineural tract, there are some cases, such as those involving mild hearing losses, in which the tuning fork does not supply sufficient information. The tuning fork will not provide a quantitative determination of hearing loss. For this kind of evaluation, and particularly in cases in which the hearing loss is limited to the high frequency range, it is necessary to use an audiometer. This is a comparatively inexpensive instrument; a good audiometer can be purchased for about $300 and is well worth the price and the small effort needed to acquire skill in its use. The audiometer should include enough equipment to do air conduction and bone conduction tests, and it should have a masking device on it to block out the ear not being tested. Directions for using an audiometer and for avoiding some of the pitfalls in its use are discussed in Chapter 22.

In every community at least some of the pediatricians and some of the general practitioners should have audiometers available to determine hearing levels in their patients. The availability of this instrument is especially essential in communities where there are no otolaryngologists. In larger cities where it is customary for general practitioners and other specialists to refer patients with hearing loss to otolaryngologists, it is advisable for the physician to have a clear understanding of audiometers, so that he may understand the significance of the reports sent to him by the ear specialist. For these reasons an adequate discussion of audiometry is included in this book, and the results of various types of hearing tests are interpreted.

Chapter 2

Classification of Hearing Losses

The cause of a hearing loss, like that of other medical conditions, is determined by obtaining a careful history, making a physical examination and performing certain laboratory tests. In otology, hearing tests play largely the same role as the clinical laboratory does in general medicine.

ESTABLISHING THE SITE OF DAMAGE IN THE AUDITORY SYSTEM

Despite recent great advances in otology, important gaps in our knowledge of the ear remain and so obscure the ultimate causes of some hearing losses. Fortunately, though often it is not possible to determine the cause, if the site of damage in the auditory system can be established, it is possible to decide on the best available treatment and the prognosis. When a hearing loss is classified, the point at which the auditory pathway has failed is narrowed down, and it is determined whether the patient's hearing loss is conductive, sensorineural, central, functional or a mixture of these.

In **conductive hearing loss** the damage is to be found in one of these structures: the external auditory canal, the middle ear or the eustachian tube leading to it. If it is in the middle ear, it may involve, for example, the footplate of the stapes, as in otosclerosis.

In **sensorineural hearing loss** the damage lies medial to the stapedial footplate—in the inner ear or in the auditory nerve. Most physicians have been accustomed to call this condition "perceptive deafness" or "nerve deafness."

In **central hearing loss** the damage is situated in the central nervous system at some point between the auditory nuclei (in the medulla oblongata) and the cortex. The obsolete term "perceptive deafness" in the past also

5

included central hearing loss, a subject on which present knowledge is very limited.

In **functional hearing impairment** there is no detectable organic damage to the auditory pathways, but some underlying psychological or emotional problem is at fault.

Frequently, two or more types of hearing loss are present in one patient, in which case the problem is one of **mixed hearing loss.** However, for practical purposes this term is used only when both conductive and sensorineural hearing losses are present in the same ear.

Each class of hearing loss has certain distinctive characteristics which make it possible to type the vast majority of cases seen in clinical practice. When certain basic characteristics are found, the classification usually can be made with confidence.

CONDUCTIVE HEARING LOSS

In cases of conductive hearing loss, sound waves are not transmitted effectively to the inner ear because of some interference in the external canal, the eardrum, the ossicular chain, the middle ear cavity, the oval window, the round window or the eustachian tube. Since the function of the middle ear is to transmit sound energy efficiently, and that of the eustachian tube is to maintain equal pressure in the middle ear cavity and the external canal, a conductive hearing loss may result from damage to any of these parts. In uncomplicated conditions of this type there is no damage to the inner ear or the neural pathway, and this is the principal difference that distinguishes conductive hearing loss from sensorineural hearing impairment, which affects the inner ear or the auditory nerve or both.

A diagnosis of conductive hearing loss offers the patient a much better prognosis than does one of sensorineural loss, because modern technics make it possible to cure or at least to improve the vast majority of cases in which the damage is in the outer or the middle ear. These patients, even if not treated surgically, are also the ones who stand to gain the most benefit from a hearing aid, because what they need principally is simple amplification. They are not bothered by distortion and other hearing abnormalities which may occur in sensorineural impairments.

SENSORINEURAL HEARING IMPAIRMENT

The combined term "sensorineural" was introduced to replace the ambiguous terms "perceptive deafness" and "nerve deafness." It is a more descriptive and a more accurate anatomic term. Its dual character suggests that two separate areas may be affected, and this is actually the case. The term "sensory" hearing loss is applied when the damage is localized in the inner ear. Another useful synonym is "cochlear" or "inner ear" hearing loss. "Neural" hearing loss is the correct term when the damage is in the auditory nerve proper, anywhere between its fibers at the base of the hair cells and the auditory nuclei. This range includes the bipolar ganglion of the 8th cranial nerve. Other common names for this type of loss are "nerve deafness" and "retrocochlear hearing loss." These names are satisfactory if used appropriately and meaningfully, but too often they are applied improperly.

At present it is common practice to group together both sensory and neural components, but it is possible in many cases to allocate a predominant part of the damage, if not all of it, to the inner ear or to the nerve. Because of this possibility and the likelihood that research soon will make it possible to distinguish even more cases of sensory from neural hearing loss, we shall split the term and describe the distinguishing features of each component. Such a separation is advisable, because the prognosis and the treatment in the two types are different. When we classify a case of hearing loss as sensory or neural, we also can narrow down the specific cause, since it is now known that certain conditions affect the inner ear, whereas others involve only the nerve.

A vital motive for distinguishing sensory from neural hearing impairments arises in cases of unilateral hearing loss in which there are reduced air conduction and bone conduction, along with impaired speech discrimination. In such cases it is essential to distinguish between sensory and neural types, because the neural type may be due to an acoustic neuroma which would make surgery imperative, whereas the sensory type is not nearly so urgent. Those cases which in the present state of knowledge we cannot identify as either sensory or neural and those cases in which there is damage in both regions we shall classify a sensorineural.

The prognosis for restoring hearing in sensorineural hearing loss with presently available therapy is guarded, but spontaneous remissions and hearing improvements with therapy do occur, particularly in the sensory type.

Sensorineural hearing loss is one of the most challenging problems in medicine. Into this group falls a large variety of hearing losses, many of which are little understood. This group includes also the very severe types of unilateral and bilateral deafness and most congenital cases. If to the inadequate knowledge of these conditions is added their poor prognosis, the great need for further research can be readily understood.

There are many different and complex causes of sensorineural hearing loss, but certain features are characteristic and basic to all of them. The history obtained from the patient is usually so variable, because of the great variety of causes, that it contributes far more information to the etiology than it does to the classification of a case.

MIXED HEARING IMPAIRMENT

For practical purposes, in this book a mixed hearing impairment is one in which a conductive hearing loss is accompanied by a sensory or a neural (or a sensorineural) impairment in the same ear. However, the emphasis is on the conductive hearing loss, because available therapy is so much more effective for this group. Consequently, the otologic surgeon has a special interest in cases of mixed hearing impairment in which there is primarily a conductive loss, complicated by some sensorineural damage. In this class of cases the most important are those with otosclerosis having so-called "secondary nerve" involvement.

FUNCTIONAL HEARING IMPAIRMENT

Functional hearing impairment occurs more frequently in clinical practice than many physicians understand. This is the type of condition in which the patient does not seem to hear and to respond; yet the handicap may not be due to any organic pathology in the peripheral or the central auditory pathways.

The hearing difficulty has an emotional or a psychological etiology that may be the entire cause, or it may be superimposed on some mild organic hearing loss, in which case it is called a functional or a psychogenic overlay. Often the patient really has normal hearing underlying the functional hearing impairment. A careful history usually will reveal some hearing impairment in the patient's family or some reference to deafness which served as the nucleus for the patient's functional hearing loss.

The most important challenge in such a case is to classify the condition properly. It may be quite difficult to determine the specific emotional cause, but if the classification is made accurately, the proper therapy can be instituted. Too often the emotional background of a functional hearing loss is not recognized, and patients receive useless otologic treatments for prolonged periods. In turn, this may aggravate the emotional element and cause the condition to become more resistant. Early and accurate classification is urgent.

CENTRAL HEARING IMPAIRMENT (CENTRAL DYSACUSIS)

Because there is so little information about central hearing loss, it remains somewhat of a mystery in otology. Physicians know that some patients cannot interpret or understand what is being said, and that the cause of the difficulty is not in the peripheral mechanism but somewhere in the central nervous system. In central hearing impairment the difficulty is not in a lowered pure tone threshold but in the patient's ability to interpret what he hears. Obviously, to interpret speech is far more complex than merely to respond to a pure tone threshold; consequently, the tests necessary to diagnose central hearing impairment must be designed to assess a patient's ability to handle complex information. Unfortunately, none of the tests available at present is particularly specific for this purpose, and it still requires a very experienced and almost intuitive judgment on the physician's part to make an accurate diagnosis. Aphasia sometimes is considered to be a central hearing loss, but in this book it will not be discussed, because it is for the most part outside the realm of otology.

Chapter 3

How To Classify Hearing Loss
With a Tuning Fork

The best general-purpose tuning fork to use is a 500-cycle steel tuning fork, but if a steel fork is not available, any other will do. We use a 500-cycle tone because forks of lower frequencies produce a greater tactile sensation that sometimes can be felt when they actually are not heard, or that can be felt before the tone is heard. Forks of higher frequencies than 500 cycles are attenuated too readily by the bones of the skull and do not provide as much information.

With the 500-cycle tuning fork it is possible to obtain a rough approximation of the extent of the hearing loss and an excellent idea of whether the cause is conductive (i.e., lies in the outer or the middle ear) or is sensorineural (i.e., is situated in the inner ear or the auditory nerve). In some cases it is possible even to distinguish with a tuning fork whether the damage is in the inner ear itself or in the nerve.

A tuning fork should not be struck very hard; too forceful a blow produces overtones that might give false information. Furthermore, a very loud tone may startle some patients who are especially sensitive to noise because of hyperrecruitment, a condition often present in Ménière's disease. Tuning forks should be struck on something firm, yet not too hard. The knuckle or the elbow or the neurologic rubber hammer is quite satisfactory. Tabletops and wooden chairs should not be used to activate tuning forks. In testing for air conduction the tuning fork should be held close but should not touch the ear, and the broad side of one of the prongs must face the ear (Fig. 1). It is wrong to hold the two prongs parallel with the side of the ear. Such an application often produces a dead spot, and no tones may be heard by the listener, even though his hearing may be normal, and the tone may be quite loud. This can be made clear to the examiner if he places the tuning fork to his own ear and rotates the

FIG. 1. Position of the tuning fork for air conduction testing.

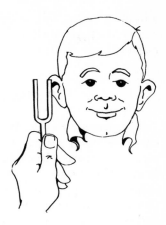

vibrating fork. The tone will appear to go off and on as the correct position is approached.

TWO BASIC TYPES OF TESTING

Two basic types of testing can be done with a tuning fork: air conduction and bone conduction. The first measures the ability of air-borne sound waves to be transmitted along the external canal, the eardrum and the ossicular chain to the inner ear. This is done by holding the vibrating tuning fork near, but not touching, the external auditory canal. The second, bone conduction testing, measures with some reservation the ability of the inner ear and the nerve to receive and to utilize sound stimuli with the air conduction passages bypassed. This is done by not utilizing the external auditory canal and the middle ear areas. The base or the handle of the

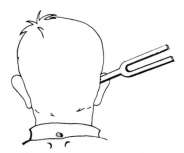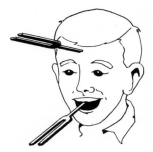

FIG. 2. Placement of the handle of the fork on the mastoid (*left*) and the forehead and the upper incisors (*right*) for bone conduction testing.

vibrating tuning fork is held directly on the skull, so that the vibrations can reach the inner ear directly (Fig. 2). The fork may be held on the mastoid bone, the forehead, the closed mandible or the upper teeth.

FACTORS IN EVALUATION

Approximate Results With the Tuning Fork. In spite of many efforts to calibrate tuning forks quantitatively so that it might be possible to measure a patient's hearing level, as yet no reliable method to achieve this has been found. The tuning fork makes it possible to obtain only a rather rough quantitative approximation of a patient's ability to hear. For example, the physician can strike the fork gently and apply it successively to the left and to the right ear, asking the patient in which ear the sound is louder. Or, the patient's ability to hear a tuning fork can be compared with the doctor's own presumably normal hearing. However, it is not possible to express the results of tuning fork tests in quantitative terms such as decibels. To do this requires an audiometer.

Transmission of Sound to Second Ear. Another important factor to remember when testing hearing with a tuning fork or an audiometer, either by air or bone conduction, is that sounds of sufficient intensity, when applied to or held near one ear, are transmitted around the head or through the bones of the skull and are heard by the opposite ear.

In air conduction testing the tone near one ear has to be quite loud to be carried around the head and heard by the contralateral ear. There is roughly a 50- to 60-db attenuation between the ears; that is to say, when a tone near one ear is 50 to 60 db or louder, it can be heard by the opposite ear. In bone conduction testing the problem is far more complex, because there is little or no attenuation by the skull for bone-conducted sound. Though a tuning fork may be held to the *left* mastoid bone, and the examiner thinks he is testing the *left* ear, actually he is testing *both* ears, because the right ear gets the sound at almost the same intensity as the left ear.

MASKING OUT THE OPPOSITE EAR

For these reasons it is necessary, especially in bone conduction testing, to mask out the opposite ear, to be sure that responses only from the ear tested are being received. This also applies to air conduction testing, particularly when there is a difference of roughly 30 db or over in hearing acuity between the two ears.

One might suppose that the opposite ear could be masked out by putting a plug in the ear or covering it with the patient's hand. Actually, this would not only fail to mask out the ear, but it would cause the tuning fork to be heard even more loudly in the covered-up or plugged ear. To convince yourself of this, you need merely strike a tuning fork and hold the handle to your upper incisors. Generally, if your hearing is normal, the fork will be heard throughout the head and seem to be louder in the plugged ear. Therefore, if you plug one ear with your finger, the fork will be heard immediately in this plugged ear. Actually, rather than masking out the ear, you are referring the bone-conducted tone to the plugged-up ear and making it hear better. A good way to mask out the opposite ear when testing one ear with a tuning fork is to have an assistant or the patient himself rub a page of stiff typewriting paper over the opposite ear. The noise made by this paper occupies the nerve pathway of that ear, and you then can be sure of getting a response only from the ear to which you are applying the tuning fork. Instead of rubbing with paper, the air pressure hose used to spray noses also can be used as a masking device. It should be done cautiously in order not to injure the eardrum. The air nozzle should be applied somewhat sideways in the ear, so that the noise gets into the canal without too much air pressure. A special noise maker, called a Barany noise apparatus, also is available. It is very inexpensive, small and is activated by winding it up and pressing the button.

USING THE TUNING FORK IN DIAGNOSIS

Now that we know the basic essentials of tuning fork testing, let us proceed to use the fork in making a diagnosis in routine office practice, bearing in mind that if only a mild hearing loss is present (that is, less than 15 db in all the frequencies), the tuning fork will not answer the purpose. It is effective only when the hearing loss is at least 15 db or more.

Regular Steps. Let us suppose a patient complains of hearing trouble in his left ear, and the otoscopic examination shows normal external canals and eardrums. What are the steps to find just where in the auditory pathways the damage has occurred, and what is the most likely cause? To determine first if there really is a hearing loss in the patient's left ear, strike the tuning fork gently, hold it to your own normal ear until the tone gets weak, and then quickly put the fork near the patient's left ear, asking him if he hears it. If he does not hear it, put it to his right and presumably normal ear, to be sure the fork is still vibrating. Finally, put it back to your own ear to be sure the tone is still on.

Obviously, if the fork is heard either in your ear or in the patient's good right ear, but he fails to hear it in his left (bad) ear, he must have some hearing loss on the left. Then, by striking the tuning fork a little harder each time and listening with your own normal ear before and after you place it to the patient's left ear, you can determine how loud the fork's vibrations must be for the patient barely to hear them. In this way a rough idea can be gained of the degree of hearing loss.

Converting this finding to decibels by an "educated guess" is surprisingly difficult. It should not be attempted even by so-called experts. If the patient seems to hear what you believe to be an extremely weak tone, almost as weak as you can hear, the chances are that his hearing loss, if it exists, is too mild to be studied with a tuning fork, or perhaps it is present only in the higher frequencies. In either case, audiometric studies are required.

Rinne Test. Now let us presume that the patient does have a moderate hearing loss in the left ear and does not respond to a vibrating tuning fork that you hear. The next step is to determine whether the damage is in the conductive area (the outer or the middle ear) or in the sensorineural pathways (the inner ear or the auditory nerve). The patient now is asked to tell you whether the vibrating tuning fork seems to be louder when it is held beside his left ear (by air) or behind his left ear directly on the mastoid bone (by bone). The tuning fork is struck hard enough so that the patient should be able to hear it fairly well, and it is held beside his left ear for about a second. Then it is quickly moved until its handle touches the left mastoid bone, where it is held for another second. Move the fork back and forth between these two points, striking the fork again, if necessary, until the patient can tell whether it is louder by air or behind the ear. This is the so-called Rinne test.

If the fork is louder behind the ear, that is, on the patient's mastoid bone, then his bone conduction is considered to be better than his air conduction, and therefore he has a conductive deafness. In other words, his sensorineural pathway is working quite satisfactorily, but something is blocking the sound waves from reaching his inner ear.

Furthermore, since the outer ear meanwhile was examined and found to be normal, the most likely diagnosis is some defect in the ossicular chain, particularly otosclerosis.

Weber Test. To confirm these findings, the tuning fork now is struck again, and the handle is placed on the patient's forehead or gently touching his upper incisor teeth. He then is asked in which ear the fork sounds louder (the so-called Weber test). In a conductive hearing loss he generally will hear it louder in his bad ear (left, in this case). Something like this happens when you plug your own ear while the fork is on your teeth; you probably will be surprised to hear it louder in the plugged ear. Plugging the ear produces a conductive hearing loss just as otosclerosis does.

Schwabach Test. Occasionally, a patient will find it difficult to lateralize the fork to either ear, i.e., to tell in which it sounds louder. This reaction does not rule out conductive deafness but suggests repeated studies, particularly with an audiometer. To complete the fork tests on this particular patient with a presumptive diagnosis of otosclerosis, the fork is struck gently and pressed against the patient's left mastoid area until he barely hears it, and then you move the instrument quickly to your own mastoid (the Schwabach test). The patient will prove to hear the tuning fork much better and longer by bone conduction on his mastoid than even you yourself can hear it. This is called prolonged bone conduction and substantiates a diagnosis of conductive hearing loss.

Further Tests. Now let us examine a different patient with normal otoscopic findings who also is complaining of left-sided hearing loss. When we compare his ability to hear by air and bone conduction (Rinne test), we find he hears much better by air conduction than by bone, in contrast with the previous patient. Furthermore, when we put the tuning fork to his teeth, he hears it louder in his good ear than in his bad ear (Weber test). Then, when his bone conduction is compared with your own (Schwabach test), you find that you can hear a tone much longer and louder than he can. It is important in this last test to mask out the good ear with noise so that the sound of the fork pressed against the mastoid of the bad ear may not be heard in the good ear. The site of damage in this patient is not in his middle or outer ear, as in the previous case, but in his inner ear or auditory nerve. He has sensorineural deafness, and the most likely cause will have to be determined by exploring the history and performing many more tests, some of which require special equipment (see Chap. 24). In Chapter 24 will be found an explanation of how it is possible with a tuning fork to decide in some patients whether the damage is located specifically in the inner ear proper; in these cases the most likely diagnosis will be Ménière's disease.

Difficult Cases. These two patients were comparatively easy to classify, and most patients are actually just as easy to test, but occasionally cases are encountered that are much more difficult, particularly when the same patient has a severe or even total loss of hearing in one ear and a partial conductive hearing loss in the other. A great deal of masking and careful interpretation of hearing tests are necessary in such cases; yet the tuning fork can provide the essential information, and each ear often can be classified properly.

Determining the site of damage can be done readily with a tuning fork, but in some instances this may become difficult, and it may be especially difficult to decide which of many possible causes applies. More sophisticated tests with an audiometer and other equipment are helpful in such instances, but the tuning fork should be used routinely to confirm or to challenge the results obtained with the more discriminating and complex equipment.

Better Service Through the Audiometer and the Tuning Fork. Few general practitioners have audiometers today, but many more would find it rewarding to purchase one and learn to perform audiometric hearing tests. It would enable them to render better service to some of their patients, just as electrocardiography refines their service to others. The technics for performing good audiometry and the pitfalls to be avoided are described in Chapter 22. If a practitioner prefers not to use an audiometer but to refer his patients to a local otolaryngologist or hearing center, he should make it a routine policy to confirm all studies done by consultants with his own tuning fork tests.

Even when a general practitioner decides to refer a case to a consultant who has more elaborate equipment and testing experience, he should not underestimate the importance of the simple tuning fork in the diagnosis of hearing loss.

Chapter 4

The Audiogram

A more detailed treatment of the subject of audiometry is to be found in Chapter 22, but since audiograms are referred to extensively in the intervening chapters, the basic information needed to interpret an audiogram is presented here. What do the numbers mean? What is zero db or normal hearing, and what, especially is −10 db of "hearing loss"? What is a high tone or a low tone loss?

Definition. An audiogram is simply a written record of a person's hearing level measured with certain pure tones. The pure tones generally used are the frequencies 250, 500, 1,000, 2,000, 3,000, 4,000, 6,000 and 8,000 cycles per second; these tones are electronically generated by the audiometer. This particular frequency range covers the speech spectrum.

Terms. With 0 db representing average normal hearing, a hearing level of 60 db means that it takes 60 decibels more sound pressure for a patient to begin hearing than it does for a person with normal hearing. Obviously, this 60 db hearing threshold level also can be called a 60 db hearing loss. Though both terms describe the same condition, the term "hearing level" is currently finding favor in otology, because it emphasizes the hearing that the patient still has left rather than the hearing that he has lost. Also, since among normal-hearing persons a −10 db level is a gain rather than a loss, the term "level" avoids the confusion of "negative losses," and provides a more positive approach in helping patients with deficient hearing.

However, the term "hearing loss" is still in common use, and since this book is concerned with the diagnosis of hearing losses, the words "loss" and "level" will both be used interchangeably to indicate the threshold of a person's hearing.

In the near future the standard of 0 db on the audiometer, now used as normal hearing, may be changed. When the new standard is in common use, the new terms "hearing threshold level" or "hearing level" will have greater validity and medical popularity; it then will become easier to adjust to them.

Reference Hearing Level. In recent years efforts have been made to change the American Standard Association reference hearing level (ASA) to conform with the reference level used in European countries, International Standards Organization (ISO). The issue has not been resolved completely, and for that reason all graphic audiograms used in this book use the two reference levels. The present ASA reference level appears on the left side, and the proposed ISO reference level appears on the right side of each audiogram. All hearing levels shown in numerals are ASA reference levels.

Horizontal and Vertical Variables in a Graphic Audiogram. Ideally, one should measure a patient's ability to hear actual speech, but this criterion has certain difficulties, and therefore pure tones commonly are used. For simplicity, only the specific frequencies indicated above were selected for routine use. They are called *octave frequencies*, because each successive tone as it goes up the scale is an octave above the one immediately below it, and for each higher octave the number of cycles per second is doubled. Octave frequencies constitute the horizontal variable in an audiogram.

Every audiogram approximates the weakest intensity at which a given patient is able to hear each one of these frequencies. This is the vertical variable in an audiogram: how well the patient hears at each frequency. Does he hear the tone as well as a person with normal hearing, or does it have to be made louder for him to hear it, and if so, how much louder? To make this comparison one must have a normal base line for each frequency.

WHAT IS NORMAL HEARING?

The threshold of a normal-hearing person at the various frequencies originally was obtained by testing a large number of young people between the ages of 20 and 29 and determining the intensities of the thresholds at the various frequencies. It was found that the thresholds fluctuated over about a 20-db range even in subjects with normal hearing. An average was reached at 0 db of hearing. Some subjects heard better than 0; many of them heard tones as weak as −10. Others did not hear a sound until it was amplified to a level between 0 and 10 db. This variation indicated that the range between −10 and +10 db could be considered as normal for the average young person.

Many people can hear at −15 db, which may be below the range that the audiometer records. Average normal hearing, or 0 db, is the reference level on the audiometer, and a hearing loss at some specific frequency is expressed and recorded as the number of decibels by which a tone must be amplified for a patient to hear it.

FORMS OF THE AUDIOGRAM

The audiogram showing a patient's hearing threshold for the standard range of frequencies can be recorded in several ways. The most common form of audiogram is a graph on which the frequencies are marked off from left to right, and the tone intensities range up and down. Figure 3, which shows such a graph, indicates the conventional marks by which the curve for the left ear can be distinguished from that for the right ear. A series of X marks connected by a dashed line denotes the left, whereas circles connected by a solid line represent the right ear. The short arrows found hereafter on some audiograms indicate that there was no response to the test tone at the output limits of the audiometer.

Figure 4 shows another form of recording these thresholds in which the intensities are recorded numerically and serially instead of being plotted. The author uses this form routinely in his practice, but since the graph form is more familiar to most readers, it is used throughout the book except in those instances in which several thresholds are recorded; in such cases the serial form is utilized. The notation NR on the serial form denotes that there was no response to the test tone at the output limits of the

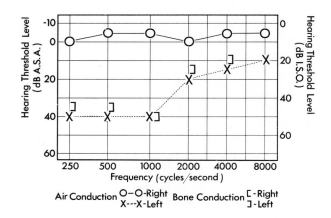

Fig. 3. *Audiometric findings:* right ear thresholds for air- and bone-conducted pure tones are normal. Left ear has reduced air and bone thresholds of about the same magnitude (no air-bone gap). Right ear was masked during all testing of the left ear.

Speech reception threshold: Right, 5 db   Left, 45 db
Discrimination score: Right, 98%   Left, 62%

Tuning fork lateralizes to right ear.

Tuning fork on left shows air is better than bone conduction (A > B), and bone conduction is reduced on the left mastoid.

audiometer. The letters WN indicate that white noise was used for masking (see Chap. 23).

WHAT THE AUDIOMETER MEASURES

Commercial audiometers are so calibrated and recording methods are so standardized that what is recorded is not a patient's ability to hear but rather his hearing *loss* in the frequencies tested. If he can hear 0 db, he has no hearing loss, but if he cannot hear until the tone is 30 db louder than 0 db, then he has a hearing loss of 30 db, and this is so recorded on the audiogram.

HEARING RECORD

NAME

AIR CONDUCTION

		RIGHT							LEFT							
DATE	Exam.	LEFT MASK	250	500	1000	2000	4000	8000	RIGHT MASK	250	500	1000	2000	4000	8000	

BONE CONDUCTION

		RIGHT							LEFT							
DATE	Exam.	LEFT MASK	250	500	1000	2000	4000		RIGHT MASK	250	500	1000	2000	4000		

SPEECH RECEPTION								DISCRIMINATION	RIGHT				LEFT				
DATE	RIGHT	LEFT MASK	LEFT	RIGHT MASK	FREE FIELD	MIC.		DATE	% SCORE	TEST LEVEL	LIST	LEFT MASK	% SCORE	TEST LEVEL	LIST	RIGHT MASK	EXAM.

HIGH FREQUENCY THRESHOLDS

	RIGHT						LEFT						
DATE	4000	8000	10000	12000	14000	LEFT MASK	RIGHT MASK	4000	8000	10000	12000	14000	

RIGHT		WEBER	LEFT		HEARING AID		
RINNE	SCHWABACH		RINNE	SCHWABACH	DATE	MAKE	MODEL
					RECEIVER	GAIN	EXAM.
					EAR	DISCRIM.	COUNC.

REMARKS

FIG. 4. Serial form used by the author in clinical practice. The special tests below the bone conduction results are described in Chapter 24.

Though the audiometer record is negative in that it measures the hearing that the patient has lost rather than the hearing which he still has, the pure tone audiometer nevertheless offers the best means yet devised for measuring hearing.

INTERPRETING THE TYPICAL AUDIOGRAM

Now let us look at a typical audiogram and interpret it.

In Figure 3, the left ear (X's connected with dashed lines) shows a level of about 40 db up to a frequency of 1,000 cycles; then the curve approaches more normal hearing (the zero line on the graph). We would say, then, that this patient hears high tones better than low tones. This is an ascending curve, and the patient is said to have a low tone hearing loss. Hearing in the right ear is normal (0 connected with continuous lines).

Frequencies are measured in cycles per second (cps). The sound intensities are measured in decibels (db), which are rather complex logarithmic units; they are discussed in Chapter 20. The reader also is referred to Chapter 24 for information on special studies, such as bone conduction, adaptation and recruitment, and speech discrimination. However, since these concepts necessarily come up in the earlier chapters on classification of hearing loss, it is necessary to define them briefly here.

Air Conduction. This denotes the ability of the ear to receive and conduct sound waves entering the external ear canal. Normally, these waves cause the eardrum to vibrate, and the vibrations are transmitted through the chain of ossicles to the oval window. When air conduction is impaired as a result of damage to the outer or the middle ear, and the sensorineural mechanism of the inner ear is intact, the maximum hearing loss by air conduction is of the order of 60 db. This is so for the reason that when the sound is louder than 60 db, it will be conducted by the bones of the skull directly to the cochlea and thus will be perceived.

Bone Conduction. To some extent this is a measure of the patient's ability to hear sound vibrations that are transmitted directly to the cochlea through the bones of the skull, bypassing the outer and the middle ear. Bone conduction is virtually unimpaired in simple conductive hearing loss. Thus, conductive hearing loss can be distinguished from sensorineural hearing impairment by tuning forks or bone conduction audiometry.

Tuning Fork Tests. An individual who enjoys normal hearing hears much better by air than by bone conduction. If a vibrating tuning fork is placed near such a person's ear, he will hear it much longer and louder than if it is placed in direct contact with some part of the skull or the teeth.

However, another person may hear the tuning fork's vibrations longer and louder when it is in contact with his skull than when he hears the sound by air conduction; this response indicates a conductive hearing loss. Such a person may hear the tuning fork by bone conduction even better than a normal-hearing person. In such cases something is obstructing transmission of air-conducted sound and preventing it from reaching the sensorineural mechanism. The interference must be in the outer or the middle ear, and the resulting hearing loss is of the conductive type.

Bone Conduction Tests. Another way to measure bone conduction is by the audiometer. It is essential to use proper masking to be certain that what is being tested is the response of the ear under study, and that the response is not in part traceable to the other ear.

Although sounds up to about 50 db directed to one ear by air conduction through an audiometer usually are heard by that ear alone, this is not the case with bone conduction. Bone-conducted sounds are heard almost equally well by both ears no matter where the vibrations are impressed upon the skull. This holds true of both the tuning fork and the audiometer. The proper way to minimize confusion when the test sound is heard by the opposite ear is to mask the latter by introducing enough neutral sound into it to occupy its auditory pathway and so prevent the test tone from reaching it.

A common way of recording bone conduction by a graph type of audiogram is shown in Figure 3. The open cusps or brackets are used to symbolize the ear as it faces the examiner. This becomes clear from a caricature of a face showing that] is the left ear and [the right.

Or the bone conduction can be recorded numerically, as in the serial type of audiogram (Fig. 4).

When the bone conduction and the air conduction curves or levels are of the same magnitude, there is *no air-bone gap*. But if the bone conduction level is better (i.e., shows less hearing loss and is closer to the normal hearing level), then there is said to be an *air-bone gap*.

Speech Reception Threshold. This is a measure of a person's ability to hear, not pure tones, but speech, using a special audiometer that controls the intensity of the speech output. One can test the speech reception threshold by means of simple 2-syllable words or sentences to determine the weakest intensity at which the subject can hear well enough to repeat the spoken words or the sentences. A normal-hearing person can hear and repeat these words at a level of about 0 to 10 db. For hard-of-hearing individuals the speech reception threshold is higher; i.e., the speech has to be made louder to enable them to repeat it. The higher the number of decibels, the greater is the hearing loss.

Discrimination Score. This measures not the weakest intensity at which the patient hears speech sounds but how well he can repeat correctly certain representative words delivered to his ear at a reasonably loud level. The normal-hearing person discriminates between 90 and 100 per cent of the words he hears. Because of distortion and damage to the sensorineural mechanism, some hard-of-hearing patients can discriminate only 30 or 40 per cent of the words spoken to them.

Recruitment. This is basically an abnormally large growth in the sensation of loudness in a hard-of-hearing person when a sound delivered to the ear is increased in intensity. To a patient with recruitment a tone that sounds soft to him becomes loud much more suddenly and rapidly when its intensity is increased, than it does to a person without recruitment. This phenomenon is especially marked in patients with sensory hearing loss and is generally absent in patients with conductive and neural hearing loss.

Abnormal Tone Decay or Pathologic Adaptation. This finding is included in audiometry because of its increasing importance as a diagnostic criterion; it occurs predominantly in neural hearing impairment. A patient who exhibits abnormal tone decay is unable to continue hearing for any length of time a tone at threshold when it is prolonged at a uniform level of intensity. Such a person's hearing fatigues rapidly. The phenomenon is called pathologic fatigue or abnormal tone decay.

A normal-hearing person continues to hear a very weak threshold tone for several minutes, but an individual with abnormal tone decay may hear the sound only for several seconds. He then will ask that the sound be made louder. When this is done, the patient will hear the sound again for a few seconds, only to lose it again quickly and request that the volume be increased—and so on.

SUMMARY

The concepts discussed and defined in this chapter are the most important ones in audiometry, and the physician who has familiarized himself with them can readily interpret the audiograms in the chapters that follow.

Chapter 5

Conductive Hearing Loss: Diagnostic Criteria

Certain findings are characteristic of conductive hearing loss. The most essential ones are that the patient hears better by bone than he does by air conduction, and that the bone conduction is approximately normal. It would seem that these observations should suffice for classifying a case as conductive. Unfortunately, they are not always reliable, because some patients are encountered who have conductive hearing loss and yet also have reduced bone conduction, as it now is measured. The difficulty is that bone conduction tests alone do not always provide an accurate assessment of the sensorineural mechanism. Other tests often are necessary, and for this reason it is essential to have a clear understanding of the symptoms and the features that characterize a conductive hearing loss.

CHARACTERISTIC FEATURES

These features are provided by the history, the otologic examination and the hearing tests.

1. The history may reveal a discharging ear or a previous ear infection. A feeling of fullness, as if fluid were trapped in the ear, may accompany the hearing loss; or a sudden unilateral hearing loss may follow an effort to clean out wax with a fingertip. There may be a history of a ruptured or perforated eardrum. Often the hearing loss is of gradual onset and is aggravated by pregnancy. The hearing loss may even have been present at birth or noted in early childhood.

2. Tinnitus may be present and most frequently is described as low-pitched or buzzing.

24

3. If the hearing loss is bilateral, the patient generally speaks with a soft voice, especially if the etiology is otosclerosis.

4. The patient hears better in noisy areas (paracusis willisiana).

5. Occasionally, the patient claims he does not hear well if he is eating foods that make loud noises when chewed, such as celery or carrots.

6. There is a hearing loss by air conduction.

7. The bone conduction threshold is normal or almost normal.

8. An air-bone gap is present.

9. Otologic examination may reveal abnormality in the external auditory canal, the eardrum or the middle ear. When only the ossicular chain is involved, the visible findings through an otoscope may be normal.

10. There is no difficulty in discriminating speech if it is loud enough.

11. Recruitment and abnormal tone decay are absent.

12. If the two ears have different hearing levels, the tuning fork lateralizes to the ear with the worse hearing.

13. The maximum hearing loss possible in pure conductive hearing impairment is about 60 db.

14. The patient's hearing responses often are indecisive when they are tested at threshold during audiometry. This is in contrast with sharp endpoints in testing for sensorineural hearing losses.

It is helpful to understand the reasons for these characteristics so that they may be logically interpreted rather than merely memorized for classifying a clinical case.

When the patient's history reveals external or middle ear infections associated with hearing loss, conductive hearing impairment may be suspected. Complaints may include a discharging ear, an infected external or middle ear, impacted wax, and a feeling of fluid in the ear accompanied by fullness. Often the fluid seems to move with a change in position of the ear. These symptoms justify a suspicion of conductive hearing loss and suggest the need of confirmatory tests. Too hasty a classification may lead to the embarrassment of a retraction. It is wise to recall at this point that fluid in the middle ear, as in secretory otitis media, produces not only a reduced air conduction threshold but sometimes may affect bone conduction as well—especially at high frequencies—even though the sensorineural mechanism is intact. The bone conduction threshold may be depressed, and yet when the fluid is surgically removed, both air and bone conduction levels quickly return to normal.

The hard-of-hearing patient's answers to the physician's questions invariably provide essential clues both to classification and etiology. Chapter 18 is devoted to this subject.

Among the distinguishing features of conductive hearing loss elicited by careful questioning are the following:

1. The patient has no difficulty in understanding what he hears as long

as people speak loud enough (because in conductive hearing loss only the threshold is affected, not the discrimination).

2. The patient often hears better in noisy areas, such as on a bus or at a cocktail party. The reason for this is that people speak more loudly in noisy places, and the patient can hear the speaker's voice better above the background noises.

3. The otosclerotic patient may say that he has trouble hearing when he chews noisy foods (because these noises are easily transmitted to the ears by bone conduction and produce a masking effect, with the result that he cannot hear air-borne speech as well).

4. Another related finding in conductive hearing loss, but most prominent in otosclerosis, is the patient's remarkably soft voice. A soft voice in the presence of insidious hearing loss immediately should suggest otosclerosis, particularly if a buzzing tinnitus is present. The voice is soft because the patient's excellent bone conduction gives him the impression that his voice is louder than it actually is. Consequently, he lowers his voice to such a soft level that often it is difficult to hear him. Tinnitus is rarely present in conductive hearing loss, except in otosclerosis, and then it is described as low-pitched—often buzzing. When otosclerosis is present, there frequently is a family history of similar hearing loss.

When inspection of the external ear canal or middle ear reveals any obstructive abnormality, a conductive hearing loss should be suspected. But before deciding on this classification, one should first rule out a possible sensorineural loss, which also may be present. Bone conduction studies can resolve this question. If otologic findings are normal, and there is a significant air-bone gap (that is, if the bone conduction is better than the air conduction), there is a conductive loss—probably due to some defect in the ossicular chain. Occasionally, fluid causing a conductive hearing loss escapes otoscopic detection because of its peculiar position, and the hearing loss is attributed to a defect in the ossicular chain rather than to the fluid.

Whenever a hearing loss is substantially in excess of 60 db, some other type of damage is almost certain to be superimposed on that which produces the conductive hearing loss. The reason for this is that even complete disruption of the sound transmission mechanism of the middle ear produces a loss of only about 60 db. For example, a complete break of this kind may occur in a radical mastoidectomy or in congenital aplasia of the middle ear.

FINDINGS IN VARIOUS TESTS

In a pure conductive hearing loss the bone conduction is normal or almost normal, because there is no damage to the inner ear or the auditory nerve. We say "almost normal" for good reason. In some cases of pure conductive hearing loss there is a mild reduction in bone conduction, especially in the higher frequencies, even though the sensorineural mechanism is normal. This observation emphasizes a significant blind spot in bone conduction tests; they are really not a completely reliable measure of the function of the sensorineural mechanism or cochlear reserve, and reduced bone conduction sometimes may be due to a mechanical obstruction.

An air-bone gap is present in uncomplicated conductive hearing loss

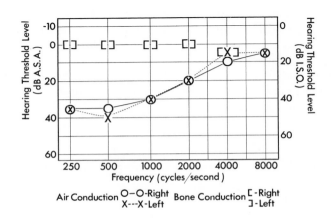

Air Conduction O–O-Right
            X---X-Left
Bone Conduction ⌈-Right
            ⌉-Left

Fig. 5. Ascending audiogram typical of conductive hearing loss. Bone conduction is better than air conduction and is normal. Discrimination is excellent.

History: 24-year-old female complaining of insidious hearing loss and buzzing tinnitus over 10 years. One aunt uses hearing aid. Has trouble hearing soft voices but understands clearly when voice is loud. Hears better at cocktail parties and noisy places. Voice is soft and barely audible.

Otologic: normal

Audiologic: vague responses during audiometry and fluctuating hearing levels. Bilateral air-bone gap present. Opposite ear masked during bone conduction tests.

Speech reception threshold: Right 30 db   Left 35 db
Discrimination score: Right 100%   Left 100%

Bone conduction prolonged and better than air conduction by tuning fork. Vague lateralization to right ear.

Classification: conductive

Diagnosis: otosclerosis. Confirmed at surgery and hearing restored.

Aids to diagnosis: The combination of being able to hear better in noisy places and the presence of a soft voice indicates a conductive lesion which was confirmed by audiometric testing (air-bone gap). Normal otologic findings suggest stapes fixation (otosclerosis).

because the air conduction threshold is reduced, but the bone conduction threshold is essentially normal. A simple and an excellent way to demonstrate this is to take a 500-cps tuning fork and strike it gently. A patient with a conductive hearing loss will hear the fork only weakly when it is held close to his ear, but he will hear it better when the shaft is placed so that it presses on the mastoid bone or the teeth. This is such a useful test that it should be used in every case of hearing loss, no matter how many other tests an audiologist or a technician may perform. In the hands of the experienced otologist the tuning fork is an essential diagnostic instrument.

If there is a conductive loss in only one ear, or if the conductive loss is considerably greater in one ear than in the other, a vibrating tuning fork pressed against the skull will be heard in the ear with the greater hearing loss. Tests depending on *lateralization*, as this phenomenon is called, are not as reliable as some other tuning fork tests, such as those comparing the efficiency of air and bone conduction.

Finally, in every case carefully done hearing tests are analyzed to confirm the classification. Air and bone conduction audiometry are fundamental but should be corroborated by tuning fork tests. If there is still

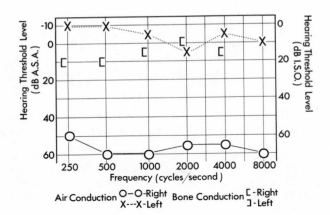

FIG. 6. Flat audiogram found in conductive hearing loss due to chronic otitis media. Bone conduction and discrimination are normal.

History: 8-year-old female with discharge from right ear since age of 6 months.

Otologic: right tympanic membrane eroded with putrid discharge in middle ear. Ossicles absent at surgery.

Audiologic: reduced air and normal bone conduction responses in right ear with left ear masked. Tuning fork lateralizes to right ear.

Speech reception threshold: Right 60 db
Discrimination score: Right 98%
Classification: conductive
Diagnosis: chronic otitis media

any doubt as to the classification, recruitment studies, discrimination and tone decay tests are performed, if possible. In this type of loss there will be no evidence of recruitment or abnormal tone decay. The patient's ability to discriminate is always excellent in conductive hearing loss. It is helpful to do all these tests routinely in every case, but this is not always possible in private practice. On the other hand, there are some audiologic centers in various parts of the country in which an entire battery of hearing tests is carried out on all patients even before they are examined and questioned. The experienced clinical physician performs only sufficient tests to make his classification or diagnosis reasonably certain. This selectivity saves the patient and the clinician considerable time and money. Despite the undoubted advantages of expensive and elaborate electronic equipment to perform hearing tests, there are many men practicing excellent

| | | | | AIR CONDUCTION | | | | | | | | | | |
| | RIGHT | | | | | | | LEFT | | | | | | |
DATE	LEFT MASK	250	500	1000	2000	4000	8000	RIGHT MASK	250	500	1000	2000	4000	8000
4/10	85	-5	-5	-10	-10	5			30	30	40	40	50	Fluid
4/10	80								0	10	5	15	20	Fluid removed
4/24									0	-5	0	0	5	

| | | | | BONE CONDUCTION | | | | | | | | | |
| | RIGHT | | | | | | | LEFT | | | | | |
DATE	LEFT MASK	250	500	1000	2000	4000	TYPE	RIGHT MASK	250	500	1000	2000	4000
4/10	85	5	-5	-10	15	20	WN	85	15	15	5	10	30
4/24								85	0	0	0	0	5

FIG. 7. Atypical audiogram in conductive hearing loss due to thick fluid in the middle ear. The bone conduction is reduced but returns to normal after fluid is removed.

History: recurrent fullness in left ear with hearing loss for past 6 months.

Otologic: eardrum not freely mobile with air pressure. No fluid level seen. Thick, clear jelly in middle ear. Removed with myringotomy and suction.

Audiologic: reduced air and somewhat reduced bone conduction thresholds in left ear. Normal discrimination. Bone thresholds returned to normal after removal of fluid. Tuning fork lateralizes to left ear.

Classification: conductive. Initial testing indicated some sensorineural involvement because of the reduced bone thresholds. Removal of the fluid allowed bone responses to return to normal.

Diagnosis: secretory otitis

Aids to diagnosis: immobile eardrum; fluctuating hearing loss with slightly reduced bone conduction; normal discrimination and lateralization to left ear suggest fluid in middle ear.

otology who use only minimal equipment, but they do exercise keen judgment and skill.

PROGNOSIS

In the vast majority of clinical cases of conductive hearing loss, the prognosis is excellent. With available medical and surgical treatment most conductive hearing losses now can be corrected. Little wonder that physicians are always anxious to classify a case as conductive rather than sensorineural or central, since in the latter types of hearing losses the absence of any established methods for restoring hearing makes the prognosis at present so much poorer.

AUDIOMETRIC PATTERNS

There is a popular impression that the different classifications are characterized by distinctly shaped audiometric patterns. One cannot be sure by merely inspecting an air conduction audiogram whether the loss is conductive or sensorineural.

However, it is true that many conductive hearing losses have audiometric patterns of a distinctive appearance. One characteristic audiogram generally is described as an ascending curve, indicating that the hearing loss is greater in the lower than in the higher frequencies. This classic audiogram, illustrated in Figure 5, demonstrates almost all the findings characteristically present in conductive hearing loss resulting from otosclerosis.

Another audiometric pattern common in conductive defects is shown in Figure 6, which illustrates the audiologic findings in chronic mastoiditis.

Not every case of conductive hearing loss presents all distinctive characteristics; some patients with conductive hearing loss give comparatively few findings. For example, Figure 7 illustrates a case of secretory otitis media in which there is a high tone loss, and the bone conduction is reduced, though the sensorineural mechanism is normal.

THE DANGER OF INCOMPLETE STUDIES

These cases illustrate the inadvisability of making a classification of conductive or any other type of hearing loss solely on the basis of the air conduction alone or even on the air and the bone conduction combined. Without a careful otologic examination some of these patients possibly may be classified incorrectly and thus be deprived of effective therapy and relief of their hearing handicap.

A well-considered analysis of all of the findings in the history, the physical examination and the audiologic studies always is essential in making a correct classification and diagnosis. A correct diagnosis cannot be achieved consistently or reliably on the basis of incomplete studies.

ESSENTIAL CRITERIA OF CONDUCTIVE HEARING LOSS

To qualify as an uncomplicated conductive hearing loss, a case must have these features:

1. The bone conduction must be better than the air conduction.
2. The air-bone gap must be at least 15 db.
3. The bone conduction must be normal or near normal.
4. The discrimination must be good.
5. The hearing threshold must not exceed about 60 db.
6. Although tests for recruitment and abnormal tone decay are rarely performed in the presence of the above features, both of these phenomena should be absent.

Chapter 6

Conductive Hearing Loss: Causes With Visible Obstruction in the External Auditory Canal

If a patient's audiologic findings show a conductive hearing loss, and an obstruction is seen in the external canal, the cause of his hearing loss may be one of those described in this chapter. Included are the following:

Congenital aplasia
Treacher-Collins syndrome
Stenosis
Exostosis
Impacted cerumen
Fluid in external canal
Collapse of ear canal
External otitis
Foreign body
Carcinoma
Granuloma
Cysts
Other causes

CONGENITAL APLASIA

When the external auditory canal is absent at birth, the condition is called congenital aplasia. It is due to a defect in fetal development. When the physician is examining an aplasia in an infant or young child, he may wonder whether the neural mechanism also is defective. However, it is helpful to recall that the outer ear and the sensorineural apparatus are of different embryonic origins. The sound-conducting mechanism of the middle ear develops from the branchial system, whereas the sensorineural mechanism is derived from the ectodermal cyst. Therefore, it is rare to find embryonic defects in both the conductive and the sensorineural systems in the same ear.

Embryonic Development. Another interesting question concerns the ability to predict from the appearance of the outer ear the likely presence of ossicles in the middle ear. The auricle starts forming in the 6th week of embryonic life and is almost complete after the 12th week. In some patients there is a small pit just in front and above the meatus of the canal. This shows the point at which the hillocks from the 1st and the 2nd branchial arches fused to form the auricle. The embryonic structure occasionally may persist as a fistula or as a congenital preauricular cyst. The eardrum and the external auditory canal start forming about the end of the 2nd month of fetal life and are complete about the 7th month. First, the eardrum is formed, and a short time later, the meatus. It is possible but uncommon to find an aplasia of the meatus with a normal eardrum and ossicles. The ossicles begin to form from cartilage during the 8th week of fetal life and are fully developed by the 4th month, though not ossified until shortly before birth.

Congenital Abnormalities. The causes of congenital abnormalities are not yet known, and the variety is great. There may be only a membranous layer closing the canal, whereas everything else is normal; or there may be no canal, no eardrum, no ossicles, and even very little middle ear. Often the aplasia is unilateral, but even in such cases evidence of a slight congenital defect may be found in the other ear.

It is not possible at present to predict preoperatively whether a functioning eardrum and normal ossicles are present in congenital aplasia. X-ray technics, though extremely useful, are not as yet quite sophisticated enough to provide complete information. This can be obtained only at surgery. However, the shape of the auricle does provide some indication of the condition of the deeper structures in the ear. Since the auricle is formed completely by the 3rd month of fetal life, a deformed auricle suggests probable deformities of the eardrum and the ossicles. The chances of improving hearing are better when the auricle is well formed.

The Question of Surgery. The question of what can be accomplished by surgery is of decisive importance in congenital aplasia. Parents are always anxious to know how much hearing is lost in children with congenital aplasia, and whether hearing can be restored.

If the aplasia is unilateral, and the other ear is normal, surgery becomes an elective procedure. In bilateral aplasia early surgery to restore hearing in at least one ear is highly desirable to permit normal speech development. If for any reason surgery is inadvisable or should be postponed for several years, a bone conduction hearing aid should be fitted on children as early as 3 months of age.

Older surgical procedures were discouraging, and consequently physicians find many cases of unilateral congenital aplasia in adults. With new surgical approaches the results are much more rewarding. It is best not to perform the surgery before the child is about 5 years old. The great variety of abnormal conditions which may be found at surgery and the distortion or the absence of landmarks make this surgery very difficult, and it should be undertaken only by trained and experienced otologists.

Studying the Extent of Involvement. Though the diagnosis of aplasia may be made by simple inspection, the extent of involvement must be determined by careful study. The taking of x-ray films can be helpful in demonstrating the presence of an external auditory canal, ossicles and semicircular canals. Newer x-ray technics with tomography can show quite clearly the shape of the ossicles but not their function (Fig. 8). The absence of semicircular canals makes the prognosis for restoring hearing very poor, since it indicates a defect in the labyrinth. Hearing studies are essential, though these are difficult to perform in an infant. Nevertheless, a reasonable estimate of the child's hearing level can be obtained by a comprehensive study, which requires good judgment and psychogalvanic skin resistance measurements, as well as tuning fork, startle reflex and many other tests. For example, if a child turns his head in the direction of a vibrating tuning fork struck not too forcefully, there is a reasonably good basis for optimism that hearing can be restored. However, if there is no response to this simple test, it does not necessarily follow that hearing is absent, but more elaborate tests then are indicated.

Prognosis. In an adult the presence of normal bone conduction when the opposite ear is adequately masked indicates a normal sensorineural mechanism and a good prognosis for restoring hearing, depending on x-ray corroboration. Children with bilateral aplasia invariably have a hearing threshold of around 60 db. Unless hearing is restored early in one of the ears, speech usually develops slowly. Such a child has no difficulty with discrimination (easily understanding speech), in contrast with a child who has a similar hearing loss resulting from sensorineural deafness.

Patients with aplasia whose hearing level exceeds 60 db are likely to have sensorineural damage, and the prognosis for restoring hearing is much poorer in such cases.

TREACHER-COLLINS SYNDROME

One type of congenital aplasia is so distinctive that it warrants separate consideration. In Treacher-Collins syndrome both auricles are deformed,

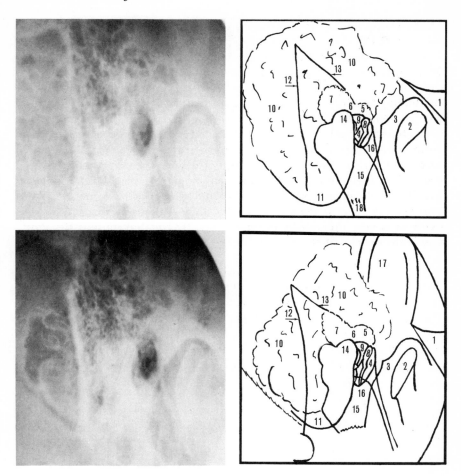

FIG. 8. Tomograms of ossicles, Mayer's position. (Dr. W. E. Compere, Jr., La Mesa, Calif.) (1) Root of zygoma. (2) Condyle of mandible. (3) Temporomandibular joint. (4) Tympanic cavity. (5) Epitympanic space. (6) Area of aditus. (7) Area of antrum. (8) Malleus. (9) Incus. (10) Mastoid air cells. (11) Mastoid tip. (12) Anterior plate of lateral sinus. (13) Dural plate. (14) Labyrinth. (15) Petrous pyramid. (16) Eustachian tube. (17) Auricle. (18) Styloid process.

and there is complete absence of both external auditory canals and ear-drums; the malleus and the incus also are deformed. In addition, the patient's eyes are slanted downward at the lateral corners in the so-called antimongoloid fashion. Congenital defects, known as colobomas, are observed in such ocular structures as the iris, the retina or the choroid. The mandible is small, and the lower jaw markedly recedes in the so-called

"Andy Gump" manner. The cheeks are pulled into the face, causing the lower eyelids and the face to droop.

Although no mental retardation accompanies this syndrome, children so afflicted present such a strange appearance that they generally are taken to be backward. A contributory factor to this impression is the marked conductive hearing loss resulting from the aplasia. Because these children hear so poorly, they are slow in developing speech, and this in turn often is attributed unjustly to lack of mental acuity. These children usually have normal sensorineural mechanisms, and their hearing can be improved by successful surgery or by the early use of a bone conduction hearing aid. Preferably, this should be provided in infancy to avoid retardation of speech development and thus to obviate many psychological problems. The hearing level is usually about 60 db for all frequencies. Preoperatively, it is very difficult to ascertain even by roentgenograms the condition of the ossicles or the presence or the absence of an eardrum.

STENOSIS OF THE EAR CANAL

Stenosis is diagnosed readily when otoscopic examination reveals com-

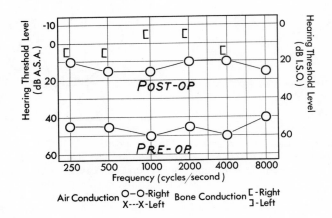

FIG. 9. *History:* 6-year-old boy with right congenital aplasia.

Otologic: left ear normal. Mild microtia of right auricle. Meatus of right external auditory canal completely occluded by firm thick skin. X-ray pictures showed normal ossicles. At surgery the aplasia was corrected, and the eardrum was found to be almost normal.

Audiologic: reduced air and normal bone conduction in right ear with masking in the left ear.

Classification: conductive

Diagnosis: right congenital aplasia with normal sensorineural function

plete obstruction of the external auditory canal leading to the eardrum. This obstruction may occur anywhere along the length of the canal. Occasionally, a skin layer, as in aplasia, is the only block present; this causes a hearing loss of roughly 40 db in the speech frequency range (Fig. 9). More often, however, there is a bony wall behind the skin, and the hearing loss then may range from 50 to 60 db in all frequencies.

Stenosis of the ear canal generally is detected on routine otologic examination in infancy. Sometimes, however, it is not picked up until the school hearing test reveals a hearing loss, after which physical examination shows closure of the ear canal.

Stenosis is not always congenital. It may be a sequel to infections, or it may result from complications from surgery on the ears, as well as from burns. In these instances the obstruction usually is fibrous.

In some instances stenosis is not complete, but it narrows the opening of the ear canal to such an extent that any small accumulation of wax or debris causes impaction and hearing loss. In such cases the canal can be enlarged and the hearing problem resolved. However, it is essential to enlarge the canal in such a manner that it does not close again.

Correction of a stenotic ear canal is always advisable, so that in the event of a subsequent middle ear infection necessitating myringotomy or ear treatment the eardrum can be visualized adequately for diagnosis and treatment.

EXOSTOSIS OF THE EAR CANAL

In exostosis of the ear canal bony projections can be seen arising from the walls of the canal. They are not uncommon in adults, but they are rare in children. Although the cause of this condition is unknown, it seems to occur more frequently in individuals whose ears are excessively exposed to water, as in swimmers.

When it is recalled that the outer portion of the external ear is cartilaginous, it seems logical that bony exostoses are found only in the bony or inner portion of the canal. Generally, these growths are small and do not of themselves occlude the lumen completely. However, they do narrow it to such a degree that any slight accumulations of water, wax or dead skin, or any infection may cause complete blockage and immediate hearing loss. Such episodes may be so frequent in some patients that surgery is necessary to prevent recurrent hearing loss and infections.

The hearing loss is generally around 30 to 40 db when the lumen of the canal becomes occluded. The loss is not as great as in complete atresia, because some of the sound waves apparently traverse the flexible material that completes the closure of the ear canal. The loss is predominantly in the lower frequencies. Upon removal of the wax or the debris hearing returns to normal. Utmost care is necessary in examining ear canals with exostoses, because trauma to the very thin skin covering them readily can produce swelling, infection and further hearing loss.

In such cases, if water enters, it is very difficult for the patient to remove it by ordinary means. The water accumulates in the pockets between the exostoses and the eardrum. The diagnosis of hearing loss due to exostoses must be based on the findings in the ear canal and the audiologic testing.

Exostoses can be removed readily with local anesthesia in the ear canal skin, elevating the skin off the bony projections, removing them and replacing the skin.

IMPACTED CERUMEN

Occurrence. Since wax glands are situated only in the skin covering the cartilaginous or outer part of the ear canal, wax is formed only in this outer area. When it is found impacted more deeply in the bony portion or against the eardrum, it usually has been pushed in there somehow. Some ear canals are so built, and the wax is of such consistency, that the

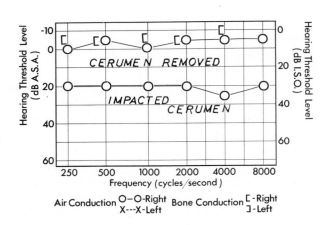

Air Conduction O–O-Right / X---X-Left   Bone Conduction ⊏-Right / ⊐-Left

Fig. 10. *History:* fullness and hearing loss in right ear for several weeks after trying to clean ear with a cotton probe.

Otologic: right external auditory canal impacted with cerumen. Removal of cerumen revealed normal eardrum.

Audiologic: mild flat hearing loss in right ear with normal bone conduction. Left ear masked. Removal of cerumen resulted in restoration of hearing to normal (upper curve).

Classification: conductive

Diagnosis: impacted cerumen

excess cerumen instead of falling out of the ear accumulates and plugs up the canal, thus causing hearing loss. This is common in infants because of their very narrow ear canals, and because mothers are likely to use large cotton-tipped applicators that push the wax into a baby's ear canal instead of removing it.

Obstruction due to excessive cerumen is of frequent occurrence among workers in industrial areas, because dirt gets into their ear canals. Individuals with an abundance of hairs in the ear canal readily accumulate cerumen, because it becomes enmeshed in the hairs and thus is prevented from falling out by itself.

Interestingly enough, the patient with impacted wax often gives a history of sudden rather than gradual hearing loss. He may say that while he was chewing or poking his finger or a probe of some kind into his ear in an effort to clean it, he suddenly went "deaf" in that ear. Of course, what actually happened was that the patient may have experienced some itching or fullness in the ear, and by probing into it with a large object he pushed the cerumen into the narrower portion of the ear canal until he caused an impaction. If the canal closes while the patient is chewing, it may be explained by the proximity of the temporomandibular joint to the cartilaginous portion of the ear canal. In such instances pressure of the joint on the soft ear canal may dislodge wax from its normal position and block the narrow lumen of the canal.

						AIR CONDUCTION							
		RIGHT						LEFT					
DATE	LEFT MASK	250	500	1000	2000	4000	8000	RIGHT MASK	250	500	1000	2000	4000	8000
		45	50	40	50	65	60		50	50	55	65	70	60
After removal of wax		20	20	20	25	40	45		20	25	35	35	45	50

						BONE CONDUCTION						
		RIGHT						LEFT				
DATE	LEFT MASK	250	500	1000	2000	4000	TYPE	RIGHT MASK	250	500	1000	2000	4000
		10	10	10	10	40			5	10	10	20	50

Fig. 11. *History:* Patient claims deafness started several months ago after attempt to remove wax from both ears. Buzzing tinnitus has been present occasionally. No vertigo. Denies family history of deafness.

Otologic: bilateral impacted cerumen. Removed. Eardrums normal.

Audiologic: bilateral reduced air conduction with near-normal bone conduction, except at 4,000 cps. Removal of cerumen closed the air-bone gap somewhat, but a residual conductive loss remained.

Classification: conductive

Diagnosis: conductive deafness caused by impacted cerumen and an underlying condition of otosclerosis.

Aids to diagnosis: Impacted cerumen does not often cause so severe a conductive loss. Stapes fixation was found at surgery, and hearing improved in left ear.

Tinnitus. If cerumen becomes lodged against the eardrum, a rushing type of tinnitus sometimes is reported. The noise stops at once when the cerumen is removed. It is not uncommon for the patient to complain of hearing his own heartbeat when cerumen becomes impacted against the eardrum. This is probably due to pressure on the ear canal obstructing some of its blood supply. The hearing loss invariably is accompanied by a feeling of fullness, and the loss usually is greater in the lower frequencies. Rarely is the loss greater than 40 db, and most often it is around 30 db.

Ruling Out an Organic Defect. Patients with hearing loss due to other causes commonly tell their physicians that wax in their ears is probably causing their hearing loss. To rule out an organic defect it is essential to inquire whether the patient had impaired hearing and tinnitus before the present episode.

Testing. A common mistake is to look in an ear, to see a large amount of cerumen and then to assure the patient that wax in the ear is his only trouble. Such a hasty diagnosis may necessitate an embarrassing retraction when after removal of the wax the hearing loss is still as bad as ever. It is well to bear in mind that the severity of the loss cannot be estimated merely from the presence of a large amount of cerumen in the ear canal. Even if there is only a small pinpoint opening through the cerumen, the patient can hear almost normally, provided that there is no organic defect. It is only when the ear canal is blocked completely that the hearing loss becomes apparent. Therefore, it is highly advisable to do at least air and bone conduction audiometry before venturing to establish the cause and the prognosis of any hearing impairment. It is also important to perform air conduction audiograms after removal of the wax to be certain that hearing has been fully restored.

Removal of Cerumen. If irrigation is used to remove impacted cerumen, the ear canal should be dried afterward; otherwise, some water may remain in the deep pit at the antero-inferior portion of the ear canal, which might cause a feeling of fullness as well as a slight interference with hearing. Figure 10 illustrates the type of hearing loss that frequently results from impacted cerumen. Figure 11 illustrates an important reason for taking a careful history and doing audiologic testing before assuring a patient that his hearing loss can be cured merely by removing impacted cerumen. Note that in this case some hearing loss still was present even though the ear canal was cleared entirely of cerumen.

The removal of cerumen requires gentleness and patience and always should be performed with good illumination. The simplest method to suit the situation should be used. Firm plugs of wax can be removed best en masse by gently teasing them out with a fine forceps. The forceps or any other instrument should come in contact only with the wax and not with the skin of the canal, which is thin and tender. Soft wax can be wiped out with a very thin cotton-tipped probe. The use of thick Q Tips to remove wax from a narrow canal serves only to push it in further and to impact it. Sometimes, it may be necessary to irrigate wax from an ear canal, but this should be avoided if the canal already is inflamed. Irrigation should not be performed in the presence of a known perforation of the eardrum, for this may cause a dry ear to flare up and result in a chronic otitis media. When irrigation is performed, the water used should be at body temperature to avoid stimulating the labyrinth and producing vertigo. The stream of water is most effective when it is directed forcefully toward one edge of the wax, so that the water can get behind the plug and force it out. The ear canal should be dried carefully at the end of the procedure.

Harsh chemicals that are supposed to soften cerumen when introduced into the ear often irritate the tender skin of the canal and cause an external otitis. Such solutions should be avoided or used with great caution.

FLUID IN THE EXTERNAL AUDITORY CANAL

The external auditory canals in some people are so angled that when water gets in, it is very difficult to remove. This may be a problem after swimming, showering or bathing, and it is becoming increasingly common in women after they spray their hair with certain lotions and after using

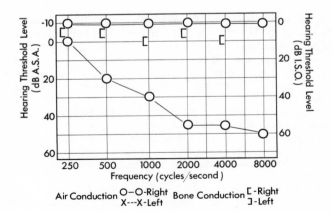

FIG. 12. Conductive hearing loss induced in right ear by filling the external auditory canal with mineral oil. Note the atypical shape of this conductive loss in that the greater loss is in the high frequencies. No recruitment is present with the ear filled with mineral oil. Hearing returned to normal after the mineral oil was removed.

shampoos. The reader may recall seeing a bather after swimming tilt his head, slapping it on one side, then jumping up and down—all this merely to get a little water out of his ear. People like this swimmer may have deformed ear canals or excess ear wax that prevents water from coming out readily. Exostoses in the ear canal also may account for this difficulty. An example of hearing loss due to fluid in the external canal is seen in

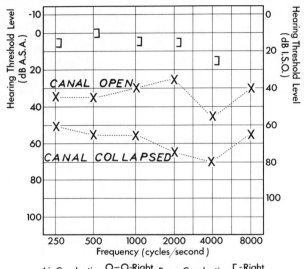

Air Conduction O—O-Right   Bone Conduction Ɛ-Right
                X---X-Left   Ɔ-Left

FIG. 13. *History:* 37-year-old male with gradually progressive hearing loss. Occasional ringing tinnitus. Maternal aunt hard of hearing.

Otologic: ears normal. Stapes fixation confirmed at surgery.

Audiologic: Right and left ears showed a moderately severe air conduction loss. The patient's responses to conversational voice did not seem to be in keeping with the pure tone responses, and a functional hearing loss was suspected. After removal of the earphones the patient reported that with the earphones in place his hearing seemed to be blocked. A stock ear mold used for hearing aid evaluations was placed in the left ear canal, the earphones were replaced, and the hearing was retested. Significant improvements in thresholds were obtained with the ear canal held open with the ear mold. Bone conduction thresholds were normal with the opposite ear masked.

Classification: conductive

Diagnosis: otosclerosis. Inconsistencies in initial pure tone thresholds and subjective responses to normal voice indicated a functional aspect to the problem presented. The patient's report pointed to the possibility of canal closure in the presence of earphones. This was confirmed, and the original moderately severe loss was found actually to be mild in degree.

Comment: In applying the earphones care must be taken not to compress the ear canals.

Figure 12. Note the high tone drop in air conduction that is so suggestive of sensorineural hearing loss, but also note that the bone conduction is normal. This example should be contrasted with a case showing fluid in the middle ear; in such a case a drop in bone conduction usually accompanies the reduction in air conduction. When fluid in the external auditory canal is the only cause, its removal restores normal hearing.

Occasionally, in children oily medicine, dropped into the canal for treating ear infections, may be trapped there for a long time and cause hearing loss. It is well worth noting that if only air conduction testing is done, as is customary in most industrial and school hearing test programs, one might conclude erroneously that the two cases presented in Figures 11 and 12 should be classified as sensorineural, because the hearing loss was most pronounced in the higher frequencies.

COLLAPSE OF THE EAR CANAL DURING AUDIOMETRY

In rare instances auditory canals may be so shaped that when pressure is directed on the pinna, the canal wall completely collapses, and conductive hearing loss results. This condition may be produced when earphones are placed over the ears during routine hearing testing. Therefore, the examiner should be careful in adjusting earphones to the ears to avoid collapse of the canal and a spurious hearing level. Usually, the patient will complain as soon as the earphones are placed over his ears, that they feel full, and he can't hear well. He also may make some effort to adjust the earphones more comfortably. The examiner should be alert to such a situation and correct it.

Figure 13 gives an example of such a situation in a patient who already had a sensorineural hearing loss. To demonstrate that there was a conductive overlay produced by the collapse of the ear canal, a plastic tube was inserted to keep the ear canal open, and the hearing level improved instantly.

If there is no collapse of the canal, and yet air conduction is reduced despite apparently normal speech reception (to judge from the patient's response to conversation), a functional hearing loss should be suspected.

EXTERNAL OTITIS

Cause. Occlusion of the auditory canal with debris or swelling due to inflammation of the surrounding skin is a common cause of hearing loss, particularly in summer and in tropical climates. The most common cause is prolonged exposure of the skin to water, especially during swimming, but inflammation may result also from excessive washing or irrigation of the ear. Trauma to the skin of the canal during the removal of cerumen or foreign bodies may be another cause of external otitis, or it may result from dermatitis, infections, allergies and systemic diseases.

Diagnosis. In diagnosing external otitis the first consideration is to distinguish it from otitis media, and this is difficult unless the eardrum is visible and appears to be normal. Occasionally, both external otitis and otitis media occur at the same time. When the eardrum is not visible, certain features aid in establishing the diagnosis. In external otitis the skin of the auditory canal generally is edematous or excoriated. Tenderness is pronounced around the entire ear, and pain in the ear is aggravated by chewing or pressing on the ear. However, in most cases of otitis media there is comparatively little swelling in the external canal unless mastoiditis is present, or there is a profuse irritating discharge from the middle ear. The pain in otitis media is usually very deep in the ear and not aggravated by movements of the jaw during eating. However, sneezing and coughing often produce severe sharp pain because of the increased pressure in the inflamed middle ear. If the discharge in an ear canal has a stringy mucoid appearance, as is found in the nose during rhinitis, it almost invariably indicates otitis media with a perforated eardrum.

Whenever a clear-cut diagnosis is not possible, therapy should be directed to both the external and the middle ears. For external otitis medication principally is applied locally to the outer ear; for otitis media it is directed to the middle ear, the nasopharynx and systemically.

Too strenuous efforts to introduce an otoscope into a tender inflamed ear canal should be avoided. In many instances a preliminary diagnosis must be based on the history and the superficial examination, as well as the clinical experience, until the infection subsides, and visualization of the eardrum becomes possible.

Treatment. Of the many successful methods of treating "swimmers' external otitis," one of the best is to insert snugly into the swollen ear canal a large cotton wick soaked in Burow's Solution diluted 1:10. The same wick should be kept in place and wetted with the same solution for 24 to 48 hours. The wick should not be allowed to become dry. This treatment merely changes the pH in the ear canal and thus inhibits the growth of certain pathogenic organisms while the ear is healing. More specific medication is indicated if this mild therapy does not resolve the infection. Too often a resistant external otitis is misdiagnosed as a fungous infection, but the fungus is usually a secondary invader, and more careful study will reveal a bacterial or an allergic problem.

The use of strong chemicals and overtreatment should be avoided, and so should excessive manipulation in a swollen ear canal. Strong medications frequently will aggravate an external otitis, and prolonged use of medication will cause an infection to persist when otherwise it would have cleared up.

After the infection has subsided in the auditory canal, and the eardrum is visualized, it is advisable to perform a hearing test to be certain that there is no underlying deafness from some other condition in the middle or the inner ear.

FOREIGN BODY IN THE EAR CANAL

Hearing loss and fullness in the ear are so often the only symptoms produced by a foreign body in the ear canal that we include it as a separate cause of hearing impairment. It is surprising how long a piece of absorbent cotton or other foreign matter can remain in a patient's ear canal without his being aware of its presence. Only when this foreign body becomes

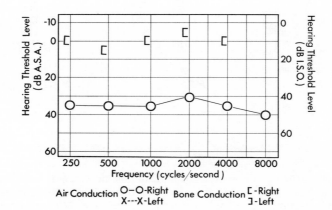

FIG. 14. *History:* 27-year-old male who complained of hearing loss in the right ear which had begun 3 months before. It started with itching and fullness in the canal. He did not seek medical attention until the ear had started to discharge 2 days before. No tinnitus.

Otologic: left ear clear. Right ear had a putrid external otitis, and behind the discharge was a thick plug of absorbent cotton and debris. The patient recalled putting the cotton in the ear about 3 months previously. The foreign matter was removed.

Audiologic: Right ear air conduction thresholds revealed a flat moderate loss. Bone conduction was normal with the left ear masked. Hearing returned to normal with removal of plug.

Classification: conductive

Diagnosis: foreign matter in ear canal

Note: For an accurate diagnosis the eardrums should be made visible by clearing out any debris that prevents inspection.

impacted with wax or swollen with moisture do fullness and hearing loss ensue, and then medical attention is sought. The hearing loss is due to the occlusion of the canal; it is usually very mild and usually greater in the lower frequencies.

The variety of foreign bodies removed from ear canals, especially in children, ranges from rubber erasers to peas. Most of these cause enough ear discomfort to attract attention before hearing loss becomes prominent, but not always. Caution always must be observed when attempting to remove a foreign body from the ear canal. Usually, special grasping instruments are essential, depending on the nature of the foreign body. In a child general anesthesia may be advisable unless the foreign body is obviously simple to grasp and to remove in one painless maneuver. It is easy to underestimate the difficulty in removing a foreign body and to

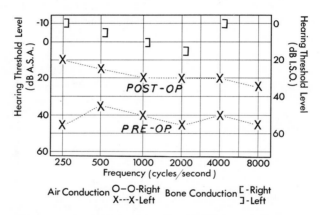

Air Conduction O—O-Right   Bone Conduction ⌐-Right
              X---X-Left   ⌐-Left

Fig. 15. *History:* Prior otologic and audiologic examinations revealed normal findings. For past year patient noted first intermittent, then gradual and constant fullness and hearing loss in left ear. No pain or tenderness in ear.

Otologic: complete atresia of left canal just inside opening. Under the thick skin was a firm bony layer that could not be penetrated with a needle. At surgery a large fibrous granuloma was removed from under the skin. The eardrum was thick and white but intact. A pathologic diagnosis of foreign body granuloma was established. The patient did not recall any event or symptom that might explain the diagnosis. X-ray films showed normal mastoid but bony occlusion in the left external canal.

Audiologic: reduced air and normal bone conduction thresholds in the left ear with masking in the right ear. Tuning fork lateralized to the left ear, and bone was better than air conduction. Postoperative air conduction responses were improved, but the air-bone gap was not closed completely. The eardrum was thick, opaque, immobile and suggestive of a long-standing external otitis.

Classification: conductive
Diagnosis: atresia with foreign body granuloma

run into unexpected problems; excessive preparation is better than too little.

Figure 14 illustrates the hearing loss and the findings in a man who was unaware that he had left a piece of absorbent cotton in his ear 3 months before. Only when shower water seemed to get trapped in his ear and cause fullness did he seek medical attention.

CARCINOMA OF THE EXTERNAL CANAL

Whenever a granuloma or a similar mass is seen in the external canal, carcinoma should be suspected and ruled out. Although carcinoma in this area is not common, the possibility is serious enough to warrant constant alertness. The most common complaints associated with carcinoma are fullness in the ear, hearing loss, and bleeding from the canal. The mass does not have to be large to occlude the ear canal. Often the symptoms have existed only for a short time, so that it may be possible to diagnose the malignancy comparatively early even though the prognosis in such cases is not always good. Hearing loss is an almost insignificant aspect of this important entity, but it is frequently the presenting symptom. Early attention to a complaint of hearing impairment may be essential to prompt diagnosis of carcinoma and early surgical intervention.

GRANULOMA

Although granuloma in the external auditory canal is comparatively rare, it warrants special comment, because hearing loss is generally the only presenting symptom. Occasionally, there may be some drainage from the ear due to secondary infection, but more often the patient complains of a gradual hearing loss for no apparent reason, or he possibly may attribute it to wax in his ear. A granuloma of the external auditory canal is seen readily by examination with an otoscope. This condition should not be mistaken for the fragile polypoid soft granulation tissue that arises in chronically diseased middle ears, sometimes extending into the canal. Granulomata are usually firm or hard masses that resemble neoplasms and regenerate when they are removed. Occasionally, their cause and diagnosis are most difficult to determine; for example, in the case cited in Figure 15 the patient's chief complaint was an insidious hearing loss in his left ear, present for about a year, with no related symptom or obvious cause to account for it. The right ear was normal, but the left showed an obvious complete atresia of the external canal a short distance from the opening.

The appearance was the very picture of a stenosis with firm, thick, normal skin covering a bony undersurface. The major diagnostic feature was that the patient had had a normal audiogram and normal hearing in this same ear 2 years prior to his latest visit to the physician's office. This case illustrates the importance of considering the possibility of a granuloma as a cause of conductive hearing loss due to visible damage in the external canal.

The causes of granuloma include tuberculosis, eosinophilic granuloma, fungous infection, carcinoma, and others. Biopsies and special tests help to establish a definitive etiology.

CYSTS IN THE EAR CANAL

A large variety of cysts can occur in the ear canal and may cause hearing loss by obstructing the lumen. The common types found in the canal are sebaceous and dermoid cysts, but others also are found.

Hematomas in the auricle may become large enough to extend into the external canal and completely to occlude it, producing hearing loss. In a chronic type of hematoma that occurs in wrestlers' or boxers' ears the opening of the canal can be so constricted by an old accumulation of blood and scar tissue that the canal is closed entirely, and hearing loss results.

OTHER CAUSES OF HEARING LOSS

Other causes of conductive hearing loss with abnormal findings visible in the canal include furuncle, keloids, angiomas, papillomas, osteomas and acute infectious diseases. None of these is a very common cause, but hearing impairment and fullness in the ear may be the chief or even the only symptoms to direct attention to the condition. The audiometric findings usually show hearing losses of less than 30 db, with the lower frequencies involved to a greater extent than the higher.

Chapter 7

Conductive Hearing Loss: Causes With Abnormalities Prominent in the Eardrum

An abnormal appearance of the eardrum detected by otoscopic examination of patients with a conductive hearing loss may indicate a condition largely restricted to the drum itself. Conditions of this type are reviewed in the present chapter. More often the abnormality visible in the eardrum is produced by injury or disease of the middle ear and communicating structures; such conditions are considered in Chapter 8. Careful inspection of the drum and the external ear also may reveal evidence of surgical procedures previously performed on the patient; these cases are discussed in Chapter 9.

MYRINGITIS

The eardrum rarely is singled out for attack by diseases without involvement of the rest of the external or the middle ear. When the drum does become affected, the condition is called myringitis. In most cases this condition is the result of a little understood viral infection. The most common type of this condition is described as myringitis bullosa, in which blebs or blisters appear on the drum due to pouching out of its outer layer with fluid. These blebs appear to be clear, and when punctured, they discharge a thin clear or slightly blood-tinged fluid. Sometimes the blebs may extend to the skin of the external canal. Myringitis starts rather abruptly and causes pain and fullness in the ear along with mild hearing loss. Usually, only one ear is involved. When the blister is punctured, and the eardrum is freed of its burden of fluid, the hearing promptly improves, and the feeling of fullness diminishes.

The diagnosis occasionally is difficult, because myringitis may be confused with a bulging drum due to acute otitis media. The absence of any upper respiratory infection and the normal appearance of the portions of the drum not affected by blebs help to distinguish myringitis from a middle ear infection.

Furthermore, when a bleb is punctured carefully, no hole is made through the drum, but only the outer layer is incised, so that with air pressure in the canal or politzerization through the nose the intact eardrum moves. In contrast, after myringotomy because of the perforation the drum does not move in response to a small difference in air pressure.

Herpes zoster, which can produce a picture somewhat similar to that of myringitis, is described in Chapter 12, since the sensorineural mechanism also is affected in many instances.

RUPTURED EARDRUM

Definition. An eardrum is said to be ruptured when suddenly it is penetrated by a foreign body (like a hairpin), or when it tears from the force of a slap across the ear. Otherwise, a hole in an eardrum is called a perforation rather than a rupture. Usually, the edge of a rupture is more irregular, and it is not accompanied immediately by signs of inflammation.

Cause. Most ruptures caused by penetrating objects are situated in the posterior portion of the drum because of the curve of the external canal and the slope of the drum. Ruptures caused by sudden and intense pressure change, as by a blow to the side of the head or by an explosion, are more frequently in the antero-inferior quadrant and occasionally in the pars flaccida. Another common cause of eardrum rupture is a slap or other impact on the ear during swimming under water. Because water gets into the middle ear, infections are more likely to ensue. In all cases of ruptured eardrum the history is most pertinent, since marked pain, fullness and ringing in the ear often are experienced.

Treatment. The sole recommended treatment for ruptured eardrums is systemic antibiotics. Nose blowing should be avoided, and above all there should be no unnecessary probing into the canal. Introduction of medications into the external canal should be avoided to prevent entry of infection into the middle ear. In most cases the small rupture heals spontaneously if infection is avoided. If healing does not take place, it may be necessary to encourage healing by cauterization or by doing a myringoplasty at some future time. The hearing loss may be as large as 60 db if the rupture was due to a force severe enough to impair the ossicular chain, but usually the loss is less than 30 db and involves practically all frequencies. Figure 16 shows an example of hearing loss due to a ruptured eardrum.

A tear in the eardrum may be considered as a special type of rupture of the eardrum. This may result from a direct blow to the head that causes a longitudinal fracture of the temporal bone, extending into the roof of the middle ear. Usually, the top of the eardrum is torn, blood gets into the middle and the outer ear, and occasionally the ossicular chain also is disrupted. Occasionally, there also may be a temporary facial paralysis and a cerebrospinal otorrhea. In longitudinal fractures the roentgenograms show a fracture line extending into the middle cranial fossa from the outer ear inward toward the foramen magnum and parallel with the superior petrosal sinus. Because there is blood in the middle ear, bone conduction also is reduced but returns to normal after resolution occurs. If the fracture involves the sensorineural mechanism, bone conduction usually is affected more seriously and permanently.

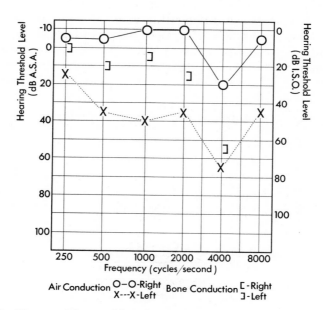

Air Conduction O—O-Right
X---X-Left
Bone Conduction ⊏-Right
⊐-Left

Fig. 16. *History:* 35-year-old male exposed to a firecracker explosion next to left ear. Intermittent ringing tinnitus. Had some exposure to gunfire in service previously.

Otologic: right, normal. Left ear had a large rupture of the eardrum without visible infection.

Audiologic: The right ear had normal thresholds except for a 20-db dip at 4,000 cps (C-5 dip). The left ear had a moderate air conduction loss and a 65-db C-5 dip. Masked bone conduction thresholds on the left ear showed a good degree of air-bone gap.

Classification: conductive

Diagnosis: acoustic trauma with ruptured eardrum. The hearing returned to a level similar to that in the right ear after a myringoplasty. The ossicles were found to be functioning.

SPARK IN EARDRUM

In industry a spark may occur and hit the eardrum, having a severe effect on hearing. Figure 17 points out what happens in such a case. Unfortunately, this is not a rare experience when men are welding, grinding, chipping or burning, and an occasional spark may find its way into the canal. It hits the drum with devastating effect. Usually, the entire drum is destroyed cleanly, leaving only the handle of the malleus hanging down. Little or no infection accompanies this trauma. The pain is severe but of short duration. The hearing loss is usually around 50 or 60 db and affects all frequencies. As in cases of ruptured eardrum, probing the canal and forceful nose blowing should be avoided after such an accident.

Myringoplasty usually is indicated, and the hearing can be restored. Wherever free sparks are produced in industry, steps should be taken to shield personnel from them. In places where this is not practical, as in some forges or foundries, it is essential to protect the ears with ear protectors and the eyes with safety glasses.

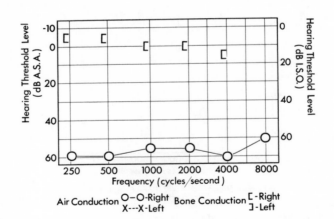

Fig. 17. *History:* patient works as a welder, and a spark flew into his right ear, causing severe burning pain and subsequent hearing loss.

Otologic: Patient was seen 24 hours after accident. Right eardrum almost cleanly and completely destroyed without evidence of inflammation. Handle of malleus visible as well as incudostapedial joint. External canal not affected visibly.

Audiologic: flat 60-db loss with good bone conduction (left ear masked) and lateralization to right.

Classification: conductive

Diagnosis: eardrum destroyed by hot spark.

PERFORATED EARDRUM

The role of the eardrum in hearing often is misunderstood, especially by laymen. Many people believe that without an eardrum it is not possible to hear at all. Some parents understandably become very much concerned when a myringotomy is suggested for their child, because they are fearful of having the hearing destroyed by a hole in the drum. There are even physicians who attribute marked hearing defects to such conditions as "hardening of the eardrum" and "too small an eardrum."

Hearing Loss

Actually, it is possible to have very little loss in hearing even though a large hole may be visible in the drum. In a recent nationwide study of school children 60 per cent of ears with dry perforations had gone undetected by hearing screening tests because the hearing loss of these children was less than 20 db. The hearing level in another 40 per cent of the ears showing perforations was better than 5 db on the audiometer. It is really not possible to predict the degree of hearing loss from the appearance of the tympanic membrane. In some cases in which the membrane is perforated and even scarred and retracted, the loss in hearing may be negligible, whereas in other instances there may be a severe hearing loss with only a pinpoint perforation. The cause of the pathology and its effect on the middle ear are more important criteria than the appearance of the eardrum.

However, the **location of the perforation** does have some **diagnostic meaning.** A persistent posterior perforation suggests associated mastoid infection, whereas an anterior perforation is not quite as serious. A superior perforation in Shrapnell's area also suggests that a fairly serious infection has been present.

A dry perforation in the tympanic membrane indicates that at some time infection probably was present in the middle ear. Only in rare instances does a perforation result from an infection in the external ear. Although the character and the location of the perforation are not reliable indications of the degree of hearing loss, yet they do play a certain role. For example, large perforations usually cause a greater loss. It would appear that the principal effect of a perforation is a reduction of the surface on which sound pressure is exerted, the effect being merely proportional to the area of the perforation. However, the relationship is not quite so simple.

Because the eardrum is effective only if it is in contact with the handle of the malleus, perforations affecting this area are especially damaging to the hearing. Perforations in the tense part of the eardrum, such as the antero-inferior portion, affect the hearing more than those in the flaccid and superior portions, since the tense part is largely responsible for the stiffness of the eardrum.

TESTING FOR HEARING LOSS

The best way to determine the hearing loss present when a perforation is found is to do an audiogram.

Caution should be exercised in correlating a perforation with the audiogram. It is quite natural for a physician who finds a small perforation in the eardrum to blame this for the presence of a hearing loss, even if the loss is as severe as 60 db; yet a perforation alone rarely produces such a marked degree of hearing loss. However, if the drum is entirely eroded, and the ossicular chain has become ineffective, a hearing loss of 60 db is to be expected. It is more than likely that there is some break in the ossicular chain when a severe degree of conductive hearing loss is found. This can be determined very simply by placing a small patch over the perforation, using Gelfoam or some other artificial material. If the hearing loss is due to the perforation, then the hearing should be restored immediately.

This therapeutic test should be used in every instance in which myringoplastic surgery is contemplated. If a hearing test shows that a temporary patch on the perforation in the drum fails to restore hearing, the otologist will know that further exploration of the middle ear is indicated to discover the major cause of the hearing loss, since a simple myringoplasty would give disappointing results.

PERFORATIONS

Demonstration. It often is difficult to be certain that a perforation actually is present in the tympanic membrane. Sometimes a large hole seems to be visible through the otoscope, but more careful scrutiny may reveal a very fine, thin, transparent film of epithelium covering the area. Such a film best can be demonstrated by gentle pressure on the ear canal with a Siegle otoscope; by moving the eardrum the light reflected from it will be visible on the covered perforation. Unless pressure is very gentle, the healed area may be broken through readily. Spraying a fine sterile powder into the ear also can outline a perforation or show an intact drum.

Healing. Perforations in the eardrum heal in several ways. Most heal with a small scar that is hardly visible. Others leave a rather thick white scar which can be seen for many years. These scars in themselves produce no measurable hearing loss.

Retracted Drum. In some ears the drum is retracted so much that it envelops the promontory like a sheet of Saran Wrap, and yet it remains intact. Or the retracted drum may have a perforation in it that is scarcely visible. The aperture can be visualized best by blowing camphor mist under pressure into one nostril while the other nostril is compressed, and the patient is asked to swallow. Through an otoscope the mist can be seen coming out of the perforation. If the eardrum is intact, often it will push out a little bit, or it may even suddenly snap out quite sharply. In the latter case the patient's hearing suddenly will improve.

Methods of Closing. Such excellent strides have been made in closing perforations in eardrums that a brief description of the methods is justified. Tympanic perforations cannot and should not be closed until the middle ear has been completely clear of infection and dry for several months; otherwise, the closure generally breaks down. A small perforation that is not marginal (i.e., does not have an edge on the annulus), generally can be closed by repeated cauterization of its rim with trichloroacetic acid. This is done to destroy the edge of outer epithelium that has grown over the rim, thus preventing the middle (fibrous) layer from closing the hole spontaneously. The cauterization is repeated every few weeks until the closure is complete. Sometimes a long-standing perforation closes of its own accord after an acute attack of otitis media. Probably, in such cases the edge of the perforation has been irritated and traumatized by the acute infection, and the trauma has stimulated growth of tissue around the edges of the perforation.

For large perforations and marginal ones myringoplasty is necessary. This is done under local anesthesia in adults. The epithelium around the edge of the perforation is removed, and either a thin piece of skin or vein is applied. This technic produces excellent results. Sometimes, in marginal perforations a sliding skin graft from the external canal is most effective. In all cases in which the preliminary closure of the perforation with Gelfoam or artificial membrane does not restore hearing, the middle ear and the ossicular chain must be explored during surgery. This is especially true in cases in which the hearing loss exceeds 30 db.

RETRACTED EARDRUM

Physicians frequently attribute a marked conductive hearing loss, such as 40 or 50 db, to a retracted eardrum, to adhesions in the middle ear, or to so-called "catarrh." In most cases these conclusions are unjustified. Rarely do any of these conditions in themselves cause a hearing loss greater than about 30 db. If the loss is materially greater, there is some accompanying defect in the ossicular chain or the middle ear.

To understand why a retracted drum usually causes only a mild loss, it should be recalled that sound waves can be transmitted through the ossicles even if only part of the eardrum is present, particularly the portion around the malleus; therefore, even some badly retracted drums cause comparatively little hearing loss. In a few exceptional cases a hearing loss much greater than 30 db is caused by retraction, and in these cases hearing returns to normal with successful inflation of the middle ear. This is demonstrated in Figure 18.

Actually, a retracted eardrum is not pulled in; it is pushed in by the greater atmospheric pressure in the external canal as compared with the pressure in the middle ear. Reduced middle ear pressure is produced most frequently by dysfunction in the eustachian tube. In children hypertrophied adenoids and allergies are the chief causes. In adults the principal causes are infections and allergies.

In any case, the eustachian tube becomes congested and blocks access of air needed to balance middle ear pressure with that in the external canal. The air already in the middle ear slowly is absorbed, and as a result the eardrum gradually is pushed in toward the promontory. Sometimes the drum is so thin that when it is retracted, it envelops the

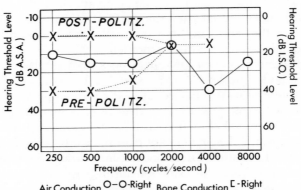

FIG. 18. *History:* 40-year-old female with insidious hearing loss for past 3 years following an upper respiratory infection. Hears better intermittently. Has occasional pulsebeat tinnitus.

Otologic: scarred eardrums with healed perforations. Drums retracted. On politzerization the left eardrum ballooned out, and hearing immediately returned to normal.

Audiologic: Air conduction thresholds revealed a mild right hearing loss and a moderate left loss with greater loss in the low frequencies. After politzerization the left ear thresholds returned to normal.

Classification: conductive

Diagnosis: retracted and scarred eardrums due to previous infections.

promontory and is hardly discernible as a drum. By forced politerization it occasionally can be distended. If it does distend, it usually is flaccid and redundant, and later it retracts again unless the cause of the original retraction has been corrected.

In retracted drums the reflected cone of light disappears, and the handle of the malleus appears to be prominent and shorter. Tinnitus rarely is caused by a retracted drum. If tinnitus is present, otosclerosis should be suspected. Since a retracted eardrum often is associated with a perforation, it is important to use forced air pressure (Siegle otoscope) to be sure that the drum is intact.

FLACCID EARDRUM

A flaccid eardrum is rarely a cause of hearing loss. The cause of the wrinkled and redundant eardrum is not always clear, but frequently it follows some long-standing malfunction of the eustachian tube, with alternate retraction and bulging of the eardrum resulting in the wrinkled appearance. Associated with a flaccid eardrum is a sensation of fullness, and occasionally the patient may report that he hears his own breath sounds in his ear. There is no general agreement on the best course of treatment, but in any case politzerization and inflations should be avoided.

THE SENILE EARDRUM

The appearance of a normal eardrum described in textbooks is always that of a young person. As human beings age, changes occur in the eardrum as they do in the eye and in the skin. The aged drum no longer reflects a cone of light, and it is no longer shiny. Its outer layer now appears to be thick and white or gray. It also loses its elasticity and becomes difficult to move with air pressure. White plaques and strands of fibrous tissue are evident in the middle fibrous layer of the drum.

How much, if any, hearing loss is caused by senile drum changes is difficult to ascertain, but it probably is almost negligible. Since the high tone hearing loss associated with aging is due to sensorineural changes, hardly any significant part of this can be attributed to the senile drum. Usually, low tone losses are negligible; if present, they are likely to be sensorineural. Many aged patients whose eardrums show marked senile changes have normal hearing. However, it is important to expect senile changes in the drums of aged persons and not to attribute hearing losses to changes which in fact have a different etiology.

Chapter 8

Conductive Hearing Loss:
Causes in Middle Ear and
Communicating Structures

Though the causes of conductive hearing loss enumerated in this chapter have their origin in the middle ear, the eustachian tubes or the nasopharynx, they frequently can be detected by transilluminating the eardrum and looking not necessarily *at* the drum but *through* it for telltale evidence of fluid, air bubbles, reflections, shadows, and the outline of the handle of the malleus. The appearance of the drum itself also may be changed by pathologic conditions behind it. What the otoscope reveals must further be interpreted by otologic experience.

CATARRHAL DEAFNESS AND ADHESIONS

One still commonly hears of a diagnosis of "catarrhal deafness." The precise pathology implied by this term is indefinite. Occasionally, it seems to refer to a cloudy eardrum, which is blamed for a marked conductive hearing loss. Many times the term is applied to any conductive hearing loss in which the drum appears to be slightly opaque or retracted. Actually, this is not catarrhal deafness but otosclerosis or tympanosclerosis with some incidental minor changes in the eardrum owing to malfunction of the eustachian tube. In all likelihood the term "catarrhal deafness" was, and may still be, intended to apply to any one of the several conditions which today are identified separately as otitis media, secretory otitis media, and slight thickening and retraction of the eardrum suggesting middle ear adhesions. In any event, a better understanding of ear physiology and pathology now makes it possible to apply more specific and meaningful terms to these conditions than "catarrhal deafness."

58

There is also some doubt concerning the role of adhesions in the middle ear as a cause of conductive hearing loss. Experience with stapes surgery, by which now the ossicular chain and the middle ear can be seen very clearly, has convinced otologists that occasional adhesions about the ossicles produce almost negligible hearing loss. Even when many adhesions have to be cut during stapes surgery, very little of the hearing impairment seems to be attributable justly to this cause. Apparently, the ossicles transmit sound waves quite readily in spite of being tied down with adhesions. However, in those instances in which the adhesions add weight and mass to the ossicular chain and drum, hearing is likely to be impaired measurably.

Figure 19 illustrates the mild type of conductive hearing loss that probably is due solely to adhesions in the middle ear. Figure 20 shows a case that was diagnosed as catarrhal deafness by several otologists and proved on surgical exploration to be tympanosclerosis. Schuknecht reported a case of hearing loss caused by a bridge of bone binding the neck of the stapes and preventing mobility (Fig. 21).

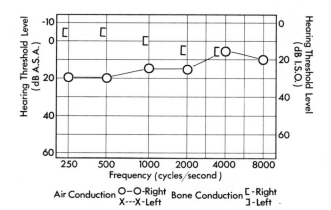

FIG. 19. *History:* 42-year-old male with a history of recurrent otitis media in the right ear as a child. Nonprogressive. No tinnitus. No familial deafness.

Otologic: Right eardrum was scarred and reflected previous infection, but it was intact and moved normally. No fluid visible. Hearing not improved after politzerizing. Exploratory surgery on the right ear revealed multiple bands of scar tissue around incus and crura, binding ossicles to promontory. Stapes footplate was mobile. The ossicles were freed of the adhesions, and hearing in the right ear returned to normal.

Audiologic: mildly reduced low- and mid-frequency thresholds with normal bone conduction thresholds in the right ear. Right ear bone thresholds were obtained with left ear masked.

Classification: conductive
Diagnosis: adhesive deafness

AEROTITIS MEDIA

Hearing loss in aerotitis media is rather mild and temporary unless complications develop. The immediate cause of hearing impairment is retraction of the eardrum, but if the pressure disparity persists, fluid may accumulate in the middle ear and further aggravate the hearing loss.

The pressure disparity between the outer and the middle ears almost invariably occurs during rapid descent in an airplane, when the atmospheric pressure increases rapidly as the plane comes down. If congestion prevents air from passing up the eustachian tube to equalize the increased pressure in the external canal, this pressure pushes in the eardrum toward the middle ear, causing sudden pain, fullness and hearing loss. It occurs most frequently in people whose eustachian tubes are congested due to infection or allergy. To prevent aerotitis media, people with upper respira-

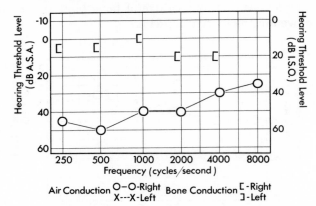

FIG. 20. *History:* Patient had had chronic otitis media for a period of 6 years, which then had cleared up and remained so for the last 10 years. The original hearing loss has not progressed. Condition originally had been diagnosed as "catarrhal deafness."

Otologic: Right eardrum was intact but was thick, scarred, and had white calcific plaques. Exploratory surgery revealed no fluid in the middle ear but layers of shalelike tympanosclerotic bone around the footplate stapes. The plate was mobilized.

Audiologic: moderately reduced air conduction thresholds with normal bone conduction threshold in the right ear. Masking used in the left ear in testing for right ear air and bone thresholds. Hearing improved with footplate mobilization.

Classification: conductive deafness

Diagnosis: deafness due to tympanosclerosis rather than to "catarrhal deafness," as originally diagnosed.

Aids to diagnosis: The severe nonprogressive conductive hearing loss with white calcific deposits is suggestive of tympanosclerosis.

tory infections and acute allergies should be cautioned against flying. With adequately pressurized airplanes aerotitis media is minimized.

If a patient is seen soon after the onset of aerotitis media, the symptoms can be relieved by myringotomy, followed by administration of an oral decongestant and politzerization. When the air pressure in the middle ear is made equal to that in the outer ear, hearing is restored, and the feeling of fullness gradually disappears. Figure 22 describes a classic example of aerotitis media with recovery. If a patient is seen several days after the onset of aerotitis media, it may be necessary to use antibiotics and apply local therapy to the nasopharynx. In all cases hearing should return to normal when the eardrum is restored to its normal position, and the middle ear and the eustachian tubes are clear.

HEMOTYMPANUM

Blood in the middle ear with an intact drum gives the latter a red hue. This is a common finding after head injury with fracture of the middle

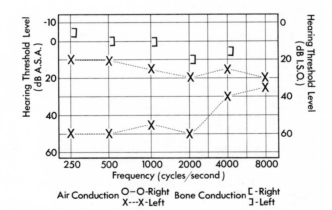

FIG. 21. *History:* progressive hearing loss for 12 years. Has worn a hearing aid in the left ear for 5 years.

Otologic: normal eardrums

Audiologic: Air conduction thresholds revealed a moderately severe loss in the left ear and a moderate loss in the right ear. Tuning fork tests indicated better hearing by bone conduction than by air conduction in the left ear.

Classification: conductive

Diagnosis: bridge of bone binding stapes visualized and corrected at surgery. (Schuknecht, H. F.: Some interesting middle ear problems, Laryngoscope 67:395-409, 1957)

cranial fossa. Sometimes a fluid level is visible. If the sensorineural mechanism has not been injured, the conductive hearing loss is generally about 30 or 40 db, usually involving all frequencies. Occasionally, the high tones are involved to a greater degree. Interestingly enough, the bone conduction shows a high tone drop (Fig. 23) and prompts the erroneous belief that sensorineural damage has occurred. As the blood is absorbed, both air conduction and bone conduction return to normal. Blood also may be seen in the middle ear for a short time following stapes mobilization surgery, and when this occurs, hearing improvement is delayed until absorption takes place.

The normal middle ear has a remarkable ability to remove fluid and debris by absorption, ciliary action of the eustachian tube, and phagocytosis. For this reason, it is unnecessary and often unwise to remove blood from the middle ear cavity by myringotomy and suction. This may only introduce infection and cause complications. Whenever a red eardrum is

		AIR CONDUCTION												
		RIGHT							LEFT					
DATE	LEFT MASK	250	500	1000	2000	4000	8000	RIGHT MASK	250	500	1000	2000	4000	8000
		20	35	35	35	20	25							
		0	10	20	10	10	10	AFTER POLITZERIZATION						
		-5	0	-10	0	5	5	AFTER ASPIRATION TO CLEAR PASSAGE						

		BONE CONDUCTION											
		RIGHT							LEFT				
DATE	LEFT MASK	250	500	1000	2000	4000	TYPE	RIGHT MASK	250	500	1000	2000	4000
	95 db	-5	-10	0	5	10							
	95 db	0	0	-5	10	10		AFTER POLITZERIZATION					
	95 db	5	5	-10	10	5		AFTER ASPIRATION TO CLEAR PASSAGE					

FIG. 22. *History:* Patient developed fullness, pain and hearing loss in right ear during descent in airplane.

Otologic: Examination 2 days following the incident showed a slightly vascular handle of the malleus and bubbles in the right ear. The drum was retracted slightly and did not move freely. The patient had received an injection of penicillin 24 hours previous to the examination, and the eustachian tube seemed to be patent. The ear was politzerized, followed by a myringotomy and aspiration.

Audiologic: Air conduction thresholds in the right ear revealed a mild loss and normal bone conduction. Hearing improved with politzerization and returned to normal after a myringotomy with aspiration.

Classification: conductive

Diagnosis: aerotitis media

Note: that politzerization alone did not restore the hearing to normal, since some fluid still remained in the middle ear.

seen, and blood is suspected of being in the middle ear, a glomus jugulare tumor should be excluded. Roentgenograms for fracture and a good history are essential.

SECRETORY OTITIS MEDIA

The cause of secretory otitis media is not yet established. In spite of considerable literature on the subject, neither the cause nor a specific cure is known at this time. Secretory otitis media seems to be increasing in incidence—a fact which has been related to the increasing use of antibiotics.

Characteristics. In any event, the major feature of the condition is the accumulation of fluid in the middle ear, usually straw-colored and some-

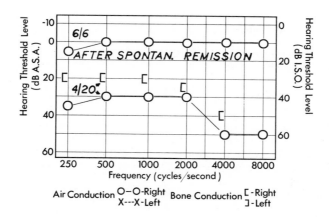

Fig. 23. *History:* 24-year-old patient who sustained a head injury causing right middle ear to be filled with blood.

Otologic: Tympanic membrane was intact but was deep red in color due to blood in the middle ear. The eardrum did not move well with air pressure. Resolution occurred spontaneously without myringotomy.

Audiologic: Pure-tone thresholds in the right ear revealed a mild air conduction loss with reduced bone conduction (left ear masked). Note the greater loss in the high frequencies and the reduced bone thresholds because of the fluid in the middle ear. Hearing returned to normal at all frequencies after spontaneous resolution.

Classification: conductive; damage in middle ear

Diagnosis: Post-traumatic hemotympanum

Aids to diagnosis: A glomus tumor must be excluded. Usually, the eardrum moves freely in a glomus tumor, and the pink color is on the promontory rather than filling the middle ear and the drum. X-ray pictures are helpful if erosion is present. Myringotomy and suction done very cautiously also are of help.

times mucoid or gellike in consistency. In many cases the eustachian tube is patent, and the fluid can be removed readily by myringotomy and politzerization. However, the fluid continues to accumulate in spite of numerous myringotomies and varied treatments, and hearing loss occurs concomitantly, usually greater in the higher tones (Fig. 24). Secretory otitis may be present in one or both ears, and it is found in babies as well as in adults.

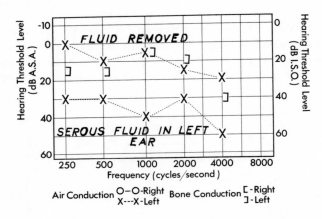

FIG. 24. *History:* 12-year-old male with recurrent episodes of painless hearing loss in left ear. These occurred in the absence of upper respiratory infections. He had a T & A and an adenoid revision, allergy studies, desensitization, autogenous vaccines, and many courses of antibiotics and nose treatments.

Otologic: The left eardrum was slightly scarred but a fluid level was seen. The eustachian tube seemed to be patent. The eardrum did not move freely with air pressure. Exploration of the middle ear showed a thick, clear, gelatinous fluid, which was aspirated. The mucosa over the promontory was thick and hydropic. A tube was used to keep open the lower edge of the replaced eardrum and left in place for several months. The patient had had no recurrence since his surgery, but not all patients respond this well after the tube is removed.

Audiologic: Pure tone thresholds in the left ear revealed a mild air conduction loss with reduced bone conduction (right ear masked). After surgery the air conduction thresholds returned to better levels than the original bone conduction thresholds at most frequencies. Reduced bone thresholds were caused by the presence of thick fluid in the middle ear.

Classification: conductive

Diagnosis: recurrent secretory otitis

Aids to diagnosis: Reduced bone conduction does not mean necessarily that a sensorineural hearing loss is present. An immobile drum, fluctuating hearing loss and a feeling of fluid in an ear should suggest that reduced bone conduction may be due to middle ear involvement rather than to sensorineural causes.

Quite often the condition suddenly stops spontaneously, and the treatment used at that particular time is likely to get the credit, but this conclusion proves to be unjustified in the long run. In some cases the secretion continues to form and causes a perforation in the eardrum. When this occurs, the findings resemble those seen in chronic otitis media, but the discharge is free of infectious elements; as a matter of fact, the discharge generally is almost sterile, and attempts to culture bacteria and viruses from the fluid have been unsuccessful.

When the mucosa of the middle ear in secretory otitis media is examined by biopsy, it is found in most cases to be thickened and hydropic. The thickened mucosa extends to the mouth of the eustachian tube in the middle ear, and perhaps this is a factor in the blockage, if present. Interestingly enough, in many patients with secretory otitis one can observe increased secretion in the nasal mucosa and in the nasopharynx as well; this suggests the possibility that secretory otitis may be more than a local middle ear phenomenon. Some ears fill with secretory fluid after removal of the soft palate for neoplasm. There seems little doubt that in such instances the condition is related to eustachian tube malfunction.

As a matter of fact, it often is difficult to distinguish secretory otitis from serous otitis. Caution in treatment is of utmost importance, and unwarranted surgical procedures should be avoided. For example, it is injudicious to perform a tonsillectomy and adenoidectomy on an infant who has secretory otitis media without positive evidence that the adenoids are the principal cause of the difficulty, in which case it would be a serous otitis. Too frequently, secretory otitis will continue to recur after a tonsillectomy and an adenoidectomy that was unjustified, thereby placing the surgeon in an embarrassing situation. When adenoids are really the major cause of secretion in the middle ears (serous otitis), other symptoms usually are present, including recurrent otitis media and mouth breathing; furthermore, the hypertrophied adenoids can be felt and visualized in the lateral area of the nasopharynx. These findings are not present if the cause is secretory otitis media.

Appearance and Treatment. The appearance of the eardrum in secretory otitis often is characteristic, and yet sometimes it is deceiving. Generally, it is easy to observe bubbles and a yellowish fluid behind the drum. Politzerization, which shows the eustachian tube to be patent, causes the fluid level to shift or even to disappear, and hearing suddenly improves (though not always does it return to normal). Only when myringotomy is performed does an accumulation of straw-colored fluid come out. With politzerization after myringotomy there is a sudden escape of fluid, and the hearing returns to normal.

Sometimes the appearance of the drum is deceiving, because the ear is so filled with fluid or has so little fluid that it cannot be observed through the drum, and thus the drum appears to be normal. An attempt to move the intact eardrum with air pressure perhaps may result in a slight movement. However, if conductive hearing loss is present, and especially if the bone conduction is reduced somewhat in the higher frequencies, myringotomy is essential, for it produces a gush of yellow fluid, and the hearing improves markedly. The length of time that the hearing loss has been present is not a factor and may even be misleading, for fluid can remain in the middle ear for many months or years.

Another Type of Secretory Otitis and Its Differentiation From Otosclerosis. Still another type of secretory otitis media can lead to the erroneous diagnosis of otosclerosis, because it is so difficult to observe

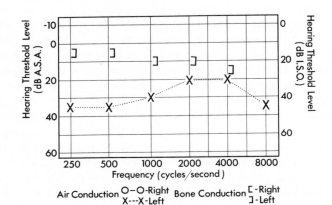

Air Conduction O–O-Right   Bone Conduction Ⅽ-Right
                  X---X-Left   Ⅎ-Left

Fɪɢ. 25. *History:* 27-year-old female with gradual onset of hearing loss in the left ear for several years. Feeling of fullness and occasional heartbeat tinnitus in the left ear. Several members in family have hearing loss. No history of ear infections. The patient had been diagnosed as having unilateral otosclerosis.

Otologic: Eardrums appeared to be normal (but did not move well with politzerization). When the eardrum was elevated, a large gelatinous mass due to secretory otitis was removed from the oval and the round windows. The stapes was found to be mobile.

Audiologic: Air conduction thresholds in the left ear were reduced mildly in the lower frequencies. Bone conduction was almost normal with the right ear masked. Tuning fork lateralized to the left ear. Bone conduction was prolonged and better than air. Hearing returned to normal after removal of gelatinous mass.

Classification: conductive

Diagnosis: secretory otitis

Aids to diagnosis: Original misdiagnosis of otosclerosis might have been avoided if the mobilization of the drum had been tested with politzerization, and if a diagnostic myringotomy had been performed. Not all cases of fluid in the middle ear cause reduced bone conduction.

abnormalities in the eardrum or the middle ear. In this type a gellike mass of clear secretion or a very thick collection of mucoid secretion is located in the middle ear so that it causes hearing loss without any abnormality being visible through the drum. This leads to a diagnosis of otosclerosis. When the middle ear is exposed with the intention of doing a stapes mobilization, a thick secretion instead is found. Its removal causes the hearing to return to normal. Such a case is shown in Figure 25. A preliminary myringotomy and the introduction of a suction tip would have revealed the mass of gellike material.

SEROUS OTITIS MEDIA AND ADENOIDS

There is understandable confusion between serous otitis and secretory otitis media. In the first place, the etiology of secretory otitis is not known, and in the second place, the two conditions sometimes are hard to distinguish clinically. Even outstanding otologists have differences of opinion concerning the differential diagnosis and the distinguishing characteristics.

Definition. For present purposes let us consider serous otitis media as a condition in which serous fluid accumulates in the middle ear because of obstruction or infection of the eustachian tubes or the nasopharynx. If the middle ear becomes infected, the condition is called acute otitis media. The fluid is a secondary phenomenon and results from pathology external to the middle ear. This is in contrast with secretory otitis media, in which the pathology seems to originate in the middle ear.

Causes. The chief cause of serous otitis in children is hypertrophied adenoids in the fossae behind the eustachian tube openings (fossae of Rosenmüller). The adenoids do not grow over the mouths of the Eustachian tubes but cause obstruction in their lumens by submucosal congestion. For this reason, it is essential to punch out this area of adenoid tissue carefully under direct visualization in doing an adenoidectomy for recurrent otitis media or hearing impairment. Merely removing the central adenoid in such cases leads to recurrent symptoms and the need for adenoid revisions.

Adhesions in the fossae of Rosenmüller usually are due to previous careless surgery and may lead to serous otitis by restricting the normal function of the mouth of the eustachian tube; the adhesions may result in hearing impairment. In such cases the adhesions must be removed meticulously under direct vision, and the tubal ends must be mobilized, care being exercised not to injure the submucosal layers and to cause further adhesions.

Nasopharyngeal neoplasms and allergies also may produce serous otitis.

Difficult Detection. The diagnosis of serous otitis as a cause of hearing loss in children often is overlooked, because the hearing loss rarely exceeds 30 db, and children generally are addressed in a loud voice. Thus their hearing difficulty is not detected until the school audiogram is performed, or until the symptom has persisted a long time. In a recent nationwide study of school children 85 per cent with visible serous otitis media

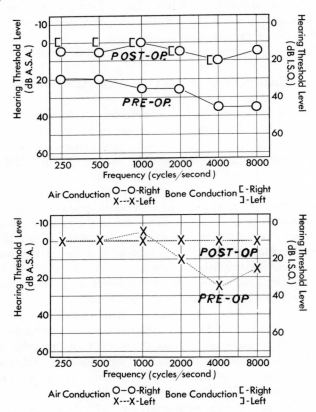

FIG. 26. *History:* 8-year-old child who failed to pass a school hearing test. No history of ear trouble. T & A performed at age 4.

Otologic: amber fluid in right middle ear. Slight amount of fluid in left middle ear, also. Eustachian tubes not clearly patent. Large mass of regrown adenoid tissue especially in lateral pharynx. No response to a year of conservative therapy. Adenoids revised and thin clear fluid aspirated through myringotomy.

Audiologic: Pure tone thresholds in the right ear revealed a mild air conduction loss with normal bone responses. The left ear had a mild loss in the higher frequencies. Hearing returned to normal after surgery.

Classification: conductive

Diagnosis: hypertrophied adenoids with serous otitis media

had hearing losses of 15 db or less, and 50 per cent had hearing losses of less than 5 db.

A fluid level and bubbles often are readily apparent through the drum. The serous fluid level shows no movement when the child's head is bent forward or backward. Sometimes the fluid is hidden or fills the ear so completely that it goes undetected even on otoscopic examination. In such a case the eardrum is immobile and does not move even with air pressure. Fullness and dullness in the ear are common complaints. Figure 26 shows a typical case of hearing loss in a child due to serous otitis that went undetected for many months until a routine school audiogram was performed.

Aim of Therapy. Simple myringotomy performed in such cases may clear up the hearing only temporarily, for the cause is still present in the nasopharynx. Therefore, therapy should be directed to the causes as well as to the immediate relief of symptoms in the ear.

ACUTE OTITIS MEDIA

Hearing loss in acute otitis media is temporary. It clears up when the inflammation subsides, and the debris in the middle ear is absorbed. Depending on the stage of the infection, the hearing loss may be as great as 50 db if the middle ear is filled with pus. Usually, all frequencies are involved if fluid forms in the ear. If there is no fluid in the ear, sometimes only the lower frequencies are involved. An interesting paradox characterizes some cases of severe otitis media in which inflammation extends to the postauricular area. A tuning fork held to the mastoid region shows considerably reduced bone conduction. The same finding can be obtained by bone conduction audiometry on the mastoid region. It seems that sound waves are conducted poorly through the inflamed mastoid bone, but the sensorineural mechanism is not affected. When bone conduction is tested on the teeth, it is found to be normal.

The hearing loss in otitis media is caused by impeded sound transmission across the eardrum and the ossicular chain as a result of the added mass in the middle ear. Tinnitus rarely is present; when it is reported, the patient says he hears his own pulse beat. Although hearing loss during an attack of acute otitis media may be a cause for concern after the pain has subsided, the immediate and urgent problem is the relief of pain. However, what is most important in the long run is to treat otitis media adequately so that it resolves without leaving any permanent hearing damage.

The Question of Myringotomy. The question naturally arises whether myringotomy should be done in all cases of acute otitis media to prevent hearing impairment. There are avid supporters for myringotomy in all cases and equally enthusiastic supporters of the concept that myringotomy rarely should be done. Probably, the best approach lies somewhere in between. Whenever a middle ear contains pus and is causing the drum to bulge, myringotomy certainly is indicated to relieve pain and to prevent hearing loss. This is in keeping with the proven surgical principle that incision and drainage are advisable whenever pus is under pressure. In most bulging drums there is an area of anesthesia in the eardrum due to the pressure in the middle ear, and if the myringotomy is done quickly in this area without pressing deeply into the drum, very little pain is experienced.

Antibiotics. In spite of the excellent results that have been achieved in the prevention and the treatment of acute otitis media by nonsurgical means, a large number of cases do progress to chronic otitis media. One of the causes for some of these failures is the use of inadequate doses or kinds of antibiotics. In many cases of otitis media a much higher blood level of antibiotic is needed than is generally recognized, because the infection has become walled off and can be reached only by very high blood levels of the drug.

Difference Between Acute and Chronic Otitis Media. Since otitis media still leads frequently to chronic otitis media and hearing loss, a fuller discussion is in order. First, we should clarify the general difference between acute and chronic otitis media. Not infrequently, a patient is referred to an ear specialist with a diagnosis of "chronic otitis media," and the otologist finds the drum to be practically normal. The history may reveal that the patient has had repeated earaches and infections almost every 3 months. This is not what is meant by chronic otitis media. Instead, otologists mean an ear that has been infected continuously for at least many months. An acute otitis media is an ear infection of comparatively short duration. If the acute otitis media does not respond satisfactorily to therapy, and the infection persists for many months, it then becomes a chronic otitis media.

If a patient has an acute otitis media that results in a persistent anterior perforation in the eardrum, and the infection clears up only to return again in a month or so, this should be considered to be a recurrent acute, not a chronic, otitis media. As a matter of fact, this very situation is most common in otologic practice. Many patients with anterior perforations whose ears have been dry either get water in them or blow their noses improperly during an upper respiratory infection, and the ear becomes reinfected. In such cases the otorrhea usually is stringy and mucoid and comes from the area of the eustachian tube. Hearing loss generally is minimal, and closure of the anterior perforation restores the hearing.

Common Causes and Prevention. The common causes of acute otitis media are upper respiratory infections and sinusitis, hypertrophied adenoids, allergies, and improper blowing and sneezing as well as eustachian tube blockage. It is notable that all of these causes are external to the ear itself, so that in most instances acute otitis media is a secondary infection, and its prevention must be directed to its causes.

To prevent otitis media and hearing loss, patients should be cautioned to refrain from indiscreet nose blowing and sneezing. Forceful blowing or sneezing while pinching both nares causes a buildup of pressure in the nasopharynx; this pressure may force small amounts of infected mucus through the eustachian tube into the middle ear, with resulting otitis media. These facts should be impressed on patients with upper respiratory infections and perforated eardrums.

Final Checking of Hearing. In all cases of acute otitis media it is important to perform hearing tests after the infection has subsided to be certain that there is no residual hearing impairment that might be permanent or that might require further treatment.

CHRONIC OTITIS MEDIA

When infection persists continuously in the middle ear for long periods of time, it is called chronic otitis media, and this is a very frequent cause of hearing impairment. The mechanism varies. There is invariably a perforation in the eardrum. In most cases the hole is in the posterosuperior portion of the drum. Occasionally, the entire drum is eroded, and much of the middle ear is visible through the otoscope. The more severe hearing losses are due to erosion of some part of the ossicular chain. The most common ossicular defect is erosion of the long end of the incus, so that it does not contact the head of the stapes. Occasionally, the handle of the malleus and even the stapedial crura are eroded. In some ears the entire incus has been found to be destroyed. Scarlet fever and measles are notorious causes of severe erosion of the ossicles and the eardrum.

Another cause of hearing loss in chronic otitis media is discharge in the middle ear. This naturally adds a mass which impedes transmission of sound waves. Strangely enough, a patient may say he hears much worse after the ear is cleared of discharge, and the audiogram often will substantiate this complaint. This result may be explained in several ways, but one of the more reasonable theories is that the discharge blocks sound waves bound for the round window niche and thereby permits some semblance of normal phase difference for sound waves hitting the inner ear. To make this clear, it may be pointed out that sound waves in normal ears selectively enter the oval window rather than the round window because of their direct transmission through the ossicular chain. When the drum is missing, and the ossicular chain is not functioning properly, sound waves occasionally strike both the round and the oval windows almost simultaneously, so that the waves may in part cancel each other before they can reach the inner ear. This causes hearing loss. A discharge in the middle ear sometimes may prevent this effect by blocking sound waves that otherwise would reach the round window niche. Thus the patient may hear better when his ear is moist. The same mechanism sometimes is used on purpose to improve hearing in ears that are free of infection.

However, these considerations should not lead a physician to disregard discharge in the hope of achieving improved hearing, for infection often can result in serious complications. There are more satisfactory methods to restore hearing after an infection has been controlled. When a postero-superior perforation is found in the eardrum with a putrid discharge, it generally means that mastoiditis is present. If the infection is allowed to continue, it may cause a number of complications, including erosion of the ossicles and severe hearing loss. A cholesteatoma may form that could erode the semicircular canals and the facial nerve, and even produce a brain abscess.

It is important, therefore, to cure a chronic middle ear infection as rapidly as possible. Unfortunately, systemic antibiotics do not often succeed in clearing up cases of chronic otitis media, because the chronically

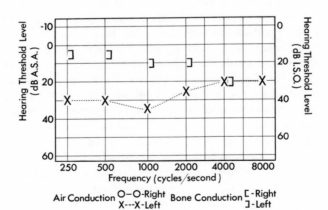

Air Conduction O—O-Right   Bone Conduction ⊏-Right
                X---X-Left   ⊐-Left

Fig. 27. *History:* This patient had a discharging left ear for many years. X-ray study showed a cholesteatoma.

Otologic: large posterior marginal perforation. The ossicular chain was not disrupted; otherwise, the hearing loss would have exceeded 50 db. Ossicular continuity was confirmed at surgery.

Audiologic: Pure tone thresholds in the left ear revealed a mild air conduction loss with a gradually decreasing air-bone gap at the higher frequencies. Right ear masked.

Classification: conductive

Diagnosis: cholesteatoma with marginal perforation

diseased mastoid cells in the middle ear have such a poor blood supply. Consequently, it is necessary to treat the ear locally, and occasionally surgery must be performed when local therapy has been unsuccessful, and complications threaten.

Figures 6, 27 and 30 illustrate several audiometric patterns that may occur in chronic otitis media.

TYMPANOSCLEROSIS

As a result of as yet undetermined causes, sclerotic changes occur in some chronically diseased middle ears. After infection has subsided, a shalelike layer of bony deposit remains over the promontory of the cochlea and around the oval window region. Occasionally, the stapes and the incus are enveloped by stratified bone that can be peeled off in layers. This condition is called tympanosclerosis, and it produces hearing loss by fixing the stapes and the incus in a manner similar to that of otosclerosis. It differs markedly from otosclerosis in that its onset follows an infection, without a familial history of hearing loss. Furthermore, it is generally unilateral. In addition, pathologic changes are visible in the eardrum in most cases of tympanosclerosis. The drums may show healed scars and are thick and yellowish white with areas that suggest sclerosis. Figure 20 describes a typical case of tympanosclerosis in which a stapes mobilization was performed. It is wise to point out that stapedectomies should be undertaken with great caution in cases of tympanosclerosis, because for some unknown reason the incidence of "dead ears" and severe sensorineural losses is high even when the surgery seems to be successful in the operating room. It even has been suggested that an operation on an ear of this type should be done in two stages, in the first removing the tympanosclerosis and in the second mobilizing the stapes or doing a stapedectomy. The hearing loss may be mild or as severe as 65 db when the fixation is complete. All frequencies usually are affected.

CARCINOMA

Carcinoma of the middle ear is rare, and frequently it is not recognized at its inception. Its onset resembles chronic otitis media, since it causes at first a mild conductive hearing loss and later an impairment of up to 60 db, as invasion of the ossicles ensues. Sometimes carcinoma occurs in an ear with chronic otitis that has been present for many years. This is even more difficult to detect, because the change takes place below the typical surface of granulation and polypoid tissue and is not visible to the examiner. Even roentgenograms may be of little help. Biopsy of all granulation tissue is advisable but not always practical in office practice. However, it should be done in all cases of long-standing granulation with recurrent polypoid formation that resists conservative therapy or continues even after surgical intervention, especially when severe pain is present. If the tissue is harder than usual or bleeds readily, a biopsy especially is indicated. Usually, the eardrum perforates early, and chronic otitis media develops, so that the appearance is not very distinctive. Figure 28 shows an unusual case of carcinoma of the middle ear. Hearing is of secondary consideration in carcinoma of the middle ear, but it may be important as a presenting symptom to alert the physician to the presence of a serious condition.

NASOPHARYNGEAL TUMORS

Unilateral conductive hearing loss is frequently the first presenting

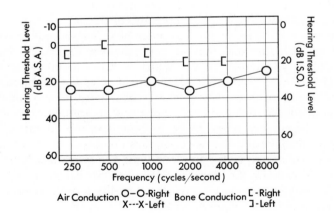

Air Conduction O—O-Right Bone Conduction ⊏-Right
X---X-Left   ⊐-Left

Fig. 28. *History:* 42-year-old woman complained of fullness and severe pain in right ear for several months. No vertigo or tinnitus. She had received antibiotics and myringotomies without satisfactory help. X-ray films showed only a mild haziness in the right mastoid but not in the left.

Otologic: The eardrum was slightly opaque but moved satisfactorily with air pressure.

Audiologic: mild conductive ascending hearing loss in right ear. Left normal.

Diagnosis: After continued unsuccessful conservative therapy the right ear was explored, and a carcinomatous invasion of the middle ear and the mastoid was found. The patient did not respond to cobalt irradiation, and radical surgery was not done.

symptom of a tumor in the nasopharynx. The mechanical cause of the resulting hearing loss resembles that described in serous otitis media: gradual obstruction of the eustachian tube. The possibility that such a serious condition may exist adds emphasis to the importance of doing a nasopharyngoscopic examination in all cases of conductive hearing loss, especially when they are unilateral. The hearing loss by air conduction is comparatively mild in the beginning and may progress to about 40 db, and that by bone conduction usually is normal. The nasopharyngeal examination shows a fullness that is sometimes clear-cut but in other cases uncertain with poor delineation, depending on the nature of the tumor. A better perspective of the tumor generally is obtained through a ·nasopharyngeal mirror below the soft palate.

In the early stages, when the hearing loss is mild, the eardrum appears to be normal. Later, retraction of the drum or serous fluid becomes visible. Whenever fluid repeatedly reforms in one ear, and multiple myringotomies are necessary, it is essential to rule out a nasopharyngeal mass.

ALLERGY

Allergy plays a rather vague role in hearing loss of middle ear origin. Undoubtedly, allergic conditions can lead to congestion of the eustachian tube and the middle ear, with resultant serous otitis media. A few cases of hearing loss have been reported that appear to result primarily from allergy in the middle ear. When the allergy is treated, hearing improves. If judgment is based on experience and a review of the literature, this type of case is not very common unless fluid is present in the middle ear.

Certainly, allergic swelling of the eardrum or the mucosa of the middle ear does occur and may produce hearing loss, but this does not happen as frequently as one might expect from the known frequency of allergies of the upper respiratory tract. Antiallergic care is of major help in clearing up many cases of serous otitis media.

Hearing loss resulting from allergy of the middle ear is necessarily mild. If it exceeds about 20 db, fluid probably is present in the middle ear, or some other causative factor is present.

X-RAY TREATMENTS

Irradiation to the region of the nasopharynx frequently produces congestion in the eustachian tube. Hearing loss along with serous otitis media often is present. The radiation may have been directed to the thyroid, the face, the skull or the nasopharynx. The hearing loss produced is mild

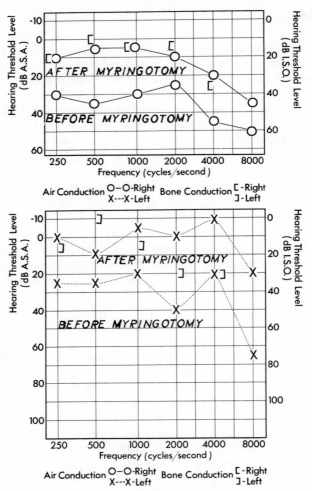

FIG. 29. *History:* 51-year-old female with acromegaly who received x-ray radiation to the pituitary gland. Several weeks later she noted insidious hearing loss and heard her own heartbeat loudly in both ears. She was treated with tranquilizers with little relief.

Otologic: normal eardrums but highly congested nasopharynx and eustachian tubes. Eardrums mobile but difficult to politzerize. Amber fluid evacuated from both ears through myringotomy, with restoration of hearing. Tinnitus disappeared.

Audiologic: Right and left ears showed mild conductive losses with normal bone conduction in the low- and mid-frequency range. After both middle ears were aspirated, air conduction thresholds returned to preoperative bone levels in the right ear, and bettered these levels in the left ear. Reduced bone conduction thresholds were caused by fluid in middle ears.

Classification: conductive

Diagnosis: otitis media due to x-ray treatment to pituitary for acromegaly

and rarely exceeds 30 to 35 db. After some months of conservative therapy the congestion subsides, and the hearing returns to normal (Fig. 29).

An extraordinary incident of conductive hearing loss due to irradiation for a brain tumor was encountered by the author. Notable was an aseptic mastoid cell necrosis that occurred more than 20 years after the treatment. The severe conductive loss was due to two factors, a large erosive defect in the posterior external canal wall and profuse serous discharge from the middle ear. The hearing could be improved slightly by occluding the perforation in the canal wall.

SYSTEMIC DISEASES

Certain systemic diseases are known to affect the middle ear and to cause conductive hearing loss. The most common of these are measles and scarlet fever. Both are notorious for the marked otitis media that they can cause, with erosion of the eardrum and the ossicles. This complication is not nearly so common now as it was years ago, but the hearing losses resulting from these conditions still are encountered in practice. Figure 30

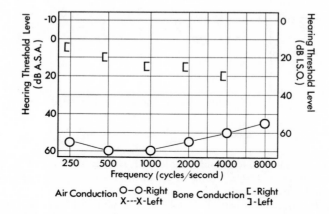

Air Conduction O—O-Right   Bone Conduction ⌈-Right
              X---X-Left   ⌉-Left

Fig. 30. *History:* 20-year-old male who had had scarlet fever as a child with right chronic otitis for 1 year. Since this time the hearing has been reduced, but the ear drained only after swimming or a bad cold.

Otologic: The entire eardrum was eroded, and the handle of the malleus was gone except for a small nubbin. The incus and the stapedial crura also were eroded.

Audiologic: Air conduction thresholds in the right ear revealed a moderately severe loss and slightly reduced bone conduction thresholds. The mild reduced bone conduction does not mean necessarily a sensorineural involvement in such a case.

Classification: conductive

Diagnosis: right chronic otitis media due to scarlet fever

shows a common example of conductive hearing loss following scarlet fever in childhood. The eardrum and the ossicles in such cases generally are eroded, and the hearing level is about 60 db.

Letterer-Siwe's disease, xanthomatosis, eosinophilic granulomatoma and other granulomata are other causes of conductive hearing loss. Though not very common, they can damage the middle ear and cause handicapping hearing loss.

GLOMUS JUGULARE

Glomus jugulare tumors are rare, but when they are present, hearing loss and tinnitus are frequently the only symptoms. This peculiar neoplasm arises from cells around the jugular bulb and expands to involve neighboring structures. In doing so it most frequently extends to the floor of the middle ear, causing conductive loss and pulsating tinnitus. The

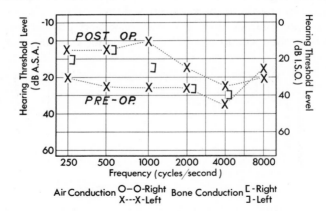

Fig. 31. *History:* 57-year-old female with sudden discomfort in left ear 6 months before. Thumping tinnitus for past 6 months. No facial paralysis. Some hearing loss. No pain.

Otologic: right ear clear. Left middle ear was red and inflamed, but eardrum moved freely. Needle aspiration produced bleeding, which was controlled quickly.

Audiologic: Left ear air conduction thresholds revealed a mild flat hearing loss. Bone conduction thresholds showed an air-bone gap at 500, 1,000, and 2,000 cps only. Left ear discrimination was 96%.

Classification: conductive with high frequency sensorineural involvement

Diagnosis: glomus jugulare tumor, surgically removed. The diagnosis actually was made before the needle aspiration, since the red color was on the promontory in the middle ear rather than in the drum. The drum moved freely with air pressure. Caution is essential in cutting into these highly vascular tumors.

hearing loss in most cases is due to pressure disparity in the middle ear with subsequent ossicular chain impairment. The pulsating tinnitus is due to obstruction of the blood supply. The key feature of a glomus tumor is its vascularity. In appearance the tumor is red or pink so far as it can be seen through the intact eardrum. As a matter of fact, a highly suggestive test for glomus is to put positive air pressure on the drum through the otoscope and watch the middle ear blanch. This is quite pronounced if a glomus tumor appears to be reddish in the middle ear. When negative pressure is applied, the middle ear blanches. The tumor is so vascular that bleeding is a major surgical consideration.

In the early stages the only symptom present with a glomus tumor is a mild conductive hearing loss, which then progresses (Fig. 31). Later, the mass causes chronic otitis media and may extend through the drum with evident granulation tissue and discharge. Whenever granulation tissue in the middle ear bleeds markedly, one should suspect a glomus tumor. X-ray films to show erosion and a careful biopsy are helpful in the diagnosis. Retrograde jugularography is useful to show an early tumor and its extent.

As in any expanding neoplasm, early diagnosis of a glomus jugulare tumor makes surgical cure more effective. Since conductive hearing loss is not only the earliest symptom but for a long time the only symptom, the physician is obligated to establish the cause for every case of unilateral conductive hearing loss. A pink looking middle ear or bleeding granulation tissue always should suggest the possibility of a glomus tumor.

Chapter 9

Conductive Hearing Loss: Effects of Ear Surgery

Details and procedures of middle ear surgery are beyond the scope of this book, but the physician who examines the ear of a patient with conductive hearing loss may discover evidence of previous ear surgery, and he should be prepared to evaluate the relation of the patient's hearing deficit to past otologic surgical procedures. A brief review of these interventions and the visible traces they are likely to leave is therefore in order.

MYRINGOTOMY

Incision and drainage through the eardrum is called myringotomy. The incision or puncture which some physicians prefer is made in the bulging part of the eardrum or in the postero-inferior quadrant, to avoid injuring any middle or inner ear structure in case the incision goes too deep. This might occur if the patient moved inadvertently during the procedure. In unusual instances the long end of the incus and even more rarely the stapedial crura are injured during myringotomy. Figure 32 is a case report in which such an injury occurred in childhood and remained undiagnosed until surgery was performed many years later.

In most instances myringotomy leaves only a very small scar which is absorbed over a period of months, and the eardrum returns to normal. Occasionally, permanent scar tissue is left, which indicates previous ear infections with myringotomies. The hearing is not damaged by a myringotomy in itself or by the scar tissue it occasionally leaves in the eardrum.

HEARING LOSS ASSOCIATED WITH EAR SURGERY

When ear surgery is performed nowadays, prime consideration is given to preservation or restoration of hearing. Of course, in surgery for mastoiditis or chronic otitis media the principal objective is to remove the infection, but the type of surgery performed is determined to a great degree by efforts to preserve hearing. A number of surgical procedures produce visible changes in the eardrum and the external ear that potentially are associated with hearing impairment. The physician has an opportunity to see these visible changes, such as a postauricular scar, and he should be acquainted with the hearing losses that normally might be associated with such evidence of past ear surgery. Some surgical procedures leave little or no recognizable scarring, and even a skilled otologist may be unable to state with certainty that the ear has been operated on. Most instances of stapes surgery fall into this category.

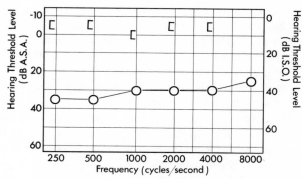

Fig. 32. *History:* 16-year-old male with right ear hearing loss following an ear infection at age 7. Ear was lanced at that time. There have been no further infections, and the hearing loss has not progressed. No tinnitus.

Otologic: eardrums almost normal with only slight evidence of scarring. At surgery the end of the incus was found to have been fractured and to have healed with fibrous union. This damage probably was caused by a myringotomy knife. A polyethylene tube was used to improve the incudostapedial connection.

Audiologic: Right ear air conduction thresholds revealed a mild flat hearing loss, with normal bone thresholds.

Classification: conductive

Diagnosis: ossicular disruption

Aids to diagnosis: Normal bone conduction thresholds are an important criterion in the diagnosis of ossicular defect (for example, not depressed as the result of fluid or stapes fixation).

Therefore, it is important to obtain a careful history of any previous surgery by direct questioning of the patient.

SIMPLE MASTOIDECTOMY

Extremely common several years ago, simple mastoidectomy now is almost a rarity. Better management of otitis media by the general practitioner and the pediatrician practically has obviated the need for this emergency procedure. It was done most commonly in children who had severe otitis media that extended to the mastoid bone and caused postauricular swelling, pain and tenderness, as well as hearing loss. Hearing loss was present because of the middle ear infection, not the mastoiditis.

A simple mastoidectomy consists merely of making a postauricular incision, removing the mastoid cells and creating an opening into the tympanic antrum that leads to the middle ear. This opening then allows pus to drain out of the middle ear from the operated area, thus relieving the pressure. Essentially, this procedure is a modified type of incision and drainage for pus under pressure. Since the middle ear is not disturbed deliberately, and the eardrum usually remains intact (after the infection subsides), hearing usually returns to normal. It is common to find patients who have retained normal hearing after having had several simple mastoidectomies with large postauricular scars.

Unfortunately, not all patients who have had simple mastoidectomies or myringotomies have normal hearing. Some have persistent hearing loss because of surgical mishaps and others because of persistent perforations in the eardrum; still others have mild hearing losses due to retraction of the eardrum or to middle ear adhesions.

The chief evidence of a previous simple mastoidectomy is the presence of a postauricular scar with a normal or almost normal eardrum and good hearing. Even if the eardrum is perforated, but the hearing level is better than about 20 db, the surgery probably was a simple mastoidectomy that left an intact ossicular chain.

MYRINGOPLASTY

Whenever a perforation is found in an eardrum without any active infection, it is now possible to close the perforation. If the hearing loss is due entirely to the perforation, the closure should restore the hearing. The improvement in hearing that can be expected by closing the perforation can be determined preoperatively by artificially patching the hole with a small piece of cigarette paper, fish skin, Gelfoam or silastic film. Audiograms obtained prior to and after the patching show the amount of hearing improvement that can be expected from permanent closure of the graft. If no improvement occurs, it means the perforation is not the sole cause of the hearing loss, and the middle ear and the ossicular chain should be inspected. In either event it is advisable to close the perforation, but the patient should be advised of the prognosis prior to the surgery. In cases in which the hearing loss is not due to the perforation, a simple myringoplasty is inadequate as far as the hearing is concerned. It then becomes necessary to reflect the eardrum upon itself and to explore the middle ear in addition to closing the perforation in the drum.

Figure 33 describes a case of simple myringoplasty.

The appearance of the eardrum following myringoplasty varies greatly. It is important to obtain a history of this type of surgical procedure from the patient; otherwise, a physician might be startled by the appearance of the eardrum and the hearing loss present and advise unjustified treatment. If a skin graft was used to close the perforation, the drum may appear to be thick and white, and redundant skin may be present so that the drum is flaccid and sometimes hardly delineated. If a vein graft was

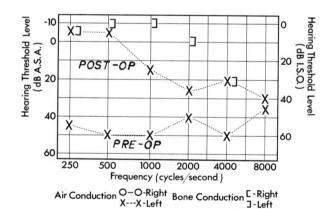

Fig. 33. *History:* intermittent discharge from left ear.

Otologic: large perforation in eardrum. Discharge was cleared up with conservative therapy, and later the large perforation was closed with a sliding flap from the external auditory canal.

Audiologic: Left ear air conduction thresholds revealed a moderate loss. Bone conduction thresholds were normal except at 4,000 cps. After the myringoplasty an air-bone gap remained at the two middle frequencies.

Classification: conductive

Diagnosis: perforated drum corrected with myringoplasty

used, the drum may appear to be stranded and scarred and sometimes thickened and discolored. The appearance of the drum often depends on the graft used, its thickness, and the manner in which it "took." When a grafted eardrum appears flaccid and retracted, and the patient complains of a fluctuating hearing loss that becomes more noticeable every time there is a feeling of fullness in the ear, gentle politzerization often can restore hearing to an improved level. Sometimes a myringoplasty heals so well that it leaves an almost normal-appearing eardrum, and the examining physician is scarcely able to detect that any surgery has been done.

OSSICULOPLASTY

The term "ossiculoplasty" is coming into greater use to denote a simple repair or restoration of the continuity of the ossicular chain. For example, in the case given in Figure 34, closure of the perforation did not restore hearing, and so at a later date the then intact eardrum was elevated, and the ossicles were examined. It then was seen that instead of a normal incus, the connection of the incus with the head of the stapes was fibrous, thin and very weak, making poor contact. This condition probably

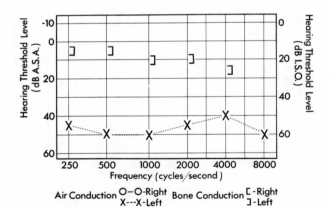

Fig. 34. *History:* 44-year-old female with a 2-year episode of left ear discharge when in her early 20's. No tinnitus. Had had a myringoplasty which did not restore hearing.

Otologic: large healed perforation. Further surgery revealed that the incus end was eroded and replaced with a thin band of fibrous tissue. The continuity of the chain was corrected with a wire prosthesis. Hearing was restored with restoration of ossicular continuity.

Classification: conductive

Diagnosis: ossicular disruption

resulted from the same infection that had caused the perforation. When the weak connection was replaced with a polyethylene joint, hearing improved markedly. The only reason that two surgical procedures were required in this case was that prior to the simple myringoplasty no therapeutic test of closure with an artificial membrane had been done.

The many types of deformities and defects sometimes found in the ossicular chain may test the ingenuity of the surgeon. The defects may be congenital or acquired and may involve any or all of the ossicles. The hearing loss can involve practically all of the frequencies, and when there is complete disruption of the chain with an intact drum, the hearing loss is between 50 and 60 db.

When the eardrum is normal, and a nonotosclerotic ossicular defect is found, the etiology is quite likely to be congenital. Exceptions do occur. More commonly, however, there is a history of otitis media, and some abnormality is present in the drum. The diagnosis is not hard to make, but it is difficult to predict just which ossicle is involved.

Whenever a patient has a 50- to 60-db hearing loss involving all of the frequencies, and patching of the perforation does not improve the hearing, there is a good possibility that the ossicular chain is disrupted (if otosclerosis is excluded). If the hearing loss is only about 30 db and other circumstances are the same, it is more likely that the ossicular chain is intact, that some fracture, or joint damage has occurred, and that the joint union is either fibrous or weakened (again, if otosclerosis is absent). It is needless to emphasize that the middle ear should be examined whenever there is any doubt that simple myringoplasty can restore hearing.

RADICAL MASTOIDECTOMY

Radical mastoidectomy is performed in selected cases of chronic otitis media and mastoiditis in which it is not advisable or possible to clear up the infection conservatively and at the same time to preserve the ossicular chain and the eardrum as well as the hearing. Usually, in such cases there is a cholesteatoma and erosion of the eardrum and the ossicles. Surgery can be done through an endaural or a postauricular incision. The mastoid cells are exenterated, and the malleus and the incus are removed. Of course, the stapes is carefully left in place. Because there is no ossicular chain or drum, the hearing level in ears after such surgery is about 55 to 60 db, involving all frequencies. The appearance of the middle ear varies, but usually skin covers a large mastoid cavity, no eardrum is present, and one can see into the anterior part of the middle ear where the eustachian tube opening lies. These ears have a tendency to collect debris and cerumen and require frequent cleaning.

In some patients with radical mastoid cavities it is now possible to improve hearing by tympanoplastic surgery that partly reconstructs the middle ear.

MODIFIED RADICAL MASTOIDECTOMY AND TYMPANOPLASTY

There is now a choice of procedures intermediate between simple and radical mastoidectomies. Aimed at the eradication of infection in the mastoid bone and the middle ear together with the preservation of hearing, these are called modified radical mastoidectomies or, more recently, tympanoplasties. The latter term has broader coverage, for it applies also to procedures on previously operated ears, now dry, for the purpose of restoring hearing. An entire field of reconstructive middle ear surgery has opened up with the new, improved knowledge of hearing and middle ear infection. For this reason, in the presence of hearing loss, more and more tympanoplasties are being performed on previously operated ears. Even in some radical mastoid cavities it is now possible to improve hearing by reconstructive surgery.

Among the most common procedures used are those involving the positioning of a polyethylene tube or wire connecting the stapes with either a newly grafted eardrum or a small remaining section of the malleus. If any part of the incus is still present in an infected ear, it can be used for a connection with the stapes footplate, and reasonably good hearing may be so obtained.

Most modified radical mastoidectomies and tympanoplasties are done through an endaural incision rather than postauricularly. Very little scar is left following endaural surgery, and this is seen as a fine line slightly above the tragus and directed upward toward the temple. The posterior portion of the ear canal usually is removed, and thus a larger canal than normal is left. The eardrum, usually present, generally is not normal, for it has been scarred by infection and in most cases has been grafted to close a perforation.

FENESTRATION

Many ears were fenestrated in the past, but this complicated procedure is being superseded by stapes surgery. It is important to recognize a fenestrated ear, to be able to care for it, and to know the procedures available to improve hearing in an unsuccessful fenestration or in one in which the hearing has regressed.

Fenestrations were done in cases of otosclerosis with excellent bone conduction, and they usually were performed endaurally. The object was to circumvent the fixed stapes and to allow sound waves to impinge directly on a new window, bypassing the fixed oval window. The new window was made in the horizontal semicircular canal and was covered with a skin flap from the posterior canal wall continuous with the eardrum. Because of the depth and the difficulty of access to the operative site, the eardrum necessarily was dislocated, and the incus and the head of the malleus were removed. On otoscopic examination the external auditory canal is found to be enlarged, and the eardrum is seen to be pushed back into the middle ear. Part of the mastoid bone also has been removed, so that a large cavity is visible. Because of the disruption of the ossicular chain and other factors, it was not possible to obtain consistent hearing levels better than 15 or 20 db in most fenestrated ears. Figure 35 shows a typical successful result. Bone conduction had to be very good with a large air-bone gap to warrant fenestration. Occasionally, hearing regressed due to closure of the fenestration.

In some of these cases it now is possible to improve hearing by stapes

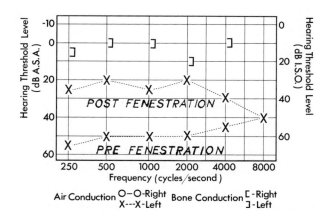

Air Conduction O—O-Right
X---X-Left
Bone Conduction ⊏-Right
⊐-Left

FIG. 35. *History:* gradual hearing loss and buzzing tinnitus over 10 years. Sister also hard of hearing. Soft voice and hears better in noisy room.
Otologic: normal
Audiologic: Left ear air conduction thresholds revealed a moderate flat loss. Bone thresholds were normal. Fenestration surgery reduced the air-bone gap, but because the ossicular continuity had been disrupted during this operation and the hearing pathway altered to go through a fenestration in the lateral semicircular canal, hearing rarely improved beyond the 15-db level.
Classification: conductive
Diagnosis: otosclerosis corrected with fenestration surgery

surgery. In such cases the stapes may be mobilized, and a polyethylene tube or a steel wire is attached under the malleus and connected with the vein graft or over Gelfoam. Another good procedure is to run a wire with a tissue plug from the malleus to the newly formed oval window.

In cleaning debris from fenestrated ears care should be exercised by the physician while he is working deep in the ear. Vertigo is induced readily by pressing near the fenestrated area.

MIDDLE EAR PROSTHESES

There are patients whose conductive hearing loss is greatly improved by inserting a prosthesis into the middle ear. We are not referring to an electronic hearing aid but to a small insert that improves the transmission of sound to the inner ear. The eardrum must be absent or have a large perforation so that the prosthesis can be inserted. Usually, the ossicular chain is not functioning, and the prosthesis simulates the chain

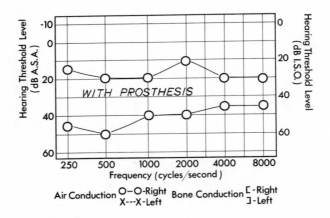

FIG. 36. *History:* Right ear drained for many years and finally cleared up with treatment.

Otologic: Right eardrum had a large perforation. The middle ear was dry. The round window niche was visible, and an artificial prosthesis with a plastic drum and nylon rod applied to the bony promontory near the round window restored hearing. This procedure was effective for periods up to 2 weeks.

Audiologic: Right ear air conduction thresholds revealed a moderate loss with poorer thresholds in the lower frequencies. Hearing was greatly improved with the prosthesis in place.

Classification: conductive

Diagnosis: right conductive hearing loss due to perforated drum and malfunctioning ossicular chain.

and the eardrum. The excellent results obtained with prostheses are sometimes as startling as that shown in Figure 36.

There are many different kinds of prostheses. The basic principle is to replace the drum and the ossicular chain so that sound waves are conducted directly to the area of the oval window. One type of prosthesis covers the round window opening so that sound waves cannot strike both the round and the oval windows simultaneously, thereby nullifying their effects in the inner ear and causing a hearing loss. Ointments can be used as a prosthesis in some of these cases. Aquaphor ointment commonly is used. If the patient's eardrum is gone so that the round window niche is visible, a patient's hearing sometimes may be improved markedly by carefully applying a plug of Aquaphor ointment over the round window niche. In appropriate cases this ointment maintains the hearing improvement for several weeks; occasionally, the patient can teach himself to replace the ointment. The patient also can be taught to insert and to remove many of the mechanical prostheses used in the middle ear. However, it is important to avoid introducing infections in using a middle ear prosthesis; therefore, frequent otologic examinations are advisable.

Prostheses are used whenever a patient's hearing cannot be corrected surgically for one reason or another.

Chapter 10

Conductive Hearing Loss: Causes With Normal-Appearing Eardrums and Middle Ears

This chapter describes the following causes of conductive hearing loss in which the external auditory canals, the eardrums and the middle ears appear to be normal on otoscopic examination:

1. Congenital ossicular defects
2. Acquired ossicular defects
3. Otosclerosis
4. Paget's disease
5. Van der Hoeve's syndrome
6. Invisible fluid
7. Malfunction of the eustachian tube

CONGENITAL OSSICULAR DEFECTS

A variety of defects may arise in the ossicular chain during fetal development, and usually they produce a conductive hearing loss of 50 to 60 db despite a normal appearance of the eardrum and the middle ear. The handicap, if bilateral, usually is discovered by the time the child is 3 years old, but the discovery may be long delayed if the defect affects only one ear.

A congenital ossicular defect should be suspected when a young patient with a normal-appearing eardrum "has had a hearing loss all his life," when it is conductive and in the range of 40 db or more, and particularly when it is unilateral, nonprogressive and nonfamilial. Tinnitus is almost never a complaint.

If the hearing loss is bilateral, careful questioning will disclose that speech development was delayed, and that the patient reacted to the handicap in one of two ways: poor school work or some behavior problem rather obviously related to the child's inability to hear and to respond. Though the nonprogressive character of the hearing loss is of considerable diagnostic importance, the hearing may fluctuate during upper respiratory infections, allergies and similar conditions, as is true also of hearing losses of other etiologies. However, in the case of ossicular defects, the hearing level always returns and is maintained at the original level.

Figure 32 shows an audiogram of a patient whose hearing loss is highly suggestive of congenital ossicular defect. Reference to this audiogram at this point serves to emphasize the importance of a careful and critical appraisal of the otologic findings in conjunction with audiology, especially

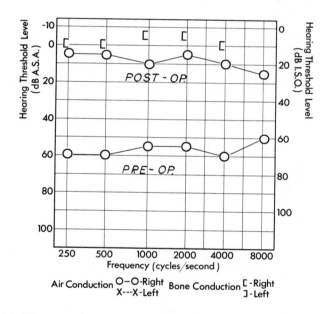

FIG. 37. *History:* 50-year-old male who had normal hearing until an industrial head injury. He lost consciousness, but there was no fracture of the skull. No tinnitus or vertigo but a marked right ear hearing loss resulted from the injury.

Otologic: normal eardrums and middle ears. Exploration revealed a complete dislocation of the end of the incus from the head of the stapes. Continuity was restored and hearing improved.

Audiologic: Air conduction thresholds in the right ear revealed a moderately severe hearing loss. Bone conduction thresholds were normal. The air-bone gap was maximal for a conductive lesion. Tuning fork lateralized to the right ear, and air was better than bone conduction.

Classification: conductive (maximum)

Diagnosis: ossicular disruption due to head trauma

a more meticulous inspection of the drum, in order not to miss this diagnosis.

In cases in which an ossicular defect is suspected, the procedure of choice is to elevate the eardrum, as in stapes surgery, and to examine the ossicular chain. When these defects are present, they can be found in almost every part of the chain. One of the most common examples is congenital fixation of the stapes. Another frequent observation is congenital absence of the long process of the incus, as a result of which the incus does not connect with the head of the stapes. General malformation of the stapedial crura also has been found to be responsible for some hearing loss. There are still other congenital defects that challenge the ingenuity of the surgeon who attempts to establish a functional continuity of the ossicular chain.

ACQUIRED OSSICULAR DEFECTS

It is possible for the ossicular chain to be disrupted or damaged

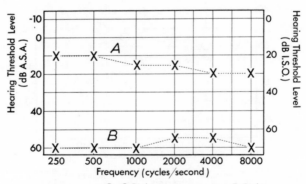

FIG. 38. *History:* Patient had good stapedectomy result (A). Fifteen months postoperative she received a sharp blow to the left ear and the side of face. Sudden deafness followed (B). No vertigo was experienced.

Otologic: Exploration revealed the polyethylene tube prosthesis was dislodged and lay free in the middle ear. This was removed and replaced with a steel piston and wire around the incus.

Audiologic: Post-traumatic air conduction thresholds represented a 35 to 50 db reduction in hearing from those obtained after a successful stapedectomy. Hearing was restored with a new prosthesis.

Classification: conductive

Diagnosis: dislocated prosthesis

without causing visible changes in the tympanic membrane. This is not found commonly but always should be borne in mind as a possibility. Figure 37 shows an interesting example of ossicular damage following head injury in an industrial accident. A similar lesion can be produced during myringotomy in childhood if the myringotomy knife penetrates too deeply and damages the incus. After the operation the eardrum may heal normally without any scarring, but the damage to the incus remains.

Figure 38 shows another interesting case in which a patient heard well following a stapedectomy until one day she received a sharp blow to the operated side of her head. Her hearing suddenly dropped. Examination of the middle ear showed that the polyethylene tube had been dislodged from its proper position by the blow. Another patient showed a contrary experience. Here the patient failed to gain better hearing from a stapedectomy and vein graft. A sudden and hard stop in a descending elevator several months later caused her hearing to return immediately. Apparently, the polyethylene tube was knocked into a better position, and the hearing improved. In all these cases the change in hearing was sudden in contrast with the long history of deafness in congenital defects and otosclerosis.

Occasionally, there is a fixation of the malleo-incudal joint or of the malleus itself. This may occur after a mild infection without evidence in the eardrum, or there may be no known cause. Two ossicles may become so fixed that they do not transmit sound waves, and a marked hearing loss may result in spite of a normal stapes and oval window.

In rare instances the incus or the stapedial crura may be broken by a blow to the head, and healing takes place by fibrous rather than bony union (Fig. 32). In such cases the hearing loss may be comparatively mild. The hearing loss resulting from ossicular defect generally involves all frequencies, and tinnitus is absent. The precise diagnosis seldom is made until the ossicular chain is examined surgically. The vast majority of these defects can be repaired and the hearing restored.

One other type of ossicular defect with normal otoscopic findings requires discussion. It is the damage which may be done either to the end of the incus or to the stapes during stapes surgery. In some cases in which stapes mobilization is attempted by pushing down on the end of the incus, or in which a wire prosthesis is too tight, the incus is weakened or split off. This impairs the efficiency of the incudostapedial joint and may cancel the benefits of successful mobilization or even make hearing worse. Fracture of the head of the stapes or its crura is another cause of acquired ossicular defect. In some such instances an initial hearing loss of 30 db may be increased to 50 db. The bones rarely heal sufficiently for the hearing to improve noticeably, and stapedectomy or replacement of the crura and the end of the incus with an artificial stapes then becomes necessary.

Stapedectomies also may be unsuccessful because, after removal of the stapes and replacement with an artificial stapes, the prosthesis may slip or make poor contact, or the oval window may close over, and the hearing loss may become worse than it was before surgery.

OTOSCLEROSIS

When conductive hearing loss is present in an adult, and the eardrum and the middle ear appear to be normal through the otoscope, the most likely diagnosis is otosclerosis. There are other possible causes, but they are comparatively uncommon. The cause of otosclerosis is unknown, but for some undiscovered reason there occurs in some people a gradual fixation of the stapedial footplate in the oval window because of pathologic changes in the cochlear bone. Actually, the name "otosclerosis" is misleading, for it is really not a sclerotic process; it is more like a vascularization in the bone with formation of spongy bone. Such changes have been reported nowhere else in the body, only in the bony labyrinth. In view of

		AIR CONDUCTION												
		RIGHT							LEFT					
DATE	LEFT MASK	250	500	1000	2000	4000	8000	RIGHT MASK	250	500	1000	2000	4000	8000
6/1955		35	35	30	20	10	5		35	40	30	20	5	5
4/1956		45	40	40	20	10	10		40	40	30	20	10	10
6/1957		50	50	50	25	15	15		40	45	35	20	15	15
4/1959		55	55	50	40	20	25		45	45	40	35	30	25
4/1962		60	55	50	50	40	35		50	55	50	45	45	40
2/1964		60	55	55	60	65	50		55	55	55	55	60	45

		BONE CONDUCTION											
		RIGHT							LEFT				
DATE	LEFT MASK	250	500	1000	2000	4000	TYPE	RIGHT MASK	250	500	1000	2000	4000
6/1955		0	0	0	5	5			0	0	0	5	5
4/1959		0	5	5	10	15			0	5	10	10	15
2/1964		0	10	20	25	30			0	10	25	20	35

SPEECH RECEPTION THRESHOLD					DISCRIMINATION SCORE					
					RIGHT			LEFT		
DATE	RIGHT	LEFT MASK	LEFT	RIGHT MASK	% SCORE	TEST LEVEL	LEFT MASK	% SCORE	TEST LEVEL	RIGHT MASK
6/1955	30		35		100	70		100	75	

FIG. 39. Progressive hearing loss in otosclerosis. Patient refuses surgical intervention and gets along well with a hearing aid. Note that bone conduction is becoming reduced even though this patient was 38 years old at the time of the last audiogram.

the high incidence of otosclerosis and the confusion surrounding its diagnosis, and on account of the large number of surgical operations being performed for it, a comparatively elaborate description is devoted to the subject in this section.

CLINICAL OTOSCLEROSIS

Actually, there are many more people with otosclerosis than there are patients who seek medical advice for their hearing loss and receive the benefit of diagnosis. For instance, it has been shown that otosclerosis is found at autopsy in the ears of many individuals who in life gave no evidence of hearing impairment. This happens when otosclerotic changes affect areas of the bony labyrinth other than the oval window. It is only when the oval window and the stapes are involved that hearing loss develops, and then it is called clinical otosclerosis. For the purposes of this book we shall call it simply otosclerosis, because the condition does not concern us clinically until hearing impairment develops. Fixation of the stapes may occur over a period of many months or even years. The hearing gradually diminishes as the footplate becomes more fixed. Figure 39 shows a serial audiogram of a patient with otosclerosis whose hearing level has been followed repeatedly for years as her hearing loss progressed.

EXTENT OF HEARING LOSS

In some cases the hearing loss stops progressing after reaching only a very mild level. We do not know yet why this occurs. More frequently, the hearing deteriorates until it stabilizes at about 50 to 60 db. The hearing deficit classically starts in the lower frequencies and gradually progresses to the high ones. Eventually, all frequencies are involved. In numerous patients the high tones continue to deteriorate even more than the low frequencies due to superimposed sensorineural deafness.

CHARACTERISTIC FEATURES

There are many intriguing and challenging features about otosclerosis. For example, it is far come common in females than in males, and it is generally first noted around the age of 18. Quite often the hearing loss is accompanied by a most annoying buzzing tinnitus; both symptoms usually are aggravated by pregnancy. The tinnitus commonly subsides over a period of many years.

Psychological Aspects. Of particular interest is the strange psychological complex almost invariably present in otosclerotic patients. Some of them become suspicious and feel people are talking about them. Many become introspective and have marked personality changes. They creep into their own shells. Some try to appear to be lighthearted and even humorous, but the attempt lacks conviction. Perhaps these symptoms are related to the gradual onset of otosclerosis; yet no comparable reaction is seen in hearing loss from other causes, though these also may have a gradual onset.

It has been suggested, without any proof, that otosclerosis is a psychosomatic disease. Certainly, the psychological aspects of otosclerosis are of paramount importance. One of the vital reasons for trying to restore hearing early with surgery is to head off adverse psychological changes.

Familial Aspects. Otosclerosis is familial to some extent. It often is found in several people in the same family. On the other hand, many patients with otosclerosis deny any hearing loss in their families for as many generations as they may recall. It is not possible to predict on genetic principles who in a family will exhibit clinical otosclerosis, but on theoretical grounds marriages between members of two families in both of which there are clear-cut cases of otosclerosis seem to be inadvisable. Nevertheless, the risk does not warrant an extreme position, and one should not stand in the way of a man and a woman who wish to get married after they have been made aware of the facts. None of their offspring may develop a hearing loss. Certainly, there is no justification for a therapeutic abortion in a pregnant woman with otosclerosis merely because her hearing loss might be aggravated during pregnancy. Some older textbooks took a contrary view, but such a stand is unwarranted in the light of the present knowledge of otosclerosis.

Effect of Excellent Bone Conduction. A prominent feature in otosclerosis is that the patient speaks in a very soft and modulated voice. As previously pointed out, this is easily explained by the fact that these patients have excellent bone conduction. Attention also has been called to the observation that the patient may complain that his hearing gets worse when he chews crunchy foods like celery. This, too, is related logically to these patients' excellent bone conduction, which causes the crunching noise to interfere with hearing conversation.

DIFFERENTIATION

During pure tone audiometry patients with otosclerosis often are uncertain whether or not they really hear the tone when they are being tested at threshold. In contrast, patients with sensorineural deafness are sure when they hear and when they do not.

In spite of the classic symptoms that otosclerotic patients present, many cases are still misdiagnosed as catarrhal deafness, allergic deafness, adhesive deafness or deafness due to eustachian blockage. Because of these errors in diagnosis the author deliberately has emphasized in discussing these nonotosclerotic conditions that they produce only mild hearing loss, and that they rarely are accompanied by tinnitus or a family history of deafness. Whenever a patient with normal otoscopic findings has conductive hearing loss exceeding 35 db in the speech frequencies, the cause in all likelihood is otosclerosis or ossicular defect, even though there may be a marked allergic history and changes in the nose, or slight retraction of the eardrum, or even a demonstrably blocked eustachian tube. An important point to remember is that few if any causes other than otosclerosis produce progressive conductive hearing losses of more than 35 db accompanied by tinnitus and a familial history.

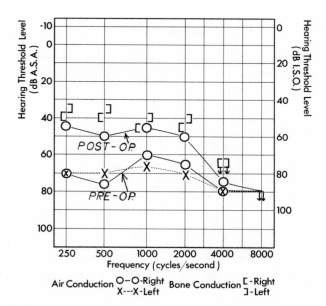

FIG. 40. *History:* 24-year-old female with insidious hearing loss only 3 years from onset. Marked roaring tinnitus and some imbalance. No familial deafness. Voice normal.

Otologic: ears normal. Right stapedectomy improved the hearing after removing a thick white otosclerotic fixed footplate.

Audiologic: Pure tone air conduction thresholds revealed a severe bilateral loss. Bone conduction also was reduced. Preoperative tuning fork tests showed bone better than air conduction in both ears and no lateralization. Postoperatively, air equaled bone conduction on the right ear. Pre- and post-discrimination scores in the right ear were in the low 40% range. The air-bone gap in the right ear was closed with surgery. (A similar result was obtained later in the left ear.)

Classification: mixed hearing loss

Diagnosis: otosclerosis and secondary nerve involvement. The presence of mild imbalance is not uncommon in this type of otosclerosis with sensorineural involvement.

Variable Progress in the Hearing Loss of Each Ear

Otosclerosis sometimes does occur unilaterally, with normal hearing in the other ear. The progress of the hearing loss in each ear, when otosclerosis is present in both ears, may differ widely, so that most of the time a patient complains that she hears better with one ear than with the other. This difference may change, however, and the patient often says, "My left ear used to be the better ear, but it has fallen off so much that the right ear is now the better one." This subjective experience, corroborated by hearing tests, may determine which ear should be operated on when an attempt is made to restore hearing by stapes surgery.

Other Types

The most characteristic type of otosclerosis has been described, but there are many other types that the otologist almost can classify mentally.

			AIR CONDUCTION										
		RIGHT							**LEFT**				
DATE	LEFT MASK	250	500	1000	2000	4000	8000	RIGHT MASK	250	500	1000	2000	4000	8000
9/17/56		90	95	85	90	NR	NR		85	NR	NR	NR	NR	NR
10/31/56		Right stapes mobilization												
1/31/57		45	50	45	75	65	65							
2/10/57								Left stapes mobilization						
2/18/57									60	70	70	70	75	NR

			BONE CONDUCTION								
		RIGHT							**LEFT**		
DATE	LEFT MASK	250	500	1000	2000	4000	TYPE	RIGHT MASK	250	500	1000	2000	4000
9/17/56		40	30	40	50	55			15	35	35	50	45

SPEECH RECEPTION THRESHOLD					DISCRIMINATION SCORE					
					RIGHT			LEFT		
DATE	RIGHT	LEFT MASK	LEFT	RIGHT MASK	% SCORE	TEST LEVEL	LEFT MASK	% SCORE	TEST LEVEL	RIGHT MASK
2/18/57	58		86		44	88		68	98	

Fig. 41. *History:* 67-year-old female with insidious deafness for over 30 years. Refuses to wear hearing aid and communicates only in writing. No familial history of deafness. No tinnitus or vertigo.

Otologic: normal

Audiologic: There is severe sensorineural hearing loss, but patient has an air-bone gap. Reduced discrimination. Hears tuning fork well by teeth.

Aid to diagnosis: The excellent results obtained by stapes mobilization emphasize that these ears were not "dead" but have hearing beyond the audiometer's limits.

One is the so-called "malignant type," which is most disturbing. It may occur in young patients and is noted for a rapidly progressing hearing loss which, often in 1 or 2 years, reaches serious proportions and is accompanied by diminished bone conduction as a result of sensorineural involvement (Fig. 40). Frequently, these cases are not seen until the sensorineural damage is already so pronounced that the otosclerotic origin is largely obscured, and surgery is of doubtful value.

As yet the relationship between otosclerosis and sensorineural deafness is not known, but the latter is such a frequent companion of otosclerosis that there is undoubtedly some connection. For this reason, some otologic surgeons advise doing stapes surgery as early as possible in otosclerosis to obviate not only any adverse psychological changes but perhaps to fore-

				AIR CONDUCTION										
	RIGHT							LEFT						
DATE	LEFT MASK	250	500	1000	2000	4000	8000	RIGHT MASK	250	500	1000	2000	4000	8000
4/39		25	15	25	20	15	15		45	35	35	45	60	65
8/40		25	15	20	20	40	25		40	35	45	45	60	65
4/42		25	25	20	20	45	25		40	40	50	50	65	65
10/43		35	40	30	50	65	30		45	50	50	60	75	60
10/52		70	65	75	85	95	NR		65	55	50	70	90	NR

				BONE CONDUCTION									
	RIGHT							LEFT					
DATE	LEFT MASK	250	500	1000	2000	4000	TYPE	RIGHT MASK	250	500	1000	2000	4000
4/39		0	5	10	25	20			5	0	30	55	NR
8/40	10	10	20	30	30				5	10	35	NR	NR
10/52	10	10	25	NR	NR				5	10	35	NR	NR

Fig. 42. *History:* 59-year-old male first noticed beginning impairment in hearing in the left ear at the age of 44. Hearing loss gradually progressed with increasing discrimination difficulty and occasional tinnitus. Diagnosed as having far advanced Paget's disease at the age of 46. Tinnitus started in the right ear 6 months after diagnosis was made. Wearing hearing aid in left ear since age of 52. Had periods of fleeting imbalance for the past few years. Speech normal. Skull roentgenograms revealed a narrowing of the left internal auditory canal and no visualization of the right canal. Neither cochlea could be made out clearly.

Otologic: Both eardrums were slightly opaque.

Audiologic: Air and bone conduction thresholds measured over a period of 13 years show a slowly progressive deafness with greater loss in the higher frequencies. An air-bone gap always was present in the lower frequencies but not in the higher frequencies. No recruitment was found.

Classification: low frequency conductive loss and subsequent sensorineural involvement in the middle and the higher frequencies.

Diagnosis: Paget's disease

stall sensorineural damage. Factual information regarding this relationship is not yet available but certainly should be forthcoming in the near future.

Another type of otosclerosis is shown in Figure 41. This is hardly recognizable as otosclerosis, and yet the patient has all the classic history and symptoms with the exception that the hearing loss is greater than 60 db, and sensorineural deafness also is present. Many features of this type of otosclerosis are discussed in Chapter 12, but it should be emphasized that this is definitely otosclerosis, and that the hearing can be improved greatly by surgery, as seen in the audiogram. Also note that the absence of any response to audiometric testing does not mean necessarily that the ear is "dead." It means merely that the threshold is beyond the limits of the audiometer. Another unusual but severe type of otosclerosis occurs when there is obstruction not only of the oval window but also of the round window. Here again the bone conduction is reduced severely, along with the air conduction loss.

The cases of otosclerosis just described that have a sensorineural component are not considered to be purely conductive but rather cases of "mixed hearing impairment." Because the conductive element predominates, they are included in this chapter.

PAGET'S DISEASE

The hearing loss in Paget's disease may either be conductive or sensorineural. Conductive hearing loss occurs as a result of stapes fixation when calcium deposits prevent normal movement of the stapes footplate. These deposits form in the annular ligament of the stapes at its attachment to the oval window and present a hearing loss pattern similar to that which occurs in otosclerosis (Fig. 42).

Sensorineural deafness takes place apparently because of a serous exudate into the labyrinth, resulting in damage to the sensorineural mechanism. Occasionally, there is narrowing of the internal auditory meatus and pressure on the auditory nerve, causing neural deafness, and by this time the sensorineural hearing loss already has become quite severe. Other findings in patients with Paget's disease are well known, and a very large head in these patients has become a pathognomonic sign.

VAN DER HOEVE'S SYNDROME

Van der Hoeve's syndrome is a combination of a generalized bone affliction, osteogenesis imperfecta (Lobstein's disease), with blue sclera and deafness. In this condition cartilages throughout the body are softened, and the teeth become transparent in a few of these patients. There seems to be a hereditary factor present, and it is common to find several members of the same family having deafness and blue sclera. Although the audiologic findings closely resemble those of otosclerosis, the impression during stapes mobilization surgery in several cases suggests that the stapes fixation is of a different consistency than that found in otosclerosis.

THE EUSTACHIAN TUBE

ACTION OF THE EUSTACHIAN TUBE

The eustachian tube generally is straight, but sometimes it has a slight curve and a little twist where the bony portion from the middle ear joins the cartilaginous portion in the nasopharynx. In addition, the openings of the tubes are wide in the nasopharynx and in the middle ear, but the lumen narrows down quite considerably at the bony cartilaginous junction. Normally, the eustachian tube is not open, because the mucous membrane lining the lumen is in contact except when swallowing, sneezing, yawning or forceful nose blowing. Behind the opening of the eustachian tube in the nasopharynx is a deep fossa called the fossa of Rosenmüller. Excessive growth of adenoid tissue in this area often compresses the tube and prevents normal aeration. Congestion and infection in the nasopharynx and the adenoid region also can cause closing of the tube by upward progression along the tubal mucosa and the submucosal areas.

Functions. The eustachian tube normally has two important functions. One is to allow drainage from the middle ear into the nasopharynx, and the other is to maintain equal air pressure on both sides of the eardrum. Since the eustachian tube normally is closed, and the mucous membrane of the middle ear aborbs air, though slowly, it is essential that the eustachian tube be opened at intervals to maintain the pressure equilibrium. This is done during swallowing, not only when eating, but continually during the day and night as saliva and mucus collect in the pharynx and stimulate the swallowing reflex.

METHODS OF EVALUATING FUNCTION. A simple way to demonstrate that the tube opens during these acts is to hold a vibrating tuning fork in front of the nostrils. It will be heard only weakly until swallowing, and then it will be much louder as the sound waves travel up the eustachian tube into the middle ear.

Another method of determining whether the tube is functioning and opening properly is to use Politzer's method. A large nasal tip on a pressure bottle containing camphor mist (or only air) is inserted snugly into one nostril while the other is compressed, and the patient is told to say, "Kick" (or "Cake"). Pronouncing the k-sound causes closure of the nasopharynx by lifting the soft palate, and the air or the mist then is forced up the eustachian tube, causing the eardrum to push out slightly. It is important to watch the eardrum through an otoscope during this procedure. The normal eardrum will move out very slightly and then return immediately to its original position. Abnormal results may include a slow return of the eardrum to its initial position, persistent pouching out of large blebs, or failure of the drum to move at all. These irregularities indicate abnormal conditions in the tube and the middle ear. Caution must be exercised not to use too much air pressure, as this may rupture a weakened eardrum. The whole procedure is contraindicated if infection is present in the nose or the nasopharynx.

Other methods of evaluating the function of the eustachian tube include direct examination through a nasopharyngoscope and catheterization. The method of Politzer is especially helpful if a small perforation is suspected in the eardrum but cannot be visualized through the otoscope. The forced-up camphor mist can be seen coming out of the small perforation, thereby pinpointing its site.

THE EUSTACHIAN TUBE AND HEARING LOSS

No part of the auditory system has been incriminated more wrongly and mistreated more than the eustachian tube. This was understandable in the days before there was a clear understanding of the physiology of hearing, of the function of the eustachian tube, and of otosclerosis. At the present time, however, there should be no reasonable excuse for blaming or mistreating the eustachian tube when actually the cause of the hearing loss lies elsewhere.

Malfunction of the eustachian tube causes only conductive hearing loss. If sensory hearing impairment is present, the eustachian tube should not be the target for treatment even though politzerization or tubal inflation may give the patient a subjective sense of well-being and an apparent hearing improvement for a few moments. Such treatment often delays the patient's actual auditory rehabilitation.

In general, simple blockage of the eustachian tube causes only a comparatively mild hearing loss not exceeding about 25 db; most of the time it is much less than that. The loss is greater in the lower frequencies than in the higher. The most common causes are acute upper respiratory infections and allergies of the nose, in which the eustachian tube becomes boggy and obstructed due to congestion and inflammation. This condition makes the ears feel full, and the individual appears to be slightly hard-of-hearing. If the obstruction in the tube persists, the air in the middle ear is absorbed by the mucosal lining, and the eardrum becomes slightly retracted; thus the hearing loss is aggravated, so that it may reach a measurable level of about 25 db. If fluid forms in the middle ear, there may be an even greater level of hearing loss, but in this case the emphasis is in the higher frequencies. This frequency change is due to the addition of the fluid mass to the contents of the middle ear. When there is fluid in the middle ear, the bone conduction also may be slightly reduced, and this reduction may suggest a false diagnosis of sensorineural hearing loss. However, removal of the fluid restores both air and bone conduction to normal.

There are exceptions to these generalizations. When the tube has been closed for many months or years, the drum may become retracted so completely that it becomes "plastered" to the promontory, a condition which causes a hearing loss of about 40 db; or if the fluid is thick and gelatinous, the loss may be slightly greater and exceed 40 db. In general, however, the eustachian tube obstruction per se causes only a mild loss in hearing. The loss increases only when complications arise in the middle ear, such as the presence of a fluid mass and retraction of the drum. Therefore, it is safe to conclude that with rare exceptions if the hearing loss exceeds 25 db, and the eardrum and the middle ear appear to be practically normal, the fault does not lie in the eustachian tube. The cause is more likely to be found in the ossicular chain and especially in the stapes. Hearing loss associated with eustachian tube blockage most frequently is found to be due to other causes, most of them not related to the tube itself.

One of the signs of eustachian tube obstruction is observed during politzerizing. The air may go up the eustachian tube quite well and distend the eardrum, but instead of the eardrum returning immediately to its normal position, as it does in a person with normal tubal aeration, it stays slightly puffed out and returns slowly. In such cases the eustachian tube in all likelihood is not functioning normally.

INJURIES TO THE EUSTACHIAN TUBE

Trauma to the eustachian tube is not a frequent cause of hearing loss, but during wartime a number of patients were seen whose eustachian tubes were injured by gunshot or shrapnel wounds to the face. The damage generally is unilateral and can be visualized through the nasopharyngoscope.

The scar tissue forming during healing following trauma to the eustachian tube narrows the tube and causes recurrent or persistent attacks of serous otitis media. In such instances it is important to avoid harsh manipulation inside the tube, which eventually would aggravate the constriction. Repeated myringotomies and the use of oral and local decongestants are the best alternatives in most cases. Patients usually complain of fullness in the affected ear and of some hearing loss, which clears up when the fluid is removed from the middle ear.

PATULOUS EUSTACHIAN TUBE

In rare instances a patient complains of a loud swishing sound in his ear whenever he inhales through his nose, and he also may state that his ear feels full, and that he is slightly hard of hearing. The examination of the mouth of the eustachian tube through a nasopharyngoscope reveals the opening to appear to be much larger and far more patent than normal. Such a condition is called a patent or patulous eustachian tube. The cause is not always clear, but emaciation and marked weight loss sometimes are factors.

Patients with a patulous eustachian tube are far more disturbed by their symptoms than are those with an obstructed tube. It can be most annoying to a patient to hear a swish in his ear each time that he breathes; obviously, the condition is aggravated by exercise. The patient generally is of a nervous temperament, and he eventually may become obsessed with this symptom. Another complaint is that he hears his own voice as if he were in a resonant chamber. This is called autophonia. The symptoms stop when breathing is done through the mouth. Another unusual observation is to see the eardrum move in and out on respiration. Although the patient may believe that he has difficulty in hearing in the involved ear, actually there is no hearing loss, and this condition basically is not a hearing defect. Although many treatments have been suggested for this abnormality, there is no one specific cure for this annoying symptom.

HYPERTROPHIED ADENOIDS

Hypertrophied adenoid tissue is the most common cause of mild conductive hearing loss in children. School surveys in several states agree that about 3 per cent of the children have significant hearing losses in at least several frequencies. Well over 80 per cent of these are conductive and due to hypertrophied adenoids. Other factors that can cause this condition are secretory otitis, cleft palate, allergies, nasopharyngitis and sinusitis, but even in some of these conditions hypertrophied adenoids are a contributing factor.

Since audiograms are not performed routinely in children, hearing loss is probably much more prevalent than commonly is believed. Children usually are spoken to in a raised voice, and as a result hearing losses seldom are noted until they approach 30 db. These losses come about insidiously in many children and may be present for many months or even years before they are distinguished from childhood inattention. Adenoidectomies often are performed because of mouth breathing or chronic ear infection without a preoperative audiogram; it seems reasonable to speculate that routine audiograms would reveal a substantial number of hearing losses in such children. In uncomplicated cases hearing loss may subside under either conservative or surgical treatment without its existence ever having been noted by either the parent or the physician. Routine audiograms clearly seem to be indicated in all children with recurrent attacks of otitis media, chronic inattention, history of mouth breathing and earache due to hypertrophied adenoids.

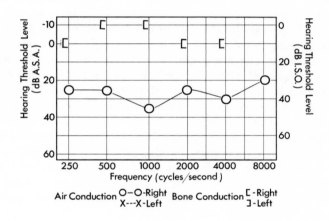

Fig. 43. *History:* 6-year-old child with recurrent earaches and hearing loss for the past year. Mouth breather. Patient had had 6 myringotomies, allergic desensitization, and a T & A before being seen by the author.

Otologic: both eardrums slightly opaque. Clear fluid with bubbles was present in both ears. At surgery a large mass of adenoid tissue filled the superior and the lateral nasopharyngeal recesses due either to regrowth or to inadequate previous surgery. No further ear difficulty postoperatively.

Audiologic: mild bilateral air conduction losses and normal bone conduction thresholds. Speech discrimination was good. Hearing returned to normal 1 week postoperatively.

Classification: bilateral conductive loss

Diagnosis: hypertrophied adenoids with fluid in both middle ears. Myringotomy and adenoidectomy under direct visualization help to restore hearing to normal by clearing all possible lymphoid tissue behind the eustachian tube openings. Compare this case with that in Figure 24, in which the adenoids were really not the cause of the problem, and their removal did not cure the patient.

Opinions differ widely as to the indication for an adenoidectomy in children. These differences range from the routine performance of adenoidectomies in almost all children having upper respiratory infections to the opposite extreme of never removing the adenoids unless there is complete obstruction in the nasopharynx. Such marked differences of opinion concerning the effectiveness of adenoidectomy in dealing with this problem indicate the need for reappraisal based on objective audiometric studies.

To determine the role of hypertrophied adenoids in children with conductive deafness, the author conducted such a study by obtaining reliable preoperative and postoperative audiograms. Of 100 consecutive children between 3 and 14 years of age with conductive hearing loss, 38 had previous adenoidectomies before being referred to the author, but the hearing loss persisted. All children had extensive conservative therapy for many months before adenoidectomy was done. The hearing tests and criteria were controlled accurately. The results are notable. Of the 100 children, 96 had their hearing restored or improved markedly within several weeks after adenoidectomy. The study emphasized that whenever hypertrophied adenoid tissue is present with conductive hearing loss, and adenoidectomy is indicated, it is essential to punch out all possible lymphoid tissue behind the eustachian tube openings (fossae of Rosenmüller) under direct visualization with special retractors in order to restore normal function to the eustachian tube and to correct the hearing loss that is present. Figure 43 describes a typical case encountered in this series.

Chapter 11

Sensorineural Hearing Loss: Diagnostic Criteria

An important and challenging problem confronting physicians, particularly otologists, is sensorineural hearing loss. Not only are there millions of people with this type of loss, particularly industrial workers and older citizens, but, more important, the hearing loss generally is irreversible, and it often affects the personality adversely. Its psychological effect on the personality places sensorineural hearing loss in the foreground of medical importance.

CLASSIFICATION

The damage to the auditory pathway may take place both in the inner ear (sensory loss) and in the auditory nerve (neural loss). We emphasize that the damage may be in both areas (as the name sensorineural indicates), because it is possible to pinpoint the diagnosis in many cases of sensorineural hearing loss specifically as being either of sensory or of neural type. If it can be established that the major damage to the auditory pathway is in the inner ear, the case is classified as a sensory hearing loss. If the chief damage is in the fibers of the 8th nerve proper rather than in the inner ear, it is classified as a neural or nerve hearing loss.

LIMITED INFORMATION

Knowledge about sensorineural lesions is comparatively limited. The precise cause or the detailed pathology of an embarrassing number of

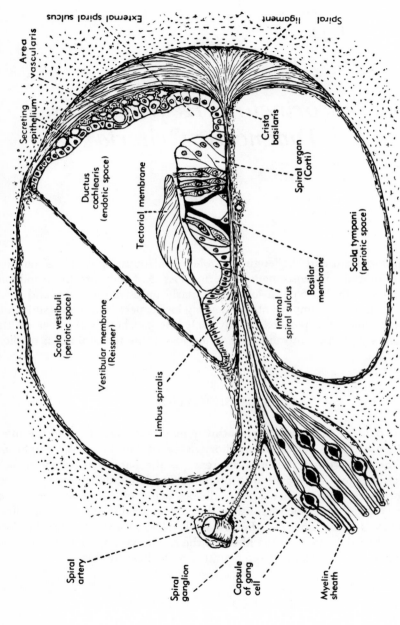

External spiral sulcus

Spiral ligament

Area vascularis

Crista basilaris

Secreting epithelium

Spiral organ (Corti)

Ductus cochlearis (endotic space)

Tectorial membrane

Scala tympani (periotic space)

Basilar membrane

Scala vestibuli (periotic space)

Internal spiral sulcus

Vestibular membrane (Reissner)

Limbus spiralis

Spiral artery

Spiral ganglion

Capsule of gang cell

Myelin sheath

Fig. 44. A cross section of the organ of Corti. (*Top*) Low magnification. (*Bottom*) Higher magnification. (After Rasmussen, A. T.: Outlines of Neuro-Anatomy, Dubuque, Iowa, W. C. Brown, 1947)

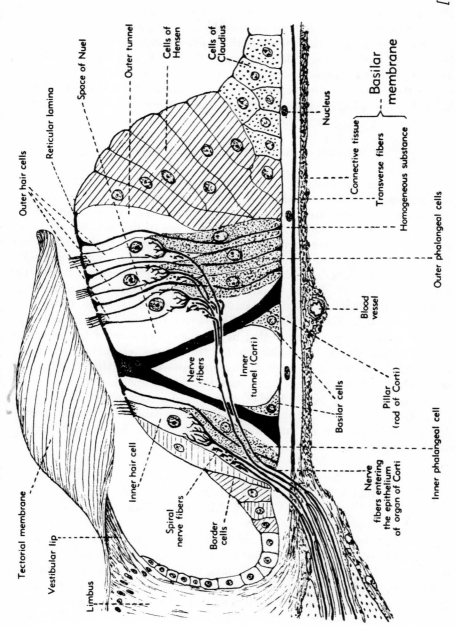

clinical cases is not known, and, what is worse, little or nothing can be done about them. It is difficult for investigators to explore the very small and intricate cochlea, deeply imbedded in the temporal bone. Temporal bones from patients whose hearing characteristics have been studied are available only infrequently—hence the problem of correlating clinical findings with pathologic observations. Animal experiments, although they are helpful, provide limited information and must be interpreted with caution.

COROLLARIES TO CLASSIFICATION

Though it is not possible to specify the causes of all clinical cases of sensorineural hearing loss, the mere fact of classifying them as sensorineural imparts important information. In the first place, such classification is a recognition that the site of the damage is not in the middle ear. This strongly contraindicates medical or surgical therapy to the middle ear. There is no logical ground for eustachian tube inflation, stapes surgery, or removal of adenoids and tonsils when the diagnosis is sensorineural hearing impairment. In the second place, the prognosis is not nearly as optimistic as it is when there is a conductive type of loss. Many times the hearing deficit is irreversible, and it behooves the physician to tell his patient in a forthright manner that he is unlikely to recover his hearing. The physician also is in a position to tell the patient whether his hearing loss is likely to be progressive or nonprogressive, and what therapy is worthwhile. For example, he can assure the patient that his deafness will not progress if it can be established that it is of a congenital type or possibly due to intense noise exposure. On the other hand, it is likely to grow progressively worse if it is due to presbycusis. So the mere classification of a hearing loss provides helpful information.

RELATION OF PATHOLOGY TO NEURAL
AND ANATOMIC MECHANISMS

Prominent investigators such as Guild, Rasmussen, Fernandez and Schuknecht recently have extended the knowledge of sensorineural hearing loss and broadened the understanding of the neural and the anatomic mechanisms underlying such phenomena of abnormal hearing as poor discrimination, recruitment and pitch distortion. Since these symptoms are prominent in sensorineural hearing loss, it seems fitting to crystallize the available information for the purpose of visualizing as clearly as possible the pathologic conditions likely to be present when these findings are encountered in practice.

It will be recalled that the organ of Corti in the inner ear contains approximately 15,000 to 20,000 hair cells resting on a basilar membrane. These hair cells are arranged in long rows conforming to the spiral shape of the organ of Corti. From Figure 44 it is evident that there are two rows of hair cells, the outer and the inner, and there is a tunnel between them. The inner row consists of a single line of cells, but the outer row has about 3 lines. There are also various types of supporting cells in the inner ear. Their function is not completely known, but they do have some relation to the nerve fibers as well as to the inner ear. It seems to be true that as long as there are adequate supporting cells in the inner ear, the nerve fibers do not show degeneration. However, if the hair cells and the supporting cells are damaged, the nerve fibers supplying them have a tendency to degenerate, so that many cases of sensory hearing loss progress to the sensorineural type.

The hair cells are supplied by fine peripheral axons that originate in the spiral ganglion and spread to the inner and the outer rows of hair cells. It should be noted that the nerve fibers leading to the inner hair cells contact only one or possibly a few hair cells and then go directly to the ganglion. On the other hand, the longer fibers going to the outer hair cells supply a number of these cells and course up and down the outer rows of cells a certain distance. This difference seems to play some role in the phenomena of recruitment and loudness. Though it is customary to say that the nerve fibers supply the hair cells, it must be remembered that these are afferent fibers functionally. They carry nerve impulses away from the hair cells to the brain.

Likewise, it is important to note that there is also an efferent bundle of Rasmussen. This is not an afferent but an efferent nerve pathway that carries impulses to the ear from the brain. This has been discovered lately and is receiving wide attention. This efferent tract has some role in the inhibition of impulses.

Schuknecht conclusively has demonstrated that whenever the cochlea is damaged directly, the outer hair cells seem to be the first to be injured. This may result from such causes as direct injury to the head, noise-induced hearing loss, and drug toxicity. Interestingly enough, the maximum hearing loss (threshold shift) that occurs even when all the outer hair cells are lost is about 50 db. A partial loss of outer cells causes a threshold shift of less than 50 db. The hearing loss exceeds 50 db only when the inner hair cells also become damaged. When all the hair cells are lost, no stimuli are available to excite the nerve endings, and consequently there is no sensation of hearing, though the nerve itself may be entirely intact.

The relation of the hair cells to the nerve is the basis for explaining the phenomenon of recuitment, which is most evident in two particular causes of hearing loss: noise-induced deafness and Ménière's disease. It is found also in patients whose hearing has been damaged by certain drugs.

The precise explanation for recruitment of loudness in its varying forms is still not clear. The essential element for loudness recruitment seems to be damage to the hair cells that is disproportionately large compared with the nerve fiber supply. The mechanics of recruitment is that enough hair cells are damaged to reduce the threshold, but enough remain so that when the sound gets loud enough, a normal number of nerve fibers are excited as if all the hair cells were present. Although this explains most types of recruitment, it does not provide a satisfactory explanation for the phenomenon of hyperrecruitment, in which the sound in the damaged ear is not only as loud as that in the normal ear but to the patient may seem to be even louder. This suggests that the number of nerve impulses ascending the auditory nerve is even greater per unit of time than in the normal ear. Patients with hyperrecruitment are those who complain habitually that noises are very bothersome and exceptionally loud.

Another interesting characteristic of some patients with damage to the inner ear and marked recruitment is their ability to detect very small changes in sound intensity, smaller than those which even the normal ear can detect. The ear seems to become ultrasensitive to loudness. This phenomenon technically is called reduced intensity difference-limen or, briefly, reduced difference-limen. Its occurrence has a logical explanation similar to that of recruitment of loudness.

At this point it is well to clarify certain facts about the ability of present-day hearing tests to detect damage to the sensorineural pathway. Though an audiogram may show a zero decibel hearing level, which is considered to be normal, it does not mean necessarily that the sensorineural mechanism is undamaged. Crowe, Schuknecht and others have shown that many nerve fibers can be destroyed without affecting hearing for pure tones. As a matter of fact, as many as 75 per cent of the auditory nerve fibers supplying a certain cochlear area can be sectioned without creating a very noticeable change in hearing threshold level. This may seem hard to believe, but it is a fact and must be evaluated in the interpretation of hearing tests and in visualizing auditory pathway damage. It also should be borne in mind that when octave bands are measured, it is only assumed that we know actually what lies in the many frequencies between the octave points measured. This is especially true in the large area between 4,000 and 8,000 cycles.

CHARACTERISTIC FEATURES

Reduced Bone Conduction; Need for Complete Examination. Since the damage is sustained by the areas that analyze sound waves and transmit nerve impulses, certain features result that are characteristic of sensorineural hearing loss. Of course, the basic feature is that the patient has difficulty in hearing a vibrating tuning fork by bone conduction. It would seem reasonable to assume that this reduced bone conduction alone would be sufficient to warrant classifying hearing loss as sensorineural, but in practice this assumption does not prove to be consistently reliable. There are equivocal cases of conductive hearing loss in which bone conduction is reduced; these make it essential to do a complete otologic and audiologic examination in all cases of hearing loss to be certain of their classification. Though a sensorineural classification may be tentatively entertained when a hard-of-hearing patient hears a tuning fork louder and longer by air conduction than by bone conduction, nevertheless, a careful history, ear examination and further audiologic studies are necessary to establish the classification and to determine the cause.

Impaired Discrimination. In comparing the histories of patients with conductive hearing losses and those with sensorineural hearing losses, one clinical difference immediately becomes evident. In addition to not being able to hear adequately, the patient with sensorineural hearing loss has the further problem of impaired discrimination. Though he may hear people speak, he may be unable to distinguish words with similar vowel sounds but different consonants. This is predominant when the speech frequency range is involved, but it may be observed also when only the higher frequencies are affected. In a conductive hearing loss the patient has no difficulty in understanding if the speech is loud enough. In contrast, the patient with sensorineural hearing loss may mistake one word for another, though it is said in a loud voice. One of the most prominent complaints in these cases is the inability to understand speech, especially on the telephone: voices do not seem to be clear, and people sound as if they are always talking with false dentures or cigarettes in their mouths. This is in part because the reproductive system in the telephone receiver is of limited "fidelity" at higher frequencies. Foreign and unaccustomed accents are a special problem to these patients. Music and voices that compete with conversation make understanding especially difficult.

Varied Causes and Clinical Pictures. The broad classification "sensorineural" incorporates such a variety of causes and clinical pictures that it is possible to describe its characteristics only in a general sense. Since presbycusis causes sensorineural deafness, this common condition helps to recall certain features of this type of hearing loss. However, it should be remembered that almost every conceivable type of onset and degree of hearing loss, unilateral and bilateral, can occur with defective hearing so classified.

GENERAL CHARACTERISTICS

General characteristics of sensorineural hearing impairment are:

1. If the deafness is bilateral and of long duration, the patient's voice generally is louder and more strained than normal. This is particularly notable when the voice is compared with the soft voice in otosclerosis.

2. If tinnitus is present, it usually will be described as high-pitched or as hissing or ringing.

3. The air conduction threshold is reduced.

4. The bone conduction threshold is reduced to about the same level as the air conduction, so that there is no air-bone gap. Often the tuning fork held to the skull is not heard at all even when it is struck hard.

5. The discrimination score is reduced decidedly when the speech frequencies are involved and to a milder degree when only the high frequencies are involved.

6. The patient finds it more difficult to understand speech in a noisy than in a quiet environment.

7. When the discrimination score is reduced, the patient will discriminate as well or slightly better when the intensity of the speech is increased (in contrast with some cases of sensory hearing impairment due to Ménière's disease).

8. In most cases there is little if any evidence of abnormal tone decay (adaptation).

9. Recruitment generally is absent; if present, it is not marked and is found only in the region just above threshold (noncontinuous and incomplete).

10. The vibrating tuning work lateralizes to the better hearing ear in patients who have a significant difference in hearing level between the two ears.

11. Responses to audiometry are usually sharp and clear-cut.

12. Otologic findings are normal.

13. Little or no separation is found between the interrupted and the continuous Bekesy audiograms.

14. If the hearing loss originally was sensory but has progressed to a sensorineural loss, some characteristics of sensory hearing loss may persist, such as mild recruitment and diplacusis.

15. The prognosis for recovery of sensorineural hearing impairment with treatment is poor, with rare exceptions.

ASPECTS OF CRITERIA

Loudness of Voice. Many of these criteria have interesting backgrounds. For instance, the loudness of voices depends on many factors, such as personality, the distance from a listener, the eagerness to be heard, the amount of background noise, what the individual has been taught to regard as socially acceptable, etc. Individuals control the loudness of their voices mainly by hearing themselves speak. This they do by both air and bone conduction to varying degrees. It is a sort of feedback system whereby the individual hears his own voice, and if it seems too loud, he lowers it, or if too soft, he raises it. In otosclerosis the patient hears his own speech chiefly by bone conduction, because it is far better than the air conduction, and so he has a tendency to keep his voice soft; otherwise, he thinks he is shouting. Furthermore, in otosclerosis the patient does not have the urge to raise his voice above the background level, because he hardly hears the background noise.

In sensorineural deafness of long standing involving both ears, the patient cannot hear his own voice either by air or bone conduction. When he fails in his continued efforts to hear his own voice and thus to obtain the feedback control to which he has become accustomed, his voice often becomes louder and more strained.

Strangely enough, not all patients with severe long-time sensorineural deafness develop loud and strained voices. We have seen patients who, in spite of having become progressively deaf as adults until no residual

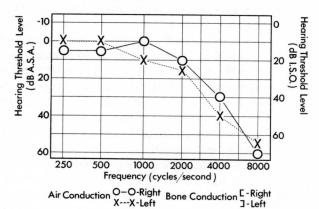

Air Conduction O—O-Right   Bone Conduction ⊏ -Right
X---X-Left   ⊐ -Left

Fig. 45. *History:* 64-year-old industrialist complaining of difficulty in understanding people speak, especially at important meetings. He finds it necessary to resign as Board Chairman of a large corporation because of his hearing handicap.

Otologic: normal

Audiologic: Patient has typical high tone hearing loss of presbycusis. Discrimination score is 86%, but he has more trouble in a noisy background.

Classification: sensorineural deafness

Diagnosis: presbycusis

Aid to diagnosis: Two years later the pure tone threshold dropped slightly, but the discrimination score fell to 58%, indicating more neural damage.

hearing was left, yet have been able for many years to maintain almost normal speech levels. Speech and voice therapy and occasionally their own conscious efforts have enabled these patients to fix a certain loudness reference level for their own voices similar to what they used when they had normal hearing. However, it becomes strikingly evident that such patients do not lower or raise their voices in different noise environments as most normal-hearing people do. Some of them will inadvertently speak loudly in a quiet room and softly in a noisy one.

Speech Discrimination. Another intriguing aspect of sensorineural hearing loss concerns discrimination of speech. In otologic practice the physician frequently sees patients such as the one described in Figure 45. The only complaint this important industrialist had was that he could not discern what was said at meetings or in groups of people in which several spoke at the same time. On the basis of accepted criteria, it would appear that this patient must have some psychological difficulty, since his hearing in the speech range is normal, and his discrimination score is good. Yet is such a conclusion warranted? Is it not more likely that criteria and tests simply are not designed to detect and to appraise this simple type of situation? Many people who have losses chiefly above 2,000 cps complain of "hearing trouble" when they actually mean discrimination trouble. In a routine otologic evaluation tests usually are not made of the circumstances under which they have noted this handicap, as in noisy areas and in multiple conversations, or on the telephone. It is not correct to attribute such difficulties to some psychic cause. Actually, such cases are merely mild examples of the common type of sensorineural hearing loss involving a bilateral high tone loss and measurable reduction in discrimination. The chief reason for the reduced discrimination of the patient reported on in Figure 45 is his inability to distinguish certain consonants that fall into the frequency range of his hearing loss. Since consonants give meaning to words, and the patient has trouble distinguishing certain consonants, he misunderstands certain key words and thus at times misinterprets the speaker. If the speaker fails to enunciate well, or if noise masks already weak consonants, the patient with high tone loss will have even greater difficulty in understanding conversation. This type of discrimination difficulty is different from that encountered in the sensory type produced by Ménière's disease, in which there is marked distortion and fuzziness of speech sounds that gets even worse when the speech becomes louder.

Tests and Their Shortcomings. In sensorineural deafness another shortcoming of hearing tests occurs in interpreting discrimination testing. In some cases of mild high tone loss discrimination testing shows an excellent score of 90 per cent despite the patient's complaint that he has difficulty in understanding speech. It must not be concluded that the patient's complaint is unwarranted. Rather it should be realized that the discrimination test was done under very quiet conditions in a sound-treated room and with a tester who enunciated very clearly and spoke slowly through an expensive amplification system. Under such conditions the patient undoubtedly does well and has no complaints. But in everyday experiences such favorable conditions are rare. Usually, there is some loud distracting noise to mask what the speaker says. Furthermore, few people speak slowly and enunciate clearly. If the speech is coming through an amplifier, it often is distorted and even muffled. It is no wonder that the patient has complaints under such circumstances.

When a physician talks to a patient, he easily may fail to evaluate fully the patient's discrimination difficulty because he communicates so well. A tendency to underrate the patient's difficulty should be watched, for most patients visit a physician only after such symptoms have long persisted and become quite enervating. To brush aside the patient's complaint on the strength of a brief face-to-face conversation is to show a lack of understanding of hearing and psychological problems that gives the patient ample motive for dicouragement.

Testing bone conduction with a tuning fork in a case of sensorineural deafness sometimes may confuse the physician. Occasionally, the physician sees a patient with about a 60-db hearing loss who absolutely denies hearing a tuning fork by bone conduction regardless of how hard it is struck. Does this mean the nerve is dead? It cannot be completely dead, or there would be no hearing by air conduction. It must be borne in mind that bone conduction is not always a reliable test for sensorineural function, and also that the ear is about 50 to 60 db more sensitive to air conduction than to bone conduction, so that the fork would have to produce a very loud tone to be heard by the deafened patient. Most forks are unable to reach this intensity even when they are struck very hard.

In patients with unilateral sensorineural hearing loss the tuning fork placed on the skull or the teeth is heard more loudly in the good ear. This is a result of the reduced bone conduction in the ear with sensorineural hearing loss. The physician also will observe that he can hear the fork on his own skull (if his hearing is normal) much better than does the patient with sensorineural hearing loss. When testing for this, it is necessary to mask the patient's good ear with noise so that the vibrations conducted through the skull to the good ear will not be reported by the patient erroneously as having been heard in his bad ear.

Recruitment and Perception of Intensity. Recruitment is the outstanding feature of sensory rather than sensorineural hearing loss. However, there may be some degree of recruitment in sensorineural hearing loss, particularly if the loss originally started as sensory and progressed to involve the nerve endings. In such cases the recruitment is mild, and the abnormal increase in loudness occurs near threshold. It rarely continues into the high intensities to equal the loudness in the normal-hearing ear; when it does, this is spoken of as "complete recruitment." When the loudness in the recruiting ear exceeds that of the normal ear for the same tone, the condition is called "hyperrecruitment."

It has been pointed out previously that during audiometry the patient with conductive hearing loss waivers in his responses as if he is uncertain whether or not he hears around threshold, whereas in sensorineural cases the responses are more decisive and sharp. The reason is that the patient with sensorineural loss often has a keener ability to detect small differences in intensity than either a normal-hearing patient or one with conductive hearing loss.

Almost Symptomless Types. Some types of sensorineural hearing loss are almost symptomless and are detected only by audiometric examinations. The dips and the early high tone hearing losses are typical.

MEDICAL TREATMENT

Some comments are in order about the medical treatment of sensori-

AIR CONDUCTION													
		RIGHT							**LEFT**				
DATE	LEFT MASK	250	500	1000	2000	4000	8000	RIGHT MASK	250	500	1000	2000	4000	8000
7th day post-op.		60	55	45	50	50	70		60	55	40	50	45	NR
9th day post-op.		15	10	20	25	20	30		25	15	15	25	10	20
16th day post-op.		10	5	5	0	5	25		5	0	5	5	5	10

BONE CONDUCTION												
		RIGHT							**LEFT**			
DATE	LEFT MASK	250	500	1000	2000	4000	TYPE	RIGHT MASK	250	500	1000	2000	4000
7th day post-op.		35	45	40	40	50			35	40	35	45	55
9th day post-op.		10	10	15	15	20			10	15	15	10	15
16th day post-op.		0	0	0	0	5			5	0	5	0	0

Fig. 46. A 28-year-old woman had undergone a tonsillectomy. During the first 6 days following surgery she took 200 tablets of aspirin for what she called "terrific pains." On the 7th postoperative day she complained of hearing loss, recurrent tinnitus and a recurrent sensation of unsteadiness. Examination showed normal eardrums. Audiometer studies indicated bilateral, symmetrical, severe hearing loss by both air conduction and bone conduction and evidence of recruitment. The aspirin was stopped, and the hearing showed considerable improvement 2 days later. The patient was aware of the improved hearing, and the tinnitus ceased altogether. Vestibular tests performed the same day showed no evidence of vestibular disturbance. Audiometric studies revealed normal hearing 9 days after the first hearing test. (Walters, J. G.: The effect of salicylates on the inner ear, Ann. Otol. 64:617, 1955)

neural deafness. An oft-repeated maxim is that sensorineural deafness is irreversible. Damage to the auditory nerve fibers cannot be cured. Although the generalization may be true, the catch lies in the term "damage." In numerous cases of sensorineural deafness the patient gets better, mostly spontaneously, but medication may be of some help. What the maxim really means is that there is no cure for permanent damage to the auditory nerve. It is not true that all sensorineural damage is permanent. The simplest example of the reversibility of sensorineural damage is auditory fatigue following exposure to gunfire. There can be a marked sensorineural hearing loss which gradually reverts to normal. There are many other cases of sensorineural hearing loss that have all the characteristics of being permanent, and yet they may improve dramatically, often with medication or even without. Sensorineural deafness can be very severe and yet return to an excellent level. Such a case is demonstrated in Figure 46. The chief lesson to be learned from such examples is that it is possible for some cases of sensorineural hearing impairment to improve, but at present there is not sufficient knowledge to forecast when this will happen; nor is there any specific therapy known to promote the return of hearing consistently in many cases. One generalization may be of partial value. The cases more likely to be reversible are those of sudden onset rather than those which develop slowly over a period of months. The onset of hearing loss of the sensorineural type is rather important in

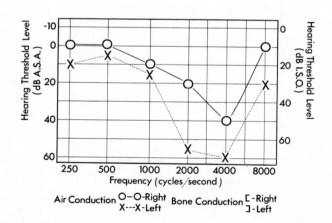

FIG. 47. Exposure to small-arms gunfire. Complete recruitment present at 2,000 cycles.

R.	L.
60	70
80	80

Classification: sensorineural
Diagnosis: repeated acoustic trauma

establishing its possible cause. In Chapter 12 is a chart showing the known and likely causes of sensorineural hearing loss of sudden and insidious onset. Examples of each cause in the list are found in the ensuing chapters.

The classic example of sensorineural hearing impairment is presbycusis, for it invariably occurs bilaterally and almost to the same degree. Occupational hearing loss is another common example. The unilateral losses are always interesting and challenging, because it is often difficult to be certain of their cause. But in those instances in which there is no well-recognized illness or injury to account for the unilateral loss, the cause is difficult to establish. Sensorineural hearing impairment frequently is attributed to such factors as viruses, vascular spasm, vascular embolus, thrombosis, or even severe emotional trauma.

A sensorineural hearing loss may occur unilaterally, or more commonly bilaterally either simultaneously or at different rates in each ear. A sudden onset of hearing loss almost always motivates the patient to seek a

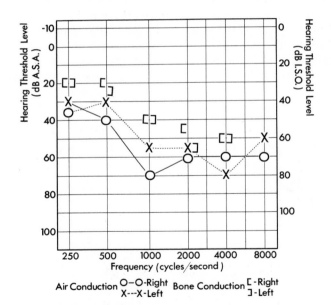

Fig. 48. *History:* 37-year-old male with insidious deafness for 10 years. No tinnitus or vertigo. A brother and a sister had had successful stapes surgery. Patient uses hearing aid successfully.

    Otologic: normal

    Audiologic: bilateral sensorineural deafness with no significant air-bone gap. Hears tuning fork only by teeth.

    Classification: sensorineural deafness

    Diagnosis: unknown

physician's advice as quickly as possible. The patient with hearing loss of gradual onset infrequently seeks help until he has experienced many difficulties in communication or has developed disturbing tinnitus or vertigo.

CHARACTERISTIC AUDIOMETRIC PATTERNS OF SENSORINEURAL HEARING IMPAIRMENT

The audiogram considered to be the classic example of sensorineural hearing impairment is the high tone loss shown in Figure 45. As a matter of fact, an audiogram of this shape has come to be called a "nerve type audiogram," because it is found so often in perceptive deafness, especially in presbycusis.

Another audiometric pattern characteristic of sensorineural hearing impairment is the high tone dip shown in Figure 47. This is caused frequently by exposure to intense noise. Initially, this type of loss is sensory rather than sensorineural. Then, as the damage grows more extensive, and the supporting cells and nerve fibers become affected, the classification becomes sensorineural, but the classic subjective symptoms of sensorineural hearing loss are not so well defined. The same explanation applies to still other audiometric patterns found in sensorineural loss. For instance, Figure 48 shows an audiogram of unknown etiology.

Although these patterns, especially the first, are highly suggestive of damage in the sensorineural mechanism, it must be remembered that other possibilities exist. For instance, an audiometric pattern similar to that shown in Figure 45 can be obtained after merely dropping oil into an ear canal, and this scarcely affects the sensorineural mechanism. The ascending curve and the flat audiogram certainly are more common in conductive hearing loss. So it becomes even more evident that a diagnosis cannot be made reliably solely on the basis of the air conduction audiogram.

The paramount audiometric characteristic of sensorineural hearing loss is that the bone conduction curve is not normal and usually assumes the same shape and level as the air conduction curve. The Bekesy audiograms show no singular features. Continuous and interrupted Bekesy tracings usually reveal little or no separation. Neither marked recruitment nor abnormal tone decay is present.

Chapter 12

Sensorineural Hearing Loss: Causes

The clinical pictures and causes of sensorineural deafness are so numerous and varied that it is hardly practical to describe even all the types seen in the author's practice alone. Different causes often produce the same clinical profile, and a single cause may produce a variety of clinical pictures. In many cases of sensorineural deafness the cause is speculative or completely unknown. To complicate the problem even further, physicians now are beginning to realize that in some patients with histories and audiologic findings highly suggestive of peripheral sensorineural deafness, the temporal bones at autopsy show scant damage in the cochlea or the nerve, and they are unable to account for the hearing loss on the basis of any visible pathology.

To provide the reader with a comprehensive perspective of sensorineural deafness, we have included as many as possible of the characteristics of the conditions commonly encountered in practice, and to make this chapter more effective, the cases are classified by causes and on the basis of whether the deafness is insidious, sudden, unilateral, bilateral or congenital. However, it should be borne in mind that patients are not always certain or able to give reliable information about the onset of their deafness. Therefore, it may be necessary for the reader to search this chapter more thoroughly in the event that he does not find the cause of a particular case in one of these sections.

Many cases that the reader might expect to find in this chapter (because it includes perceptive deafness) will be found in Chapter 14, which breaks down the classification further into sensory and neural.

For reasons of convenience, several causes of sensorineural deafness are treated in detail in other chapters (Chap. 27, Hearing Loss in Children, and Chap. 26, Prevention of Occupational Deafness), but because theoretically these causes belong in this chapter, they are mentioned briefly here, with directions for the finding of further details.

CLASSIFICATION

With these qualifications the present chapter includes all causes that damage both the inner ear and the auditory nerve, or that first attack the inner ear and later involve also the auditory nerve. The conditions of this general description can be classified as follows:

Causes of Sensorineural Deafness With Gradual Onset

1. Presbycusis
2. Occupational deafness (see Chaps. 14 and 26, which are devoted to this subject)
3. Sensorineural aspects of otosclerosis
4. Sensorineural aspects of Paget's and van der Hoeve's diseases
5. Effects of hearing aid amplification
6. Neuritis of the auditory nerve and systemic diseases
7. Unknown causes

Causes of Sudden Bilateral Sensorineural Deafness

1. Meningitis
2. Infections
3. Functional deafness
4. Ototoxic drugs
5. Multiple sclerosis
6. Unknown causes

Causes of Sudden Unilateral Sensorineural Deafness

1. Mumps (see Chap. 27, Hearing Loss in Children, for details)
2. Head trauma and acoustic trauma
3. Ménière's disease
4. Virus infections
5. Vascular disorders
6. Following ear surgery
7. Following general surgery and anesthesia
8. Unknown causes

Causes of Sensorineural Congenital Deafness (For all these causes see Chap. 27, Hearing Loss in Children.)

1. Heredity
2. Rh incompatibility with kernicterus
3. Anoxia
4. Viruses
5. Unknown causes

CAUSES OF SENSORINEURAL DEAFNESS WITH
GRADUAL ONSET

PRESBYCUSIS

The most common cause of sensorineural deafness is presbycusis, the gradual reduction in hearing with advancing age. The hearing loss takes place in a well-defined manner. It occurs gradually over a period of years, with the very highest frequencies affected first and the lower ones gradually following. Both ears are affected at about the same rate, but sometimes the loss in one ear may progress faster than the other. Whenever an older patient is encountered who has a hearing loss much greater in one ear than in the other, a diagnosis of presbycusis should not be made without reservation, for in all likelihood some other cause is present.

Development. Actually, the process of presbycusis starts quite early in life. Children can hear up to about 20,000 cycles per second. But many adults can hear only up to 14,000, 12,000, or 10,000 cps. With advancing years the ability to hear the higher frequencies becomes less acute, and by the age of 70 most people do not hear frequencies above 6,000 cps.

Since human beings make very little use of frequencies above 8,000

					AIR CONDUCTION									
		RIGHT							LEFT					
AGE	LEFT MASK	250	500	1000	2000	4000	8000	RIGHT MASK	250	500	1000	2000	4000	8000
53		0	0	5	15	25	40		0	0	0	10	20	35
58		0	0	10	15	30	45		0	0	5	10	25	40
63		5	0	10	15	55	60		0	0	10	15	40	55
67		5	0	10	20	60	75		5	0	10	20	55	65
74		10	10	25	35	65	75		10	5	15	30	65	70

FIG. 49. *History:* Routine audiograms were done on this patient while he was being treated for allergic nasal discomfort. At age 63 he started to complain of discrimination difficulty. No tinnitus or vertigo.

Otologic: ears clear

Audiologic: This is a longitudinal study of gradual progressive deafness due to aging. Important here are the comparatively small change in pure tone thresholds at 500, 1,000, and 2,000 cps between the ages of 63 and 74, and the dramatic change in discrimination ability during that same period.

Discrimination score: Age 63   Right 92%   Left 90%

Age 74   Right 60%   Left 56%

Bone conduction thresholds were at the same level as the air thresholds at all frequencies for the years covered.

Classification: sensorineural hearing loss

Diagnosis: presbycusis

cps, they do not become aware of any loss in hearing until the frequencies below 8,000 cps are affected. These frequencies start to become affected around the age of 50. The rate at which presbycusis advances, and the degree to which the individual becomes affected varies widely. To some extent heredity plays a role, for early or premature presbycusis often is found in several members of the same family.

There is perhaps a form of early presbycusis in which the inner ear structures may be affected in such a manner that only the frequencies between 2,000 and 6,000 cps become involved before there are any changes in the higher ranges. This is not a common condition, but when it occurs, deafness does not progress to a marked degree before the higher frequencies also become involved. It should be noted that this picture closely resembles that of the hearing loss caused by intense noise exposure.

A Typical Case and Average Values. Figure 49 shows the typical manner in which presbycusis develops in one individual. This is a longitudinal study, since the same man has been examined for about 20 years. In all presbycusis cases in which 6,000 and 8,000 cps are impaired, there is always a greater loss in the higher frequencies, such as at 10,000 and 12,000 cps. It is possible to find middle-aged people with marked presbycusis, whereas quite elderly people may be found who have very little hearing loss for pure tone thresholds. Presbycusis should not be confused with hereditary progressive nerve deafness, which, starting at a

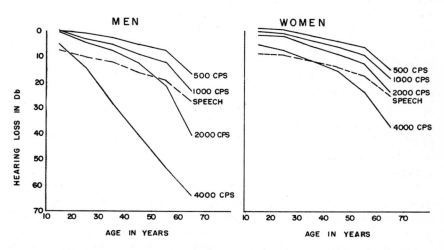

Fig. 50. Average hearing loss by decades for men and women from age 10 to 70. Median loss in right ear and median loss in left ear were averaged. (Adapted from data collected by Research Center, Subcommittee on Noise in Industry, American Academy of Ophthalmology and Otolaryngology, Wisconsin State Fair Survey, 1954)

much earlier age and becoming quite severe, is undoubtedly inherited. Figure 50 shows the average hearing loss in each frequency that can be expected with aging in the general population. These are average values to be used for statistical purposes; they do not hold necessarily for specific individuals.

A Complex Phenomenon. Despite its simple definition and predictable development, presbycusis actually is a complex phenomenon. Even its CLASSIFICATION is complicated. In the early stages of presbycusis only the epithelial elements in the cochlea may be affected, and it then would be classified as sensory hearing impairment. Later the nerve elements also are involved, putting it into a sensorineural classification. Eventually, in the last decade of life, the cortex and the central pathways become involved, and the condition then takes on the aspects of central hearing impairment or central dysacusis. In still other cases of presbycusis the nerve fibers seem to be damaged, making it chiefly neural hearing impairment. So a single etiology, presbycusis, can produce hearing impairment that may fall into one of four different classifications. For our purposes we classify the condition chiefly as sensorineural, its most common form.

THE CAUSE of presbycusis also is complex and not well understood. The simplest hypothesis is based on arteriosclerosis. However, this theory is not borne out by studies, most of which show no pertinent vascular changes in the ear to explain the clinical findings of sensorineural deafness. Still under debate are the factors that predispose to presbycusis or that produce the damage to the hearing mechanism. A recent study in Africa showed that elderly natives who had spent their lives in an atmosphere free of the everyday noises to which most human beings are exposed in modern society show little clinical evidence of presbycusis. This led the investigators to propose that presbycusis really may be the damage produced by exposure to the everyday noises of modern civilization. The proof of this concept is yet to be established, for there are many other incidental circumstances to be taken into account. On the basis of comparable physiologic studies of the eyes, the skin, the brain, etc., one would expect a natural wearing down of the hearing mechanism function with age.

It is helpful at this point to emphasize one distinction between presbycusis and noise-induced hearing loss. If the higher frequencies are on a more normal level than the lower ones, the cause is not likely to be presbycusis, except rarely in the unusual type of mild epithelial damage.

The clinical picture of the sensorineural type of presbycusis, as it is seen in our offices, is rather characteristic. The patient is usually over 50 years of age and generally over 60. His chief complaint, if he can express himself accurately, is not that he has difficulty in hearing, but that he had gradually noted that he occasionally misses what has been said to him. At first this happens only in noisy gatherings such as cocktail parties or when several people are speaking at the same time, particularly if the high-pitched voices of women are prominent. As the loss continues to progress, his symptoms become more apparent. Now he may miss what is being said on the radio and television or at church or meetings. If the patient is a business man (or a woman doing secretarial work) this will cause many difficult situations in cross conversation. He will complain that he hears someone is speaking, but he cannot distinguish what is being said, and generally he has to ask with embarrassing frequency, "What did you say?" This difficulty may be even worse when the speaker talks quickly or drops his voice or has false dentures or talks with a cigarette in his mouth, and it is even more marked when the speaker has a foreign accent and poor enunciation. The audiogram by this time shows that all the high frequencies have become affected, and the loss has extended into the speech range at 2,000 cycles. The hearing threshold level usually has reached about 20 db.

The patient's difficulty in understanding speech is similar to that in advanced cases of occupational hearing loss; certain consonants fall into the high frequency range, and the patient has trouble distinguishing one from the other. He hears the vowels but cannot differentiate certain consonants. For example, he cannot tell whether the speaker said, "Yes," "Yet," "Jet," "Get," or "Guess." This inability to understand what is being said generally is mistaken for inattention or, in the case of an aging parent or a boss about ready to retire, for "brain deterioration" or "signs of old age."

WAYS OF HELPING. The psychological problems faced by the senior citizen as the result of his hearing difficulty are a major handicap and demand better understanding by physicians and people generally. Though we as physicians have no cure for presbycusis, this does not mean that we cannot help the patient who has discrimination difficulty. It reassures the elderly patient with presbycusis when we explain to him that his chief difficulty is not in his brain but merely in the hearing mechanism of his ears. His microphones are not working properly, and this is the reason that he cannot make out what is being said at the dining room table or during conversations in the living room.

If members of his family can be made to understand this situation, they will obviate countless strained situations that breed insecurity, depression and introversion in the senior citizen. Families deliberately should speak softly, slowly and clearly to parents or grandparents with handicapping degrees of presbycusis. Every effort should be made for the speaker and the listener to be in the same room, so that the older person can see the face of the speaker. In this way consonants that cannot be heard are seen on the lips, and conversation can be carried on much more readily and easily. The plight of the oldster who has exiled himself to the proverbial rocking chair because of poor communications needs attention. His insecurity should be bolstered and not aggravated. It is difficult to adjust to the loneliness of old age after a successful career, and each family and physician must strive to help the senior citizen to communicate better.

If the loss in the speech frequencies is greater than 25 db, a hearing aid sometimes can be of considerable benefit to the elderly patient. Although the hearing aid does not improve the patient's discrimination, it helps him to hear with greater ease and less strain. Unfortunately, some elderly patients cannot adjust readily to using an aid and have to be helped by repeated educational talks and reminders to understand that their cooperation is essential for improved communication.

TINNITUS is not often a problem in presbycusis. Occasionally, a patient will complain of ringing or hissing head noises, and sometimes these may become even a severe complaint. In the absence of specific therapy symptomatic treatment may be needed to reduce his excessive reaction to head noises.

BONE CONDUCTION. A common audiologic finding in presbycusis is inordinately poor bone conduction. The bone conduction threshold is usually much worse than the air conduction, and often the bone conduction cannot even be determined with a tuning fork or an audiometer. This does not mean necessarily that the patient's sensorineural mechanism is incapable of responding. It may mean that there is something in the skin or in the bone conduction of the head that prevents him from hearing the vibrating tuning fork or the audiometric oscillator. Frequently, by placing the tuning fork on the patient's teeth or false dentures, he will hear it much better than when the fork is pressed against the skull. Bone conduction testing in older patients is a particularly poor indication of their sensorineural potential.

THE EARDRUM. In elderly patients a change in the appearance of the eardrum also is often seen. The cause of sensorineural hearing loss must not be attributed to a thick, scarred or white eardrum. This does not solve his difficulty and may lead him only to look for treatment of his eardrum while his real problem is disregarded.

A STRIKING FEATURE of presbycusis is a complaint of difficult hearing without any corresponding reduction in audiometric threshold. Even the discrimination score sometimes is not reduced as much as the patient's complaints would lead one to expect. This is characteristic of elderly patients with presbycusis. In the central type of presbycusis and pure nerve damage the results of tests are even more out of line with the patient's complaints.

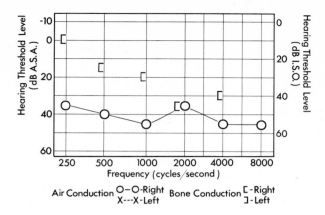

Fig. 51. *History:* 22-year-old female with right ear deafness for 2 years. Occasional ringing tinnitus. No vertigo.

Otologic: normal

Audiologic: left ear normal. Right ear air conduction thresholds revealed a moderate and essentially flat loss. Bone thresholds were reduced, but an air-bone gap existed at all frequencies except at 2,000 cps. The right ear had complete recruitment with diplacusis. There was no abnormal adaptation. Right ear discrimination was 86%. Masking used in the left ear for all right ear tests.

Classification: mixed hearing loss

Diagnosis: unilateral otosclerosis with secondary sensorineural involvement.

Aids to diagnosis: The presence of an air-bone gap, good discrimination and negative otoscopic findings indicate middle ear damage; specifically, stapes fixation. The presence of recruitment, diplacusis and reduced bone conduction indicate sensorineural involvement. Otosclerotic stapes fixation was confirmed at surgery, and hearing improved.

Loudness Balance Tests for Recruitment (Preoperative)

1,000 cps		4,000 cps	
L	R	L	R
−5	45	10	45
10	40	25	45
25	45	40	55
40	50	55	60
55	65	70	65
70	80		
85	90		

Since this is the first chart in which loudness balance testing appears, an explanation is provided as follows: The columns of figures indicate first that, on pure tone threshold testing, the left ear at 1,000 cycles had a threshold of −5 db, and the right ear had a threshold of 45 db. When subsequently the intensity of the tone presented to the left ear was raised, and the patient was asked to match the loudness of the tone in the right ear with that in the left, it was noticed that the threshold difference tended to disappear. At 85 db for the tone in the left ear, the intensity required to produce equal loudness in the right ear was 90 db. Thus the threshold difference, which was 50 db, compares with a difference of only 5 db when the tone intensity was increased to 85 db (left) and 90 db (right), respectively. This is a measure of recruitment.

If the tone loudness in the 2 ears matched exactly at the same intensity, this condition would be called *complete recruitment.* If the tone sounded even louder in the bad ear than in the good ear at the same intensity, it would be called *hyperrecruitment.*

OCCUPATIONAL DEAFNESS

For details see Chapters 14 and 26.

OTOSCLEROSIS (SENSORINEURAL SEQUELAE)

Otosclerosis is basically a disease of the cochlear bone. When it reaches the oval window and the stapedial footplate, it can cause the classic clinical picture of conductive hearing loss which is known as clinical otosclerosis.

Bone Conduction. Unfortunately, the clinical findings are not always quite as classic or so simple. Many cases of otosclerosis, even in their incipient stage, do not have normal bone conduction. One feature of the reduced bone conduction associated with clinical otosclerosis is so common that it sometimes is called the Carhart notch. This is a 10- or 15-db reduction in bone conduction at 2,000 cycles. Its cause has been attributed to some defect in the transmission of bone-conducted sound of this frequency through the patient's skull due to the fixed footplate. When hearing is restored by surgical technics, the reduced bone conduction often improves to about 5 db.

In most cases of otosclerosis in the author's experience, bone conduction is rarely normal for all frequencies. There always seems to be some reduction in bone conduction at 2,000 and 4,000 cps and even at some other frequencies. The frequent association of otosclerosis with reduced bone conduction has created a latent suspicion in the minds of many otologists that there must be some relationship between the two. As yet, no experimental or valid clinical relationship has been established.

Sensorineural Damage. There is little doubt in the author's mind that otosclerosis often leads to sensorineural damage. In my experience, cases of otosclerosis in which bone conduction and the sensorineural mechanism remain normal for years are in the minority. High tone hearing loss, associated with reduced bone conduction, and even recruitment in the early stages are definite manifestations of this sensorineural damage. In many cases the early perceptive effects seem to be only in the cochlea. However, in others the picture is one of sensorineural deafness associated with otosclerosis. In unilateral cases with sensorineural damage it often is possible to demonstrate complete recruitment (Fig. 51). Even the so-called Carhart notch may in some instances represent a sensorineural loss rather than a mechanical defect. This is especially true in cases in which the hearing and the bone conduction do not improve markedly after surgery, or in which the improvement is only to 5 or 10 db. The normal level for such an individual probably was −10 db, and actually he has a 15-db sensorineural hearing impairment in that frequency. Though there is impressive evidence that otosclerosis can cause sensorineural deafness, there is as yet no proof that surgical correction of hearing prevents the development of sensorineural hearing impairment.

DIAGNOSTIC CLUES. The onset of sensorineural deafness associated with otosclerosis is generally very insidious. It may appear long after the con-

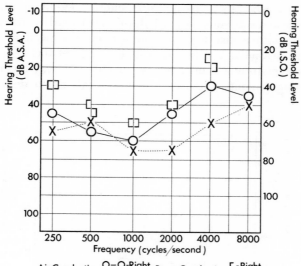

FIG. 52. *History:* 50-year-old female who has a soft speaking voice and uses a hearing aid in the left ear. Insidious hearing loss for several years. Initially, had buzzing tinnitus, which gradually has disappeared. Two sisters have hearing loss. No vertigo or ear infections. Patient says she is getting satisfactory results with her hearing aid.

Otological: normal

Audiologic: Very little air-bone gap is present, but the patient hears better with the tuning fork on the teeth than by air conduction. Dental bone conduction is also better on the teeth than on the mastoid, where there is little or no response.

Discrimination score: Right, 88%; Left, 84%.

Classification: mixed hearing loss

Diagnosis: otosclerosis associated with sensorineural deafness

Aids to diagnosis: Soft voice, satisfactory hearing aid usage, familial history of hearing loss, fairly good discrimination, and bone conduction better than air conduction by tuning fork, all point to the possibility of initial conductive involvement.

An exploration was done on the left middle ear, and the footplate was found to be markedly fixed, with otosclerosis in the oval window. Mobilization was achieved, and the patient said that she heard better. There was a 10-db improvement at most frequencies postoperatively.

ductive hearing loss has been recognized. Occasionally, otosclerosis and sensorineural loss appear simultaneously (Fig. 52). In a few such cases the diagnosis of otosclerosis may seem to be farfetched, but it is established definitely at surgery, and hearing sometimes can be improved. The important clues in such cases are that bone conduction is definitely present and better than air conduction (especially with the tuning fork in contact with the teeth); there is also reasonably good discrimination. The typical history of a soft voice also is helpful, particularly if the patient gets better results with a hearing aid than would be expected in a case of sensorineural deafness. The fact that many cases of this type have been diagnosed successfully and operated on should in no way be misconstrued as encouraging patients with sensorineural deafness to demand middle

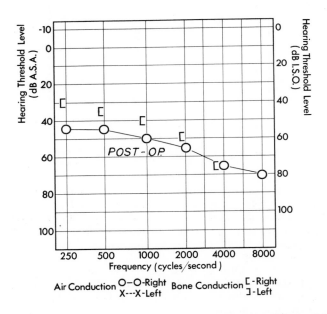

Air Conduction O–O-Right   Bone Conduction ⌈-Right
                X---X-Left   ⌉-Left

Fig 53. *History:* Patient had had a right stapedectomy followed by vertigo, fullness, and tinnitus. Hearing worsened after surgery. There is a family history of otosclerosis.

Otologic: normal

Audiologic: left ear normal. Right ear air conduction thresholds are reduced moderately, as are the bone thresholds. Right ear discrimination is 66%. There is complete recruitment with diplacusis.

Classification: mixed hearing loss

Diagnosis: otosclerosis with postoperative labyrinthosis

Aids to diagnosis: Although this picture is highly suggestive of Ménière's disease, the history points to postoperative labyrinthosis as the etiology.

ear surgery for possible otosclerosis. A diagnosis of otosclerosis must be made positively by hearing tests and history, not by surgical exploration.

SURGICAL COMPLICATIONS. So many patients with otosclerosis have had stapedectomies, and so many of these have had some postoperative labyrinthitis with high tone hearing loss and reduced bone conduction, that it is now common to see cases like that in Figure 53. In all likelihood, this patient had good bone conduction preoperatively and reduced bone conduction postoperatively. Seeing this patient for the first time post-operatively, a physician may wonder why surgery was done in the first place, since he can find little or no air-bone gap, and the diagnosis now is sensorineural deafness. The new examiner always should bear in mind that the bone conduction may not be the same now as it was preoperatively and may have been caused by some surgical complication.

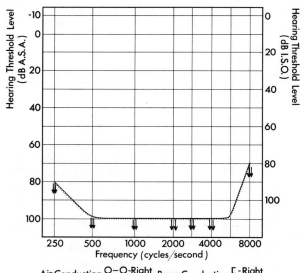

FIG. 54. *History:* 70-year-old female with hearing loss for over 30 years. Wears a hearing aid in the right ear and seems to get along with some residual hearing. Other members of her family have long-term deafness. Both this patient and other members of the family have a history of having blue sclera and repeated fractures of the long bones.

Otologic: ears normal

Audiologic: no response to air conduction audiometry and only tactile response to bone conduction at the lower frequencies.

Classification: mixed deafness

Diagnosis: van der Hoeve's disease

Aids to diagnosis: Deafness, blue sclerae, fragile bones and the heredi-tary features establish the diagnosis.

PAGET'S AND VAN DER HOEVE'S DISEASES

Both Paget's and van der Hoeve's diseases can affect the auditory nerve pathway. In the early stages, usually only conductive hearing loss is produced, but as the disease progresses, the sensorineural mechanism becomes affected, often quite severely. The specific reason for this involvement is not completely clear, but there generally are degenerative processes in the inner ear and the nerve fibers. Sometimes the auditory nerve may be constricted by a narrowing of the internal auditory meatus caused by the disease. A toxic effect on the inner ear such as that which probably exists in some cases of otosclerosis also warrants consideration in Paget's and van der Hoeve's diseases. In some cases of this condition the conductive and the sensorineural deafness seem to start simultaneously and to progress in parallel. An interesting case is described in Figure 54. Note the characteristics of van der Hoeve's disease as a cause of hereditary deafness—blue sclera and fragile bones that sustain repeated fractures.

		AIR CONDUCTION												
		RIGHT							LEFT					
DATE	LEFT MASK	250	500	1000	2000	4000	8000	RIGHT MASK	250	500	1000	2000	4000	8000
5/10/52		25	55	60	70	90	AID	ON	15	40	50	50	45	
6/ 7/54									70	NR	NR	NR	NR	
6/21/54							AID	OFF	50	70	85	85	75	Ring. Tin.
9/ 5/54									30	55	60	55	50	
10/ 2/54							AID	ON	25	50	60	55	50	
11/20/54									60	85	95	85	70	
12/ 4/54							AID	OFF	30	50	60	60	50	Sudden
4/ 2/55							AID	ON	25	60	85	80	80	Ring.
4/ 8/55							AID	OFF	15	50	60	60	50	Persist. Ring.
9/ 4/56		25	50	65	70	85	AID	ON	55	NR	NR	NR	NR	
9/14/56	AID ON		50	65	70	85			60	90	NR	NR	NR	
10/13/56		15	45	60	65	85	AID	OFF	20	50	60	70	60	
1/20/57		20	45	65	70	90			25	45	65	70	70	
4/ 6/57		15	40	60	75	NR	AID	ON	55	NR	NR	NR	NR	
9/ 2/57		20	45	70	70	NR	AID	OFF	NR	45	40	75	NR	

FIG. 55. *History:* In 1950 at age 5 this boy was seen first for a hearing loss that parents had noted since he was age 3. Child had a mild speech defect and developed speech slowly. The diagnosis was congenital deafness of unknown origin. A hearing aid was placed on his left ear, and he did very well until he noted worse hearing in left ear several years later. After numerous studies were done to rule out other causes, the hearing aid was removed, and his hearing improved. Each time the aid was used for many days the hearing got worse but then improved when the aid was taken off. Finally, it was recommended that the aid be worn on the right ear, and the patient noted no adverse effect.

Diagnosis: sensorineural hearing loss due to noise-induced hearing loss.

Note that even the low frequencies were affected in this case.

HEARING AID AMPLIFICATION

In a few cases a person who has used a hearing aid has noted marked aggravation of his hearing loss only in the ear in which he uses the aid. There seems to be no doubt about this causal relationship, but it is a rare incident, and in no way does it justify advising against the use of hearing aids. Apparently, only a few ultrasensitive ears are affected. The hearing loss, usually associated with the use of a powerful hearing aid, is of a peculiar type. Ordinarily, in a typical picture there would be a temporary or even a permanent threshold change as the result of amplification by the aid. This is not what we generally find, as is shown in the interesting case described in Figure 55. Although the hearing returned to its previous level after the hearing aid was removed, it took much longer to return than it would have taken in a temporary threshold shift (TTS), and it did not have other classic characteristics of TTS.

Whenever a patient who uses a hearing aid complains that his hearing is getting much worse in the aided ear, amplification should be suspected as a possible cause if the loss is sensorineural. In such instances the hearing aid should be removed, and the hearing should be watched to see whether it returns to its original level. It may be necessary for the patient to use

AIR CONDUCTION

		RIGHT							LEFT				
LEFT MASK	250	500	1000	2000	4000	8000	RIGHT MASK	250	500	1000	2000	4000	8000
95	30	35	40	40	55	60	95	40	50	55	60	65	NR

BONE CONDUCTION

		RIGHT							LEFT			
LEFT MASK	250	500	1000	2000	4000		RIGHT MASK	250	500	1000	2000	4000
95	25	30	40	40	50		85	35	45	50	50	NR

SPEECH RECEPTION						DISCRIMINATION		RIGHT			LEFT			
RIGHT	LEFT MASK	LEFT	RIGHT MASK	FREE FIELD	MIC.	DATE	% SCORE	TEST LEVEL	LIST	LEFT MASK	% SCORE	TEST LEVEL	LIST	RIGHT MASK
40	85	55	95	45			65	70	4E	85	52	85	4F	95

HIGH FREQUENCY THRESHOLDS

	RIGHT							LEFT				
4000	8000	10000	12000	14000	LEFT MASK	RIGHT MASK	4000	8000	10000	12000	14000
55	60	NR	NR	NR	85	95	65	NR	NR	NR	NR

	RIGHT		WEBER	LEFT	
	RINNE	SCHWABACH		RINNE	SCHWABACH
	A>B	Poor	TO RIGHT	A>B	Poor

FIG. 56. *History:* 55-year-old male with bilateral hearing loss following attack of "flu" during an epidemic. Loss has not progressed. No tinnitus or vertigo.

Otologic: normal. Caloric examination was normal.

Audiologic: bilateral hearing loss with no air-bone gap, reduced discrimination, and poor tuning fork responses. No recruitment or abnormal tone decay.

Classification: sensorineural hearing loss
Diagnosis: neuritis of auditory nerve

the aid in his other ear, and if this ear shows the same sensitivity to amplification, a less powerful type of hearing aid might be indicated.

As in all cases of unilateral sensorineural deafness, the possibility of an acoustic neuroma always should be suspected, and all necessary studies, such as discrimination, recruitment, tone decay, caloric and neurologic studies, should be done.

NEURITIS OF THE AUDITORY NERVE AND SYSTEMIC DISEASES

Neuritis of the auditory nerve may follow such systemic infections as scarlet fever, influenza, typhoid fever and many other infectious diseases that produce high fevers. The hearing loss may be noted immediately, but the onset generally is progressive over a period of days or weeks. The type of neuritis more commonly encountered in present-day practice perhaps should more aptly be classified under "unknown etiology." There is an insidious development of sensorineural deafness very similar to presbycusis but occurring at a much earlier age and attributed to such causes as anoxia, anemia and nonspecific viruses, vague labyrinthitis of uncertain origin, and other conditions that as yet are poorly understood.

AIR CONDUCTION														
	RIGHT								LEFT					
DATE	LEFT MASK	250	500	1000	2000	4000	8000	RIGHT MASK	250	500	1000	2000	4000	8000
1951		10	20	30	85	90	NR		20	30	60	90	NR	NR
1955		80	80	100	NR	NR	NR		80	95	100	NR	NR	NR
1960		75	85	NR	NR	NR	NR		NR	NR	NR	NR	NR	NR
1961		75	NR	NR	NR	NR	NR		NR	NR	NR	NR	NR	NR

BONE CONDUCTION												
	RIGHT								LEFT			
DATE	LEFT MASK	250	500	1000	2000	4000	TYPE	RIGHT MASK	250	500	1000	2000	4000
1951		10	20	35	NR	NR			20	40	NR	NR	NR
1960		NR	NR	NR	NR	NR			NR	NR	NR	NR	NR

FIG. 57. *History:* Since the age of 18, this healthy 36-year-old male had known that he had a very mild high tone hearing loss. It was not progressing, and he participated in active military service. After the age of about 26 he became aware that his hearing was becoming worse, and in spite of extensive studies and a great variety of treatments, he continued to lose his hearing. No tinnitus or vertigo. There is no history of familial deafness.

Otologic: normal. Normal caloric responses

Audiologic: rapid progressive bilateral deafness

Classification: sensorineural deafness

Diagnosis: unknown

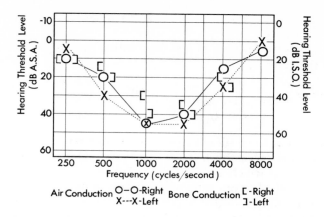

FIG. 58. *History:* 50-year-old female first noticed gradual hearing loss about a year ago and reports that it is progressing. Has had no ear infections or infectious diseases. No tinnitus or vertigo. No history of familial deafness.

Otologic: normal

Audiologic: bilateral basin-shaped loss with no significant air-bone gap. Monaural 2-frequency loudness balance tests indicate some recruitment in both ears. There was no abnormal tone decay.

Speech reception threshold: Right 38 db   Left 42 db
Discrimination score: Right 100%   Left 94%

Classification: sensorineural hearing loss

Diagnosis: unknown

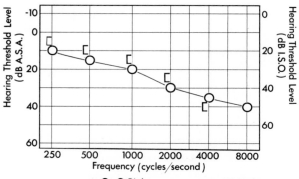

FIG. 59. *History:* 45-year-old female noted gradual onset of hearing loss in the left ear with slight ringing tinnitus. No vertigo. Blood pressure normal.

Otologic: normal

Audiologic: left ear normal. Right ear had mild to moderate loss, which is greater in the high frequencies. No air-bone gap. No recruitment or abnormal tone decay.

Classification: unilateral sensorineural hearing loss, progressive

Diagnosis: no clear-cut cause for this progressive unilateral deafness

Figure 56 shows the findings in a patient with a presumptive diagnosis of neuritis of the auditory nerve.

UNKNOWN CAUSES OF BILATERAL AND UNILATERAL
SENSORINEURAL DEAFNESS OF GRADUAL ONSET

There are almost countless cases of sensorineural deafness for which it is not possible to establish a specific cause. The following series of examples, each of which emphasizes a different factor associated with the deafness, will illustrate cases of this type (Figs. 57 to 59). Vascular problems such as hypotension and hypertension are most prominent. In addition, Chapter 14 contains examples of sensory and neural deafness not included in this chapter. As has been pointed out, causes such as Ménière's disease, noise exposure and occupational deafness may start as sensory hearing impairments and later progress to sensorineural.

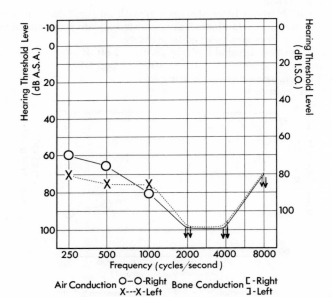

FIG. 60. *History:* 16-year-old boy who had had meningococcus meningitis at age 6. Speech shows marked evidence of deterioration. He goes to a school for the deaf but does not use a hearing aid.

Otologic: normal, but caloric responses are absent.

Audiologic: Patient has some residual hearing in low tones.

Classification: sensorineural deafness

Diagnosis: effect of meningitis on the cochlea

Comment: This boy could get some benefit from a powerful hearing aid and was urged to use one in his right ear.

CAUSES OF SUDDEN BILATERAL
SENSORINEURAL DEAFNESS

Sensorineural deafness of sudden onset is of special interest to the otologist for at least two reasons. First, the cause is hardest to establish, and second, it is not uncommon for the hearing to return spontaneously. Certain causes more often affect both ears, whereas other causes affect

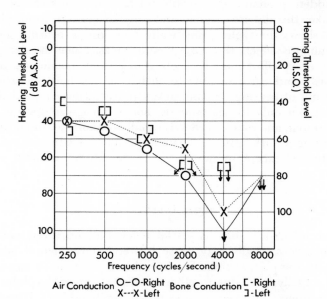

FIG. 61. *History:* 48-year-old man with bilateral otitis media and draining ears since age 6 following scarlet fever. Has had some ringing tinnitus but no vertigo. Uses a hearing aid but has trouble because of ear discharge.

Otologic: both eardrums eroded and no evidence of ossicles. A putrid discharge is present in both middle ears. X-ray pictures show sclerotic mastoids but no cholesteatoma.

Audiologic: bilateral sloping audiogram shows moderate to severe hearing loss with no air-bone gap. Poor response to tuning fork even on the teeth.

Classification: sensorineural hearing loss

Diagnosis: chronic otitis media and labyrinthitis involving the cochlea following scarlet fever.

Comment: A bone conduction hearing aid usually is not recommended in losses of this type. However, the chronic otitis precludes the use of an air conduction aid, which requires an ear mold in the ear. Use of a bone conduction aid when the ear is discharging might eliminate long periods of lack of amplification.

only one ear. The severity of the hearing loss varies, but quite often it can be very profound. The common causes of sudden bilateral sensorineural deafness are the following: (1) meningitis, (2) infections, (3) drugs, (4) emotionally induced illness, (5) multiple sclerosis and (6) unknown causes.

MENINGITIS

The sudden, profound irreversible bilateral deafness caused by meningitis makes this disease of great and singular concern to all physicians. Figure 60 shows the typical, practically total loss of hearing that results when meningitis affects the sensorineural areas. Since the damage is irreversible, every effort must be exerted to prevent meningitis or to treat it vigorously and early to obviate such complications. Occasionally, a small amount of hearing remains, and a powerful hearing aid then is of some value but only to hear sounds, not to recognize speech. Tinnitus rarely is present, and rotary vertigo is usually of short duration. Imbalance, particularly in a dark room, is common because of labyrinthine damage. Caloric studies, except in rare cases, reveal absent or poor vestibular function.

ACUTE INFECTIONS

Systemic infections, such as scarlet fever, typhoid fever, measles and tuberculosis, occasionally may cause bilateral sensorineural hearing impairment. In the past, syphilis has been blamed for many cases of deafness that actually were due to other causes. At present syphilis is a rare cause of deafness, but in some cases it can cause sudden bilateral hearing loss that is not amenable to treatment. It is important to bear in mind that, though a patient may have positive serologic findings for syphilis along with sensorineural deafness, there may not be a causal relationship. The incidence of sensorineural deafness is so high that undoubtedly some people so affected have syphilis without any relation between the two. However, scarlet fever still causes a moderate degree of sensorineural deafness, usually accompanied by bilateral acute and later chronic otitis media. Figure 61 shows a type that was much more prevalent in days prior to antibiotics. Usually, the eardrum and the ossicles also were eroded.

FUNCTIONAL DEAFNESS

Some cases of bilateral sudden deafness are due to emotional disturbances, and although there is no real damage to the sensorineural mechanism, the clinical findings so strongly resemble this diagnostic entity that it warrants emphasis here. Hysteria is the outstanding feature of such cases, and they are common during periods of marked emotional stress, as in wartime. Episodes of severe stress and tension can result in sudden deafness, with audiologic findings very similar to those found in sensorineural deafness attributable to other causes. The main distinguishing features are the history and the inconsistent audiologic findings. Since such cases sometimes do occur in civilian life, it is important to rule out functional deafness by obtaining consistent audiologic findings and an adequate history. Psychogalvanic skin resistance testing and even narcosynthesis sometimes prove to be of value in establishing a proper diagnosis. Figures 62 and 63 illustrate examples of functional deafness encountered in otologic practice.

		AIR CONDUCTION											
		RIGHT						LEFT					
DATE	LEFT MASK	250	500	1000	2000	4000	8000	RIGHT MASK	250	500	1000	2000	4000	8000
4/60		40	45	50	50	50	55		45	50	55	50	45	50
		40	45	50	45	45	55		40	45	50	45	50	50
5/60		45	50	40	50	40	55		45	50	50	55	40	55
8/60		0	-5	0	0	-5	0		0	-5	-5	-5	-5	0

		BONE CONDUCTION										
		RIGHT						LEFT				
DATE	LEFT MASK	250	500	1000	2000	4000	TYPE	RIGHT MASK	250	500	1000	2000	4000
4/60		30	35	40	40	40			35	35	40	40	40
5/60		35	30	40	45	40			30	35	40	45	45

SPEECH RECEPTION THRESHOLD					DISCRIMINATION SCORE						TUNING FORK TESTS (500 CPS.)		
					RIGHT			LEFT					
DATE	RIGHT	LEFT MASK	LEFT	RIGHT MASK	% SCORE	TEST LEVEL	LEFT MASK	% SCORE	TEST LEVEL	RIGHT MASK		R	L
4/60	10		10		98	40		100	40		AIR-BONE COMPARISON		
5/60	10		10		96	40		100	40		LATERALIZATION		
											B. C. COMPARISON TO NORMAL		

Fig. 62. *History:* 14-year-old girl whose hearing loss was suspected by teacher and confirmed by school nurse after audiometry. School work deteriorating past year. No ear infections or related symptoms.

Otologic: normal

Audiologic: Note consistent hearing loss in air and bone conduction tests taken days apart, though the speech reception thresholds are normal (10 db). The girl's normal hearing was confirmed by later testing. She had an emotional problem at school which was rectified by psychotherapy.

Classification: functional

Etiology: emotional conflict

OTOTOXIC DRUGS

With the increasing use of ototoxic drugs it is important to inquire from every patient with sensorineural hearing loss what kind of drugs he has taken, particularly in relation to the onset of deafness. The most important offenders have been dihydrostreptomycin, neomycin and kanamycin when they were used systemically and without proper precautions. Sudden deafness from these drugs occurs principally in the presence of impaired kidney function. It may occur also from overdosage. Figures 64 and 65 provide examples of the severe hearing damage that can result from the

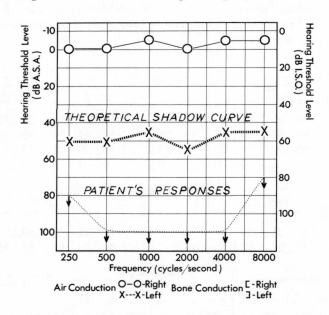

FIG. 63. *History:* 36-year-old male received a sharp blow behind left ear, lacerating the scalp but causing no unconsciousness. He claims sudden deafness in left ear following the industrial injury. No tinnitus or vertigo.

Otologic: normal

Audiologic: Patient denied hearing anything in his left ear even when the right was unmasked. This led to a suspicion of nonorganic hearing loss. All malingering tests showed good hearing in left ear and did not substantiate a sudden deafness following head injury, as the man claimed.

Classification: functional deafness

Diagnosis: malingering

Aid to diagnosis: When one ear is normal, and the other is impaired severely, a shadow curve from the good ear (if unmasked) should appear when testing the impaired ear. This did not happen, and after much testing and discussion the patient admitted he was fabricating his deafness, and eventually he gave a normal hearing audiogram in the left ear.

improper use of ototoxic drugs. These drugs are very valuable when they are properly used, and they seldom cause hearing damage under such circumstances.

MULTIPLE SCLEROSIS

Multiple sclerosis is a rare cause of deafness, but it has been reported as a cause of sudden bilateral hearing loss. Usually, the deafness fluctuates, and hearing may return to normal even after a very severe depression. The precise mechanism of this loss has not yet been established. The presence of marked abnormal tone decay during certain active periods of the disease even with an almost normal hearing level is an important finding.

UNKNOWN CAUSES

Bilateral sudden deafness occurs much less frequently than unilateral sudden deafness. Many cases of bilateral sudden deafness still remain unexplained. Their causes have been attributed to viruses, vascular rupture or spasm, or toxins, but as yet there is no certain knowledge of the precise

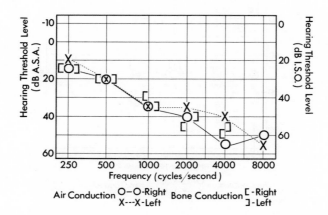

FIG. 64. *History:* 10-year-old boy with normal speech and otologic findings. Had had a kidney infection and received kanamycin. No progressive hearing loss but has constant ringing tinnitus.

Otologic: normal

Audiologic: bilateral downward sloping audiogram with reduced bone conduction.

Classification: sensorineural hearing loss

Diagnosis: injudicious use of an ototoxic drug in presence of kidney dysfunction.

mechanism. Case reports like those that follow occasionally are met in clinical practice (Figs. 66 and 67).

CAUSES OF SUDDEN UNILATERAL SENSORINEURAL DEAFNESS

Far more common than bilateral is unilateral sudden deafness. Here again there is no satisfactory evidence to establish the specific cause for a large number of such cases. The degree of hearing impairment may range from a slight drop at 4,000 to 8,000 cps to total unilateral deafness. The hearing loss in some instances may disappear completely just as spontaneously as it appeared (and the particular medication used at the time generally gets the credit). Unilateral sudden deafness is, indeed, a

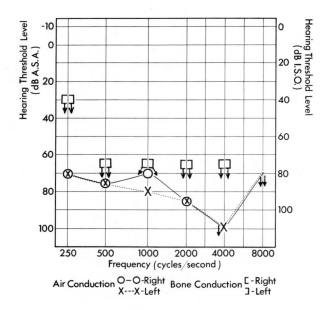

Air Conduction O–O-Right   Bone Conduction ⌐-Right
              X---X-Left   ⌐-Left

FIG. 65. *History:* 49-year-old male who received kanamycin injections daily for 4 weeks because of acute renal failure. Patient claims normal hearing before these injections.

Otologic: normal. Normal caloric responses

Audiologic: severe to profound bilateral loss with no air-bone gap. No response to speech tests except for experiencing great discomfort when speech was presented at levels above 100 db (low threshold of discomfort, an indication of recruitment).

Classification: sensorineural deafness

Diagnosis: deafness due to ototoxic effects of kanamycin

most perplexing clinical picture for the very reason that it occurs uni-laterally in such a systemic disease as mumps.

MUMPS

See Chapter 27, Hearing Loss in Children.

DIRECT HEAD TRAUMA AND ACOUSTIC TRAUMA

A blow to the head can cause sudden hearing loss in one ear by affect-ing the sensorineural mechanism. The degree of hearing loss varies with the severity of the blow and the amount of damage to the ear.

Acoustic trauma, that is, deafness caused by a sudden loud noise in one ear, may be produced by firecrackers, cap guns and firearms, and it is commonly seen in practice. Unless the noise is directed to only one ear, the opposite ear also shows a slight hearing loss. In most cases of acoustic

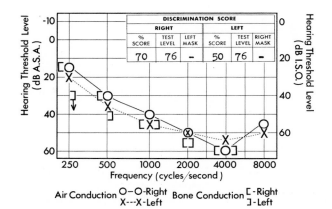

DISCRIMINATION SCORE					
RIGHT			LEFT		
% SCORE	TEST LEVEL	LEFT MASK	% SCORE	TEST LEVEL	RIGHT MASK
70	76	–	50	76	–

Air Conduction O–O-Right X---X-Left Bone Conduction Ϲ-Right Ϳ-Left

FIG. 66. *History:* This 40-year-old male noticed sudden deafness after getting chilled and sneezing repeatedly in an air-conditioned restaurant. He had a rushing tinnitus but no vertigo. Sounds became fuzzy and dis-torted. The hearing loss did not clear up with time; nor did it get worse.

Otologic: normal

Audiologic: Air and bone conduction were reduced. No abnormal tone decay. Recruitment could not be measured accurately.

Classification: unknown

Cause: unknown

Comment: Sudden deafness of this kind with chills and vasospasm is not uncommon but rarely occurs bilaterally and permanently. The patient did not respond to vasodilators or histamine desensitization. A viral cause is unlikely here.

trauma the hearing loss is temporary, lasting only a few hours or days, and the hearing returns to normal. Generally, such patients do not reach the otologist, but if they do, it is interesting to watch the return of hearing by taking follow-up audiograms. In some cases of hearing impairment due to head trauma and acoustic trauma, two types of hearing loss are present: a temporary loss and a permanent loss. As the hearing levels are observed over several days, it is noted that the temporary hearing loss disappears, and there remains a considerably reduced hearing loss that is permanent.

Usually, when the hearing loss has persisted for many weeks, it can be considered to be permanent. Since some of these cases have a medicolegal aspect, the reader should acquaint himself with the more detailed

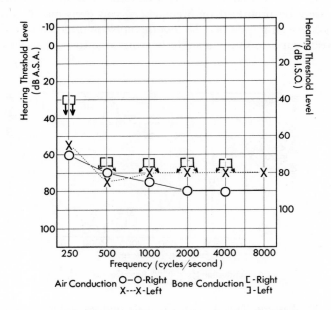

Fig. 67. *History:* This 8-year-old boy developed speech normally until the age of 5, when he awoke one morning and was severely deaf. This occurred 1 week after a severe "virus" infection with high fever that might have been encephalitis. He had no other adverse effects.

Otologic: normal. No caloric responses

Audiologic: severe air and bone conduction loss

Classification: profound sensorineural deafness

Diagnosis: unknown

Comment: Delayed deafness due to virus infection occasionally occurs and may have been the cause here following encephalitis. No treatment is available, but speech therapy is essential to preserve good speech. A hearing aid is of some use.

discussion of head trauma in Chapter 14. When the hearing loss exceeds 60 db and involves the speech frequencies, the auditory nerve fibers as well as the inner ear mechanism undoubtedly are involved in the permanent hearing loss.

In the cases of severe unilateral deafness due to head trauma, it is usually the ear on the same side as the injury that is affected. The opposite ear also may be disturbed, but usually the degree of disturbance is less. The same statement holds for acoustic trauma.

VIRUSES

In spite of there being no laboratory proof that viruses other than the mumps virus cause certain types of sudden deafness, the clinical impression seems to be convincing (Fig. 68). Although no viral studies were performed on this patient, the clinical picture was that of aphthous ulcers with stomatitis, a syndrome often associated with viral infection. The patient has had several recurrences of stomatitis since the serious complication.

		AIR CONDUCTION											
		RIGHT							LEFT				
DATE	LEFT MASK	250	500	1000	2000	4000	8000	RIGHT MASK	250	500	1000	2000	4000	8000
11/56		55	60	80	70	80	65							
1/57		45	40	55	60	NR	NR	← Right stapes mobilization.						
5/57		80	95	100	95	NR	NR	← After attack of aphthous ulcers or herpes.						

		BONE CONDUCTION										
		RIGHT							LEFT			
DATE	LEFT MASK	250	500	1000	2000	4000	TYPE	RIGHT MASK	250	500	1000	2000	4000
11/56	90wn	5	10	20	25	35							
5/57	90wn	NR	55	NR	NR	NR							

FIG. 68. *History:* Patient with bilateral otosclerosis had a right stapes mobilization followed by mild vertigo for a few days postoperatively. Patient had a fair hearing improvement, but apparently mobilization was not adequate. About 4 months later he developed either aphthous ulcers or herpes inside his buccal mucosa and on his tongue. During this period he experienced sudden vertigo and roaring tinnitus in his right ear and deafness that has not improved.

Otologic: normal, and normal caloric response

Audiologic: There was marked depression of air conduction thresholds with no measurable bone conduction responses ("threshold" of 55 db at 500 cps is a tactile response).

Classification: sensorineural deafness

Diagnosis: viral cochleitis and labyrinthitis

Herpes zoster also is known to cause sudden unilateral deafness of a severe degree. The author has seen one instance of total loss of hearing that returned to normal in a few days. The patient had a typical case of shingles on his face.

Many cases of sudden unilateral deafness that now are attributed to blood vessel spasm or rupture may prove to be due to virus infections. The peculiar reversibility of some cases of unilateral sudden deafness, even when they are very severe, is very intriguing. Though now it is customary to consider sensorineural deafness to be permanent and incurable, many cases shed doubt on this maxim. Examples are shown in Figures 46 and 69. It is hard to believe that such a long-standing hearing loss as that in the subject of Figure 69 can reverse itself. One is always

AIR CONDUCTION

| | | RIGHT | | | | | | | LEFT | | | | | |
DATE	LEFT MASK	250	500	1000	2000	4000	8000	RIGHT MASK	250	500	1000	2000	4000	8000
2/57		5	0	0	0	20	30		0	0	0	0	10	25
12/60	80wn	45	40	40	15	25	45		5	-10	-5	-5	15	20
2/61	80wn	60	50	45	15	30	40							
3/61	80wn	30	15	10	10	10	35							
6/61		20	5	15	15	5	15							

BONE CONDUCTION

| | | RIGHT | | | | | | | LEFT | | | | |
DATE	LEFT MASK	250	500	1000	2000	4000	TYPE	RIGHT MASK	250	500	1000	2000	4000
12/60	80	45	45	35	15	30	wn						
2/61	80	45	50	35	20	45	wn						

| SPEECH RECEPTION THRESHOLD | | | | | DISCRIMINATION SCORE | | | | | | TUNING FORK TESTS (500 CPS.) | | |
| | | | | | RIGHT | | | LEFT | | | | | |
DATE	RIGHT	LEFT MASK	LEFT	RIGHT MASK	% SCORE	TEST LEVEL	LEFT MASK	% SCORE	TEST LEVEL	RIGHT MASK		R	L
12/60	35	80			65	65	80				AIR-BONE COMPARISON	A>B	A>B
2/61	40	80			60	70	80				LATERALIZATION	→	
											B. C. COMPARISON TO NORMAL	Poor	

Fig. 69. *History:* 50-year-old female with recurrent attacks of hearing loss, rotary vertigo and tinnitus in right ear since 1955. Occasional vomiting with attacks. Marked diplacusis and distortion in right ear during attacks.

Otologic: normal. Normal caloric responses

Audiologic: fluctuating hearing loss. Continuous and complete recruitment at 1,000 and 2,000 cps during attacks. Normal discrimination when hearing returns to normal.

Classification: sensory hearing loss

Diagnosis: Ménière's disease

Comment: This sensory hearing loss persisted for over 2 months, and then hearing returned.

suspicious in such examples and inclined to attribute the cause to psychological factors. In these and many other cases reported in the literature, this attitude merely diverts attention from finding the real cause and explanation for this phenomenon. Viruses play an important role in sensorineural deafness.

The influenza virus has been blamed for many cases of deafness, especially during major epidemics. Here, again, it is hard to find laboratory proof, but the clinical evidence is impressive. In all likelihood, many cases described as auditory neuritis could have been due to viruses with a predilection for nerve tissue, as is true of mumps.

VASCULAR DISORDERS

Causes. The role of blood vessel spasm, thrombosis, embolism and rup-

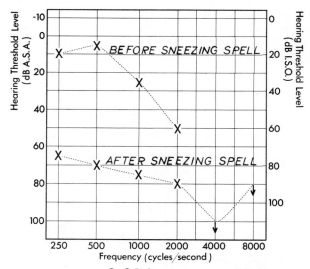

Air Conduction O–O-Right Bone Conduction Ɛ-Right
X---X-Left ꓱ-Left

FIG. 70. *History:* During a severe sneezing spell this 56-year-old man noted ringing tinnitus in his left ear, and 2 hours later his hearing became bad. The hearing continued to get worse for many months until the ear was practically deaf. He experienced no vertigo.

Otologic: normal, and normal caloric responses

Audiologic: no abnormal tone decay. Slight separation of Bekesy fixed frequency tracings. Left ear discrimination, 40%. Bone conduction poor; no air-bone gap.

Classification: sensorineural

Diagnosis: unknown

AIR CONDUCTION													
	RIGHT							LEFT					
DATE	LEFT MASK	250	500	1000	2000	4000	8000	RIGHT MASK	250	500	1000	2000	4000	8000
3/62	100	55	55	55	35	50	55		40	40	35	40	30	40
9/63	85	10	15	25	15	NR	NR	After right stapedectomy.						
1/64	100	75	75	80	80	NR	NR	Buzzing tinnitus, sounds are garbled.						
1/64	100	75	85	95	90	NR	NR	Exploration: fibrous growth						
4/65	100	NR	85	95	90	NR	NR	into vestibule.						

BONE CONDUCTION												
	RIGHT							LEFT				
DATE	LEFT MASK	250	500	1000	2000	4000	TYPE	RIGHT MASK	250	500	1000	2000	4000
3/62	100	0	5	15	10	20		0	5	15	10	20
1/64	100	NR	NR	NR	NR	NR						

FIG. 71. *History:* Four months after a successful right stapedectomy, using a teflon piston over Gelfoam, this 23-year-old male suddenly noticed a pop in his right ear, and his hearing improved. Several hours later he noted a buzzing tinnitus and distortion. The next day his hearing gradually diminished, became garbled, and was completely gone that evening. Has constant hissing tinnitus but no vertigo.

Exploratory surgery showed that the prosthesis was in good position, but a fibrous tissue mass had invaded the labyrinthine vestibule. Removal of much of the mass failed to improve the hearing.

AIR CONDUCTION							
		RIGHT					
DATE	LEFT MASK	250	500	1000	2000	4000	8000
Stapedectomy		30	35	50	40	45	60
		55	60	75	80	NR	NR

BONE CONDUCTION							
		RIGHT					
DATE	LEFT MASK	250	500	1000	2000	4000	TYPE
Stapedectomy		-10	0	25	30	30	
		10	30	50	NR	NR	

FIG. 72. *History:* 62-year-old female who had a stapedectomy in right ear and heard well for 2 days. She then developed vertigo and roaring tinnitus, and hearing deteriorated. She complained of distortion and being bothered by loud noise.

Otologic: normal

Audiologic: reduced bone conduction postoperatively with recruitment, diplacusis, lowered threshold of discomfort and reduced discrimination.

Classification: sensory deafness

Diagnosis: postoperative labyrinthitis

ture as causes of hearing loss is still not clear. It is common and logical to attribute a progressive sensorineural deafness in an older person to arteriosclerosis or thrombosis. Yet such an explanation rarely is confirmed by histopathologic studies. Although physicians continue to blame terminal blood vessels in the ear for many causes of hearing loss, they do not have proof that this is so. Other logical causes also should be considered.

Sudden unilateral deafness may be explained most reasonably on the basis of blood vessel spasm and rupture. In clinical practice one sees quite a few patients with unexplained attacks of sudden unilateral deafness of short duration—or even of longer duration, an attack that may last for several weeks—followed by a spontaneous return of hearing to normal or improved levels. Often the hearing losses are accompanied by rotary vertigo, imbalance and high-pitched tinnitus. In other cases deafness is the only symptom other than a sensation of fullness in the ear. In still

AIR CONDUCTION														
		RIGHT							LEFT					
DATE	LEFT MASK	250	500	1000	2000	4000	8000	RIGHT MASK	250	500	1000	2000	4000	8000
9/15/59		45	45	45	50	NR	NR		65	70	65	65	85	75
9/19/59									10	25	60	65	NR	75
9/21/59									55	50	50	60	90	75
9/24/59									15	15	30	45	90	75
10/ 4/59									15	15	5	30	85	75

BONE CONDUCTION												
		RIGHT							LEFT			
DATE	LEFT MASK	250	500	1000	2000	4000	TYPE	RIGHT MASK	250	500	1000	2000	4000
9/15/59		-10	-10	-10	25	50			10	0	-5	15	55

SPEECH RECEPTION THRESHOLD					DISCRIMINATION SCORE						TUNING FORK TESTS (500 CPS.)		
					RIGHT			LEFT					
DATE	RIGHT	LEFT MASK	LEFT	RIGHT MASK	% SCORE	TEST LEVEL	LEFT MASK	% SCORE	TEST LEVEL	RIGHT MASK		R	L
9/15/59			64					94	90		AIR-BONE COMPARISON		
9/24/59			34		9/19/59			42	64		LATERALIZATION		
10/ 4/59			12					60	42		B. C. COMPARISON TO NORMAL		

Fig. 73. *History:* This patient had an excellent improvement in pure tone threshold after a left stapedectomy, but she was very unhappy with the result, because she could not use the left ear satisfactorily. Speech testing postoperatively showed a real drop in discrimination, which probably was due to postoperative labyrinthosis. No satisfactory treatment for this is known to the author at present. Note that before surgery she heard 94% of the test words, but after surgery, only 60%. When the test material was presented at a higher level, the discrimination score dropped to 42%, due to distortion.

other patients both deafness and tinnitus are permanent, but the imbalance disappears.

Cases of permanent sudden deafness in one ear usually are blamed on vascular rupture or vascular occlusion, whereas those that recover are attributed to reversible vessel spasm. There are, however, some pitfalls in this explanation. For want of a better one at this time, most otologists continue to blame such cases of deafness on circulatory difficulties or virus diseases.

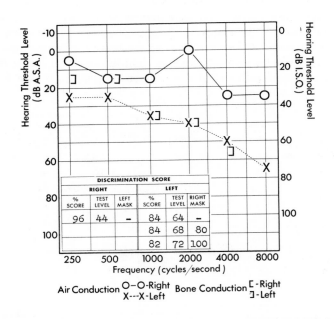

FIG. 74. *History:* 50-year-old patient who developed sudden deafness in left ear 3 months before, accompanied by distortion and buzzing but no vertigo of any sort. All symptoms except deafness gradually subsided.

Otologic: normal. Only minimal response from both ears after caloric stimulation. No spontaneous nystagmus.

Audiologic: left ear hearing loss greater in higher frequencies with reduced bone conduction. Complete recruitment in all frequencies and diplacusis. No abnormal tone decay.

Classification: sensory hearing loss

Etiology: unknown

Comment: Findings of complete recruitment and diplacusis and no abnormal tone decay localize the lesion to the inner ear. The good discrimination score which did not worsen with increased sound intensity, and the cessation of tinnitus and distortion are not in keeping with Ménière's disease. Possible causes include vasospasm and viral cochleitis.

The roles of hypertension and hypotension in deafness also are unknown. In the author's experience hypertension is rarely, in itself, the cause of either insidious or sudden hearing loss. On the other hand, hypotension seems in some cases to be vaguely associated with progressive high tone sensorineural deafness. Usually, recurrent attacks of imbalance also are present in such patients. Hypotension may predispose to sudden losses in hearing, but here again convincing proof is lacking.

A most interesting case of sudden sensorineural unilateral deafness was seen by the author recently in a patient who blamed it on an attack of severe sneezing. The findings are shown in Figure 70. We are not certain about forceful sneezing being the cause, but its effects should be considered. It would appear also that patients with certain vascular disorders, such as endarteritis, Buerger's disease, diabetes and others, should have a high incidence of sensorineural deafness, but this has not been borne out by investigations.

The degree of hearing impairment present in patients with sudden unilateral deafness varies and may be only 15 or 20 db and last only a few

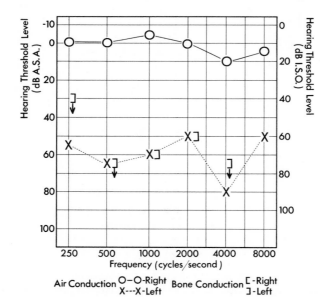

FIG. 75. *History:* 45-year-old male with sudden deafness in left ear on awakening one morning. Some ringing tinnitus but no vertigo.
Otologic: normal
Audiologic: very little recruitment present and no abnormal tone decay. Discrimination about 68% and no diplacusis.
Classification: sensorineural hearing loss
Diagnosis: unknown. This damage possibly could be of vascular origin.

moments, as most individuals probably have experienced at one time or another when they have felt a sudden fullness and ringing in one ear; or the hearing loss may be up to 50 db or even total, as described previously. Whether or not a sudden deafness is reversible seems beyond the ability of physicians to predict reliably. Nevertheless, it is wise to utilize reasonable therapy as early as possible to reverse the damage.

FOLLOWING EAR SURGERY

The increase in stapes surgery has brought with it a marked increase in the incidence of unilateral sudden deafness. Physicians already are familiar with the sudden severe deafness that may result as a complication of mastoid and fenestration surgery. The loss is sudden and occurs either at the time of the operation due to invasion of the inner ear or shortly

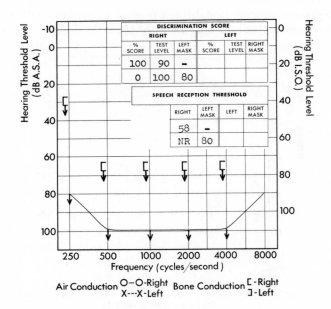

Air Conduction O—O-Right   Bone Conduction ⊏-Right
                X---X-Left   ⊐-Left

FIG. 76. *History:* 45-year-old female who for several years had experienced a pounding sensation in the right ear whenever she became nervous. Two weeks ago she developed complete deafness, accompanied by momentary severe dizziness and positional vertigo lasting 1 day. Since then she has had buzzing tinnitus in the right ear.

Otologic: normal. Normal caloric response in right ear

Audiologic: no response to pure tones or speech testing with the left ear masked.

Classification: sensorineural deafness

Diagnosis: unknown, but probably a vascular accident

after surgery due to infection. With the advent of stapedectomies otologists now are encountering sudden hearing loss in patients weeks or even months after surgery. Figure 71 is an example of a patient who became deaf in his operated ear 4 months after a stapedectomy. Surgical exploration showed invasion of the vestibule with white scar tissue from the middle ear. The hearing in another patient suddenly became bad several months after stapedectomy during a bad infection described as a virus. No unusual findings were encountered in the middle ear or the oval window during exploration, and the perilymphatic fluid in the inner ear appeared to be normal. It is important, therefore, in all cases to inquire about previous ear surgery. Surgery for tympanosclerosis in which the oval window is opened is a common cause of sudden deafness, usually noted within 1 or 2 days postoperatively.

The sensorineural deafness that can follow ear surgery need not be severe or total. More often it consists of a high tone hearing loss that did not exist preoperatively (Fig. 72). We generally attribute this to injury to the inner ear during surgery or infection postoperatively. The patient's chief complaint in such situations is reduced ability to understand what he hears. This is a justified complaint, one that can be demonstrated with discrimination tests. Sometimes a patient with a most successful return of threshold hearing following stapes surgery will appear to be most unhappy about the result and bewilder the surgeon. Figure 73 shows such a case, and the discrimination scores show that in spite of the improved threshold level this patient is far worse off postoperatively than she was preoperatively.

DEAFNESS FOLLOWING ANESTHESIA AND GENERAL SURGERY

Hearing impairment following anesthesia and general surgery has been encountered by some otologists, but evidence is unavailable as to which, if either, of these conditions is the immediate cause. It is not uncommon in otology to find patients who claim that they suffered hearing loss, or that their hearing loss was aggravated after some surgical procedure. A causal relationship may be possible, or it may be coincidental.

UNKNOWN CAUSES OF SUDDEN SENSORINEURAL DEAFNESS

Unilateral sudden sensorineural deafness is so common in clinical practice that a number of additional examples are presented to help the physician to make a better classification and diagnosis (Figs. 74 to 76).

Chapter 13

Sensory and Neural Hearing Loss: Distinguishing Sensory From Neural Etiologies

Until recently, when bone conduction was found to be reduced, a case could be classified only as sensorineural or, as it was more commonly called, perceptive or nerve deafness. With the development of improved tests based on a clearer understanding of auditory pathology it is now possible in some cases to determine whether the damage is primarily in the sensory or in the neural mechanism. The designations "sensory" and "neural" are becoming more meaningful as knowledge of ear pathology improves. The distinction is not possible in every case, because many patients actually have damage both in the inner ear and in the nerve and thus have a sensorineural loss. In some patients the hearing loss has its origin in the inner ear and satisfies all the criteria for sensory hearing loss, but later the damage extends to the nerve, and the classification then becomes sensorineural.

Even the two most prominent causes of sensory hearing impairment, Ménière's disease and noise-induced hearing loss, result in damage to the auditory nerve after long periods of time. It is not usual, on the other hand, for neural hearing impairment to progress into the secondary sensory type. Whenever a case of hearing loss, particularly a high tone loss, shows reduced bone conduction without an air-bone gap, it should be classified tentatively, as sensorineural until further tests are done to determine whether it is more specifically sensory or neural in type.

DIFFERENTIATING SENSORY AND NEURAL TYPES

In the present state of knowledge, two criteria, when available, are of

156

most value in differentiating between sensory and neural types. These are recruitment and abnormal tone decay. If a patient demonstrates marked recruitment and diplacusis, the site of his auditory damage is in his inner ear, and the hearing loss is classified as sensory. Patients with nerve deafness rarely have this marked degree of recruitment. If a patient demonstrates clear-cut evidence of abnormal tone decay, the damage is in the fibers of his auditory nerve proper, and the classification then is neural hearing loss. Cases of sensory hearing loss usually do not show abnormal tone decay. This does not mean necessarily that every case of neural deafness must show abnormal tone decay, or that every case of sensory hearing loss must show marked recruitment, but when these phenomena are present, they are pathognomonic of the type of hearing loss.

The availability of these criteria is limited. Recruitment tends to disappear when neural factors complicate sensory hearing loss. Abnormal tone decay can be elicited only when damage to the nerve fibers is only partial, whereas it cannot be elicited in those cases in which nerve fibers have presumably lost all function, as in congenital nerve deafness and most cases of presbycusis.

The tests used to establish the presence of recruitment and abnormal tone decay are described in Chapter 24. One testing procedure of increasing importance is continuous and fixed frequency audiometry, which is done with a Bekesy type audiometer. This instrument is rather expensive and at present is used principally in large hearing centers. For this reason the emphasis in this book is on the results of the tests and their interpretation rather than the details of technic.

SENSORY HEARING LOSS

The classification of sensory hearing loss includes all cases in which, according to the best information available, the damage to the auditory pathway is in the inner ear. The damage is usually in the labyrinthine fluids and the hair cells.

CHARACTERISTICS OF SENSORY HEARING LOSS

1. Some patients give a history of recurrent attacks of labyrinthine vertigo associated with fullness in the ear, ocean-roaring tinnitus and intermittent hearing loss. This history is highly suggestive of the syndrome variously called Ménière's disease, cochlear hypertension, labyrinthosis or labyrinthine hydrops.

2. In Ménière's disease the hearing loss is more likely to be unilateral,

which is sometimes a distinguishing feature from sensorineural hearing loss (except in acoustic neuroma or vascular accident).

3. In Ménière's disease, if tinnitus is present, it is described as an ocean roar; it may be likened to the sound of a seashell held against the ear. In cases of hearing loss due to exposure to loud noises the tinnitus is said to sound like a high-pitched ring.

4. Occasionally, the history will reveal exposure to intense noise accompanied by ringing tinnitus. In Ménière's disease there may be a reduction in the threshold of hearing during an attack, and a return of hearing when the attack has subsided. The hearing loss eventually becomes permanent.

5. The patient's voice is usually of normal loudness.

6. The otologic examination is normal.

7. There is a hearing loss by air conduction.

8. There is a hearing loss by bone conduction.

9. There is no air-bone gap.

10. If the hearing loss is moderate or marked in the speech frequencies, speech discrimination is reduced markedly.

11. Frequently, the discrimination score gets worse when the patient is addressed in a loud voice.

12. Recruitment is present, marked and usually continuous and complete, and occasionally there may even be hyperrecruitment.

13. Diplacusis is present.

14. The threshold of discomfort for loud sounds is lowered.

15. There is no abnormal tone decay.

16. With some exceptions, the tuning fork lateralizes to the better-hearing ear.

The reasons for some of these distinguishing features will be described, but only briefly, since practically all are discussed in the section on hearing testing.

The history is helpful, because it is distinctive in two notable causes of sensory hearing impairment: noise-induced hearing loss and Ménière's disease. The patient with noise-induced hearing loss generally will volunteer the information that his hearing loss and ringing tinnitus started after he was exposed to gunfire, exploding firecrackers or industrial noise. In Ménière's disease the hearing impairment usually will be unilateral and accompanied by ocean-roaring or seashell tinnitus and a feeling of fullness in the ear. Vertigo may or may not be a feature, and this as well as the hearing loss will be intermittent at first, though later it may become persistent. Many patients with Ménière's disease, even when it is unilateral, will not say that they do not hear, but they will complain that they are unable to distinguish the exact words they hear. *Bath* sounds like *path*, *bomb* like *palm*. This indicates a reduction in discrimination. Along with this, they will say that speech and sounds are distorted and irritating, especially if loud. A baby's cry may sound unbearably loud. (This indicates a lowered threshold of discomfort due to recruitment.)

According to most authorities on Ménière's disease, this disorder is characterized by a pathologic change in the endolymph, which then affects the hair cells. This causes damage which at first is temporary and reversible but later results in permanent damage inside the cochlea, and ultimately degeneration of the auditory nerve fibers takes place, making the final result a sensorineural hearing impairment.

If both ears have been involved markedly for many years, the patient's voice then becomes loud, because his bone conduction is affected. However, it is usually not as loud as in some cases of neural deafness of long standing, because many sensory hearing losses are unilateral and are accompanied by recruitment.

There is no air-bone gap, because the bone conduction hearing level is usually about the same as the air conduction hearing level. In Ménière's disease the patient's ability to distinguish or to discriminate between words which sound somewhat alike often gets worse instead of better when the voice is raised. Much of this is due to recruitment and increased distortion with higher intensities. The otologic findings are normal, since the damage is restricted to the inner ear.

The comment regarding lateralization with a tuning fork is of special interest. If the tuning fork is struck gently and held to the forehead or the teeth in a case of unilateral sensory hearing impairment, it will sound louder in the normal ear. However, if marked recruitment is present in the bad ear, and the tuning fork is struck hard, there is a good chance the tone will sound even louder in the bad ear than in the normal ear. For this reason, testing for lateralization in cases of unilateral hearing loss should be performed with deliberate control of the sound intensity of the tuning fork while caution is observed in technic and interpretation of results.

Distortion is an outstanding feature of sensory hearing loss. Pure tones such as those produced by a tuning fork or a piano sound raspy and of different pitch in the bad ear than in the unaffected ear—hence the phenomenon of diplacusis. This sensory distortion affects not only pure sounds but also voices and noises generally and represents a source of much irritation, frustration and emotional strain to the patient, a problem too little understood by many physicians.

Patients with bilateral sensory hearing loss are hardly ever able to use hearing aids in a satisfactory manner. The amplification provided by the aid adds to speech distortion and thus makes voices even less intelligible, especially in noisy areas.

The prognosis for sensory hearing impairment is better than it is for the neural type but not nearly as favorable as for conductive hearing loss.

In the early stages many cases of sensory hearing loss seem to be reversible. For example, there are recurrent intermittent attacks of hearing loss with Ménière's disease alternating with periods of better hearing. According to most published reports, no such optimism is warranted in most cases of neural deafness. There is, however, great need for more facts and information concerning this point.

AUDIOMETRIC PATTERNS IN SENSORY IMPAIRMENT

As in conductive hearing loss the shape of the air conduction audiogram in sensory impairment depends to a great extent on the cause and the pathology. However, two audiometric patterns are typically associated with the two common causes of sensory hearing loss.

Figure 80 of Chapter 14 shows the audiometric pattern found in a classic early case of Ménière's disease. This is described as an ascending air conduction hearing level with a reduced bone conduction curve following almost exactly the same pattern. This patient presented practically all the symptoms classically associated with sensory hearing loss due to Ménière's disease.

The other characteristic type of audiogram found in sensory hearing loss is shown in Figure 83 of Chapter 14. This is sometimes described as a C-5 dip, and in this instance the cause was exposure to intense noise. It is the audiogram of a man who was exposed to small arms gunfire, with the result that he suffered a permanent high tone loss. It is appropriate to point out that the term "C-5 dip" is not very satisfactory. The only reason it is commonly so designated is the manner in which the audiograms and the test hearing are recorded. If the tests were to be made at several hundred cycles on either side of 4,000 cps, the so-called C-5, the chances are that the dip would be found there as well. When testing is done with continuous frequency audiometry, the dips can occur at 3,000 cycles, at 5,000 or 6,000 cycles, or anywhere in between, without involving 4,000 cycles. Consequently, the term "C-5 dip" is not satisfactory and should be replaced by the term "high tone dip," which really means that the hearing is normal on either side of a sharp depression in the hearing level.

Though the range of frequencies involved in this high tone dip is comparatively small, recruitment studies generally show complete and continuous recruitment. However, no significant reduction in speech discrimination is detectable with presently available tests. This is so because speech frequencies have not become involved. As is demonstrated also in Chapter 14, a high tone dip is not the only type of threshold shift that can be produced in the early stages of noise exposure; nor is noise the only etiology of dips in the hearing level.

Obviously, in sensory as in conductive hearing loss and, as will be noted, in neural hearing loss as well, certain characteristic patterns apparently are associated with each; it does not follow that other patterns do not occur, or that one may not find a so-called characteristic pattern associated with nonclassic types of hearing loss.

The basic audiologic features, then, that should be looked for in making a classification of sensory hearing loss are: (1) reduced threshold of hearing by air conduction and bone conduction; (2) the absence of any air-bone gap; (3) marked recruitment that is generally continuous and complete; (4) reduced discrimination if the speech frequencies are involved, and still further reduction as the intensity of speech is increased; (5) lateralization of the sound of the tuning fork to the better-hearing ear, with certain exceptions; and (6) an absence of pathologic adaptation. When these features are present along with a corroborating history and otologic examination, a case can be classified accurately as sensory hearing impairment.

NEURAL DEAFNESS

When hearing impairment results from damage to the fibers of the auditory nerve per se, it is classified as a nerve or neural type of hearing impairment.

CHARACTERISTICS OF NEURAL HEARING LOSS

Certain features are characteristic of neural hearing loss.

1. The history is variable. The deafness may be sudden in onset and practically complete in one ear, as may occur in fracture of the skull involving the internal auditory meatus; or it may be gradual and bilateral, as in progressive hereditary nerve deafness. A history of familial deafness often is helpful, but it should be borne in mind that a similar history is to be expected in otosclerosis. The patient's age is of little help, because nerve deafness may occur in any age group. Vertigo is a most important symptom. If it is present, especially in the presence of a unilateral sensory hearing loss, its cause must be established: at least the presence of an auditory nerve tumor must be ruled out. Tinnitus does not aid the differential diagnosis of nerve deafness per se; if present, it is likely to be high-pitched.

2. Air conduction and bone conduction are both reduced.

3. There is no air-bone gap.

4. If the hearing loss is unilateral or more severe in one ear than in the other, the vibrating tuning fork is referred to the better hearing ear.

5. Recruitment usually is absent, but if present, it is minimal and not complete.

		AIR CONDUCTION												
		RIGHT							LEFT					
DATE	LEFT MASK	250	500	1000	2000	4000	8000	RIGHT MASK	250	500	1000	2000	4000	8000
6/12/59		15	10	0	0	20	15							
6/29/59	85	90	95	NR	NR	NR	NR	After injury to 8th nerve						
7/22/60	95	65	50	40	30	30	NR							

		BONE CONDUCTION											
		RIGHT							LEFT				
DATE	LEFT MASK	250	500	1000	2000	4000	TYPE	RIGHT MASK	250	500	1000	2000	4000
6/12/59		20	15	0	15	15							
6/29/59	85	NR	NR	NR	NR	NR		After injury to 8th nerve					

RIGHT MASKING 100 DB.
LEFT MASKING _____ DB.

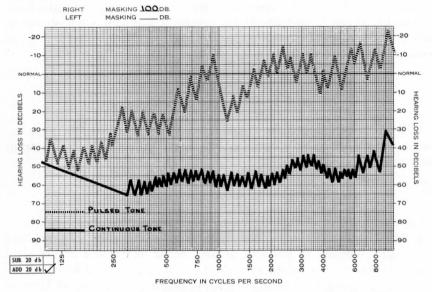

Fig. 77. *History:* 43-year-old female with recurrent attacks of severe pain in the right side of face for 5 years. No other complaints. Hearing was normal.

Otologic: normal

Audiologic: normal hearing. After accidental injection of the 8th nerve with boiling water for relief of the facial pain there were total deafness, facial palsy and absence of caloric response due to direct injury to the 8th nerve.

Classification: nerve deafness

Diagnosis: injury to auditory nerve. Severe deafness persisted for several months, and then hearing gradually returned and showed no recruitment but marked tone decay in all frequencies. Return of hearing after such a severe injury and profound loss is remarkable. The marked tone decay is evident in the large separation between the pulsed (*bottom,* upper curve) and continuous (*bottom,* lower curve) Bekesy tracings. (Harbert, F., and Young, I. M.: Threshold auditory adaptation measured by tone decay test and Bekesy audiometry, Ann. Otol. 73:48, Fig. 1, March 1964)

6. There is generally a striking disparity between the hearing threshold level and the patient's ability to discriminate speech.

7. Abnormal tone decay is present except in cases of congenital nerve deafness and presbycusis. If this feature can be elicited, it localizes the damage to the auditory nerve fibers, and this is of great diagnostic value.

8. Bekesy audiometry in the presence of abnormal tone decay generally shows a separation between the continuous tone and interrupted tone tracings, and the continuous tone tracings are of small amplitude.

The basic causes underlying some of these criteria have been traced by a study of proven cases of auditory nerve tumors. Of paramount importance is the finding of abnormal tone decay. This phenomenon rapidly is becoming recognized as pathognomonic of acoustic neuroma. Any injury that causes what one might call "partial damage" to the auditory nerve is likely to produce abnormal tone decay. A classic example is shown in Figure 77. Here, after the nerve was damaged by direct injection, all features of nerve damage were evident. It is notable also that temporary damage to the auditory nerve can occur; recovery from nerve damage is, indeed, not an uncommon clinical experience. Another example of the reversibility of nerve damage is auditory fatigue or "temporary threshold shift" (TTS). It is generally assumed that TTS, like "permanent threshold shift" (PTS), results from damage to the hair cells of the inner ear. Although there is extensive proof that this is true for PTS, there is no reliable information that it is true for TTS. As a matter of fact, if present criteria for classifying nerve deafness are reliable, and if findings from animal experiments are to be accepted, it appears that TTS is a phenomenon associated not with hair cell damage but possibly with nerve damage. Animal experiments have demonstrated that hair cells do not fatigue readily, and experiments with humans seem to indicate that TTS is really a reversible neural type of hearing loss.

Comment on Criteria. The onset of neural deafness is very variable. It may occur slowly, as in a case of acoustic neuroma, or suddenly, as a result of herpes virus.

From the little known about tinnitus, one would expect it to be an important feature accompanying neural deafness, but this is not borne out in practice. Many patients with acoustic neuromas complain little, or not at all, of noise in their ears. Even elderly patients who give evidence of a marked neural type of hearing loss do not complain of tinnitus very often. This is in contrast with patients having sensorineural hearing loss, who sometimes complain bitterly of hissing or ringing tinnitus.

The reduced bone conduction in nerve deafness is particularly marked. The vibrating tuning fork is unheard even when struck very hard. This is especially true in older patients with senile changes in the skull bones and the mastoid. Therefore it would be expected that the fork would lateralize to the better-hearing ear.

One of the earliest findings in auditory nerve damage due to pressure from a neoplasm is disturbance of the vestibular pathways. Although there may be no subjective vertigo, vestibular studies usually show abnormal findings, and such studies should be done routinely in all cases of unilateral sensorineural deafness, especially when marked recruitment is absent.

Another singular feature in nerve deafness is the great discrepancy often found between a hearing threshold level and the patient's ability to discriminate. Figure 78 shows an excellent example of a patient with a comparatively good hearing level but a disproportionately poor discrimination score. At surgery an acoustic neuroma was removed. The reason for the good hearing threshold level in spite of so much auditory nerve

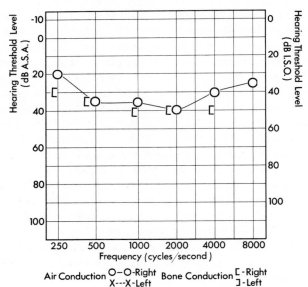

Fig. 78. *History:* 40-year-old female with occasional imbalance and feeling of fatigue. No tinnitus and no rotary vertigo. Noted progressive hearing loss in right ear for 2 years.

Otologic: normal. Vestibular studies showed no response in the right ear and perverted response of the vertical canals on the left side.

Audiologic: Bekesy audiometry—wide separation between pulsed and continuous tone tracings and small amplitude of continuous tone tracings. No recruitment but marked tone decay. Moderate pure tone loss with no air-bone gap. Right ear discrimination was 42%. Left ear masked during all testing of right ear.

Classification: neural. Damage in auditory nerve fibers

Etiology: acoustic neuroma right side, removed at surgery

damage must be borne in mind: almost three quarters of the auditory nerve can be severed before the threshold for pure tones is affected markedly. The discrimination score and the patient's ability to understand what he hears, however, are considerably affected, even though the hearing thresholds are not. It seems that the neural patterns carrying information to the auditory cortex are disturbed by the nerve damage so that the patient has great difficulty in understanding what is said. This handicap is further aggravated by anything that interferes with understanding, such as ambient noise, distortion and distraction.

As a rule, recruitment is not present in nerve damage, but it may be found occasionally when there is also some cochlear damage not recognizable by available testing methods.

AUDIOMETRIC PATTERNS IN NERVE DEAFNESS

It is difficult to describe definite characteristic patterns associated with

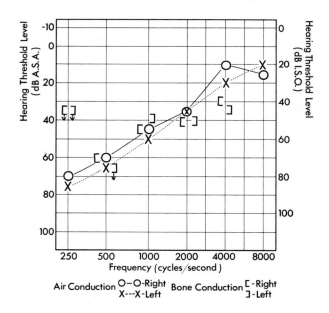

FIG. 79. *History:* 74-year-old female with insidious hearing loss for 30 years. No tinnitus or vertigo. Soft speaking voice.
   Otologic: normal
   Audiologic: moderate to severe bilateral hearing loss with greatest loss in the low frequencies. No air-bone gap.
   Discrimination score: Right, 82%; Left, 78%.
   Classification: neural hearing loss
   Diagnosis: unknown

pure nerve deafness except for such a cause as acoustic neuroma. When actual nerve deafness develops in presbycusis, this often is preceded by degeneration in the inner ear, causing the typical high tone loss. This makes it difficult to be certain precisely what the nerve deafness alone would cause. For our purposes, however, we can assume that the typical picture of nerve deafness is that of high tone hearing loss.

However, the mind should not be closed to the fact that other types of audiometric patterns besides these two are possible in nerve deafness. (For example, Figure 79 shows an ascending type of nerve deafness in a very elderly patient. The cause was never established, but the findings were highly suggestive of nerve deafness.)

Chapter 14

Sensory and Neural Hearing Loss: Causes

Certain causes of hearing impairment are known to affect the inner ear primarily and to produce findings characteristic of sensory hearing loss. Because inner ear damage frequently progresses into the nerve elements, many cases originally starting as sensory progress to the sensorineural type.

The following causes are known to produce sensory hearing impairment. All are characterized, at least in their early stages, by some degree of recruitment and hearing distortion.

Causes of Sensory Hearing Loss
1. Ménière's disease
2. Prolonged exposure to intense noise (occupational hearing impairment)
3. Acoustic trauma
4. Direct head trauma
5. Ototoxic drugs
6. Virus infections
7. Labyrinthosis following ear surgery
8. Early presbycusis
9. Congenital cochlear disease

Certain other causes are known to damage the auditory nerve per se. Abnormal tone decay becomes an important finding in some cases when there is "partial damage" to the nerve fibers, according to some investigators.

Causes of Neural Hearing Loss include the following:
1. Acoustic neuroma
2. Skull fracture and nerve injury
3. Section of the auditory nerve
4. Virus infections

SENSORY HEARING IMPAIRMENT—ITS CAUSES

Ménière's Disease

Ménière's disease presents all the classic symptoms and findings associated with a sensory hearing impairment. There is still confusion concerning the criteria for diagnosing Ménière's disease. Part of the confusion centers about the original findings of the 19th century otologist, Prosper Ménière, who reported the autopsy findings on a patient who had suffered from dizziness and deafness. Apparently, what he described and what is now considered to be Ménière's disease are not the same. However, the confusion lies mostly in terminology and the tendency of some physicians to call all cases of vertigo of undetermined origin Ménière's disease.

Terms and Definition. Recent research studies on patients with vertigo, tinnitus and deafness have revealed histopathologic findings suggesting a hydrops of the labyrinth caused by distention with endolymphatic fluid. The cause of the presence of excessive fluid is unknown, but it has now come to be associated with subjective symptoms of Ménière's disease. Because of this hydrops new names have been applied to the condition. It is variously called labyrinthosis (in contrast with labyrinthitis, which implies an inflammatory involvement) and even labyrinthine hypertension. Common clinical usage now seems to restrict the condition named Ménière's disease to patients who have recurrent attacks of vertigo, deafness and tinnitus. Although this definition may be commonly accepted and proper, actually Ménière's disease or cochlear hydrops is an abnormality of hearing and does not necessarily involve the balance mechanism, so that a diagnosis of Ménière's disease is based primarily on the history and the audiologic findings and secondarily on the vertigo and the labyrinthine findings. Many patients have Ménière's disease without vertigo. Precisely why vertigo is present at all in some cases and not in others is still a mystery, but the essential diagnostic feature is the type of hearing loss and its special criteria.

Symptoms and Their Effect on the Patient. The characteristic findings in Ménière's disease are generally clear-cut, and all are present in most cases. As might be expected in any condition, occasional borderline cases and variations are encountered. The typical history is marked by a sudden onset of fullness, hearing loss and a seashell-like tinnitus in one ear. This may last for a period of minutes or several days and then disappear. The same symptoms then may recur at varying time intervals. After several attacks the hearing loss and the tinnitus may persist. The loss may not be severe, but voices begin to sound tinny and muffled on the telephone, and it becomes difficult for the patient to follow a conversation because of the inability to distinguish between different words that have related sounds. In addition, there is distortion of sound, and the threshold of discomfort for loud noises is reduced. Fullness in the ear is common.

VERTIGO AND TINNITUS. More often, in addition to these symptoms, the patient complains of recurrent attacks of vertigo, during which either the room seems to spin, or the patient feels himself to be spinning. Everything goes around, and the tinnitus is aggravated severely during the attack. Sometimes nausea and even vomiting may occur.

The vertigo in Ménière's disease is of a specific type that involves some sort of motion. It is "subjective" when the patient has a sensation of moving or "objective" when things move about the patient. Usually, the motion is described as rotary, especially during the acute attack. Occasionally, between acute attacks patients have a mild feeling of motion whereby they seem to fall to one side and cannot keep their balance. Less often there is a strange up-and-down or to-and-fro motion. Other types of sensation such as a feeling of faintness or weakness, or seeing spots before the eyes, or just vague "dizziness" should not be attributed to Ménière's disease. The possible causes for these subjective symptoms are numerous, but Ménière's disease is not one of them. Furthermore, there must be some evidence of hearing loss being, or having been, present for the diagnosis properly to be Ménière's disease. It is true that in the very early phases hearing may be lost only during the acute attack, and that it may be normal between attacks. But even in such cases the patient will recall having experienced fullness and roaring in one ear. If these subjective symptoms are absent, and no hearing loss is present, a diagnosis of Ménière's disease should be made only with the utmost caution, and further studies should explore the possibility of some other likely cause of the dizziness.

Patients are concerned more frequently about the vertigo and the tinnitus than about their hearing loss. For an individual who works on scaffolding or drives a car or a truck, a sudden unexpected attack of vertigo beyond his control is indeed a serious problem. These patients are invariably apprehensive and gravely concerned. As a matter of fact, nervous tension is a most prominent symptom in patients with Ménière's disease. Most of them seem to be much improved and less subject to attacks when they are relaxed and free of tense situations.

The ocean-roaring or seashell-like tinnitus is also a matter of grave concern. When patients are in quiet surroundings, or when they are under tension, the tinnitus may become so alarming to them that they often are willing to undergo any type of surgery, even if it means the loss of all their hearing in the affected ear, provided that the noise can be made to disappear. Under such circumstances the otologist should not let the patient influence him to perform irrational and sometimes unsuccessful surgery for the removal of tinnitus. As yet physicians have no specific, reliable procedure to control tinnitus and consistently to preserve hearing.

THE HEARING LOSS generally is not as disturbing to the patient as the other two symptoms, but when it happens to a businessman who uses the telephone to conduct his affairs, it becomes an important issue.

THE AUDIOLOGIC FINDINGS in a typical case of Ménière's disease are

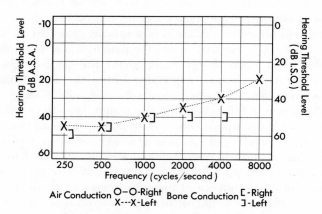

Air Conduction O—O-Right   Bone Conduction Ⅎ-Right
                X--X-Left   ꓵ-Left

Fig. 80. *History:* 37-year-old male with recurrent sudden attacks of rotary vertigo accompanied by nausea, vomiting and an ocean-roar tinnitus in the left ear. Between attacks the patient reports fullness and deafness, aggravated during attacks. Patient is annoyed by loud noise in the left ear, and voices sound fuzzy and unclear.

Otologic: normal

Audiologic: moderate hearing loss with no air-bone gap. Left ear discrimination: 60%. Binaural loudness balance studies show complete recruitment in the left ear:

	1,000 cps
R	L
0	40
10	45
20	50
30	55
40	55
50	60
60	65
70	70

During the loudness balance test the patient reported that the tone in the left ear was not as clear as the tone in the good ear. This is diplacusis and is an important symptom in inner ear pathology. The patient also has a lowered threshold of discomfort. There was no abnormal tone decay.

Classification: sensory impairment

Diagnosis: Ménière's disease

shown in Figure 80. Note the low tone hearing impairment with reduced bone conduction. If the bone conduction were not reduced, this audiometric pattern would be typical of conductive instead of sensory hearing loss. There is no air-bone gap, since both air conduction and bone conduction are reduced to the same degree. The patient's ability to discriminate in the bad ear is so reduced that he can distinguish only 60 per cent of the speech that he hears at ordinary levels of loudness. Furthermore, if speech is made louder (from 50 to 70 db), the patient distinguishes even less (contrary to expectations). This brings out one of the most important features of Ménière's disease, distortion. Distortion ex-

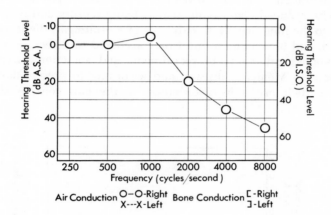

Fig. 81. *History:* 42-year-old male with sudden hearing loss and rushing tinnitus in the right ear. Symptoms present for 6 months when first seen for examination. Has slight difficulty distinguishing certain sounds. Feels occasional fullness in the right ear. No vertigo.

Otologic: normal with normal caloric responses

Audiologic: left ear normal. Right has a high tone loss with complete recruitment at 2,000 cps. No abnormal tone decay. Diplacusis with 2,000-cps tone.

Discrimination score: Right, 4%.

Classification: sensory hearing loss

Diagnosis: Ménière's disease

Aids to diagnosis: This man worked in a noisy environment, and his unilateral hearing loss originally was misdiagnosed as occupational deafness. The presence of complete recruitment, diplacusis and discrimination difficulty point to sensory hearing loss and probably Ménière's disease without vertigo. In this case the diagnosis was confirmed months later when the patient developed attacks of rotary vertigo. His hearing then changed to levels similar to those in Figure 80. Both the unilateral deafness with depression at 8,000 cps and the relatively low noise level (90 db overall) in the allegedly "noisy plant" mitigated against a diagnosis of noise-induced hearing loss.

plains many of the symptoms, not only the reduced discrimination but the tinny character that speech assumes in the patient's ears, the inability to discriminate between words on the telephone, and diplacusis.

RECRUITMENT. Another interesting phenomenon in patients with Ménière's disease is called a lower threshold of discomfort, and it is manifested by the patient's complaint that loud noises bother him. This difficulty is related partially to distortion but principally to the phenomenon of recruitment. Recruitment is a telltale audiologic finding in the diagnosis of inner ear deafness and particularly Ménière's disease. It stems from an abnormally rapid increase in the sensation of loudness, and when it is present to a marked degree, it permits the physician to classify a case with reduced bone conduction as being sensory and to localize the damage to the inner ear. In the absence of recruitment, the localization is uncertain, and the condition must be considered to be sensorineural.

Continuous and complete recruitment and sometimes hyperrecruitment occur in Ménière's disease, and according to present-day thinking they have their origin in disturbances in the hair cells. A simple but

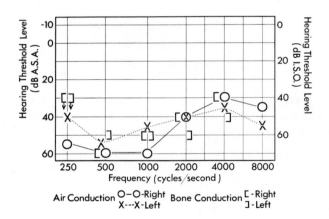

Air Conduction O—O-Right Bone Conduction [-Right
                 X---X-Left   ] -Left

FIG. 82. *History:* 31-year-old male with insidious deafness for many years with ocean-roar tinnitus and rare mild vertigo. Complains of severe discrimination problem and has great difficulty with telephone conversation. Gets no help from a hearing aid in either ear because of distortion.

Otologic: normal

Audiologic: bilateral loss with no air-bone gap. No abnormal tone decay.

Discrimination score: Right 32%, Left 36%. Discrimination is reduced when the intensity of the test material is presented at levels above 80 db. Both ears exhibit a lowered threshold of discomfort.

Classification: bilateral sensory impairment

Diagnosis: bilateral Ménière's disease

superficial test for recruitment should be done routinely in cases of reduced bone conduction by means of a tuning fork. Note in Figure 80 that this patient evidences all the phenomena associated with Ménière's disease, including marked recruitment. Abnormal tone decay is absent. The Bekesy audiogram (see Chap. 24) also is often characteristic, without a gap between the continuous and the interrupted tone.

CLINICAL STUDIES. The case in Figure 80 is typical of Ménière's disease, but there are many cases in which the diagnosis is not quite so certain. For example, Figure 81 shows a patient whose history is suggestive of Ménière's disease. In this patient, however, only the high tones were impaired, while the audiologic findings were equivocal, except for complete recruitment; and for this reason such a case may be classified as Ménière's disease. The diagnosis was established definitely as the disease progressed. Figure 82 shows a most difficult and frustrating type of case in which there is bilateral Ménière's disease. Note the comparatively mild reduction in auditory threshold but the severe discrimination loss. A hearing aid is of no value to this patient, for it generally aggravates the distortion, and he sometimes hears more poorly with it, but rarely better. The psychological effects of not being able to make out what his customers were saying and the severe tinnitus have driven this pharmacist to seek psychiatric attention.

LABYRINTHINE TESTS. Rotary vertigo may occur both in sensory and neural deafness, and when it is essential to differentiate between unilateral inner ear deafness and unilateral nerve deafness (possibly due to a tumor), labyrinthine tests are necessary. Not infrequently a patient will experience the vertigo as he is being examined in a physician's office. The patient will complain that the room, or he, is starting to turn, and that he has a severe noise in his ear. At that time, examination of the eyes shows a marked nystagmus with a slow and fast component. The type of nystagmus may be in almost any plane; it even may be oblique, and the direction also may vary. Such a strange type of nystagmus often suggests the presence of an intracranial tumor. However, careful watching usually reveals that the nystagmus soon subsides, and the vertigo stops (in contrast with most cases of intracranial involvement). Caloric studies, which should not be performed during the attack, show either diminished or exaggerated labyrinthine responses such as a hypersensitivity or a hyposensitivity with nausea and vomiting in Ménière's disease, but the direction and the type of nystagmus are normal with respect to amplitude and direction unlike the findings in posterior intracranial fossa neoplasm.

The treatment of Ménière's disease is beyond the intent of this book. However, no specific therapy is available. Many remedies have been suggested as curative, but the spontaneous remissions typical of this disease make it difficult to evaluate the effectiveness of suggested cures. The author firmly believes that destructive surgery of an ear with Ménière's disease should be performed only as a last resort and, at that, very rarely. Even though discrimination is poor with the residual hearing in the diseased ear, there is always the chance that the other ear may become in-

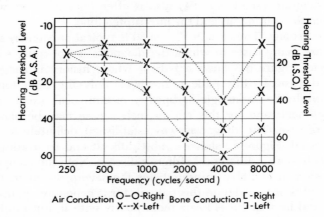

FIG. 83. Classic audiometric curves showing deafness due to exposure to gunfire. The hearing loss can continue beyond that shown in the upper threshold curve if the exposure continues, and if the noise is very intense, as indicated in the two lower threshold curves.

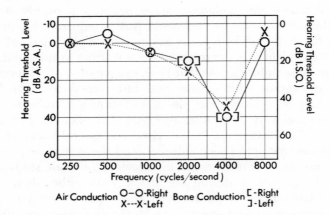

FIG. 84. *History:* 40-year-old female with ringing tinnitus for the past year. No trauma. No noise exposure, and patient denies having had any serious illness or infection. Hearing loss is nonprogressive.

Otologic: normal

Audiologic: normal thresholds except for bilateral C-5 dip

Classification: sensory hearing loss

Diagnosis: unknown but possibly viral cochleitis

volved, and thus destructive surgery in the ear first affected could produce a most serious handicap. Also the chance that a specific cure might be found at some future time should be borne in mind and should deter indiscriminate destructive surgery.

PROLONGED EXPOSURES TO INTENSE NOISE (OCCUPATIONAL HEARING IMPAIRMENT)

It is an established fact that intense noise can produce hearing loss. If the exposure is brief, such as the effect on the ear of a single pistol shot, explosion or firecracker, the sudden hearing loss produced is called acoustic trauma. If the exposure is prolonged, over many months and years, and the hearing loss develops gradually, the condition is called occupational hearing loss, industrial deafness or noise-induced hearing loss.

Two Components. Both acoustic trauma and occupational hearing loss have two components: one is the temporary hearing loss (auditory fatigue or temporary threshold shift—TTS) that is of brief duration and clears up, and the other is the permanent hearing loss (or permanent threshold shift —PTS) that remains. When we speak of occupational hearing loss, we

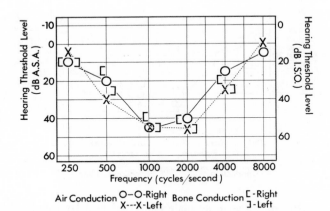

FIG. 85. *History:* 50-year-old female noted gradual hearing loss 1 year ago. No exposure to intense noise. No vertigo or tinnitus. Hearing loss is progressive.
Otologic: normal
Audiologic: Hearing loss is chiefly in the speech frequencies, and discrimination also is reduced.
Classification: sensorineural deafness
Diagnosis: unknown

really refer to the permanent loss in hearing from prolonged exposure, not the temporary loss.

Clinical History and Findings. The broad aspects of occupational hearing loss are discussed in detail in Chapter 26 because of the growing importance of the subject and because the physician will be called upon more and more to express an opinion in cases of this type. In this section are presented the clinical history and findings that the physician encounters in practice.

The pattern of occupational hearing loss is such that physicians generally do not see patients with this complaint until the impairment has become handicapping in daily communication. This means that the hearing loss is well advanced and irreversible. These two points indicate the importance of the problem of occupational hearing loss and the need for preventing it.

Noise-induced hearing loss generally develops in a well-defined manner. In the very early stage only the frequencies around 3,000 and 4,000 cycles are affected. This is the C-5 dip (so-called because 4,000 cps corresponds to C-5 (or the fifth C) in the normal audiometric testing range seen in the audiogram (Fig. 83). Note that the 8,000-cps frequency is normal. The fact that hearing at the higher frequencies remains normal is an important

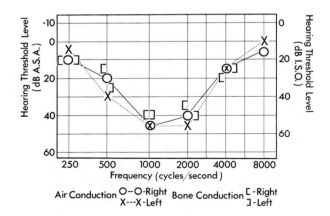

Air Conduction O—O-Right   Bone Conduction ⊏-Right
            X---X-Left   ⊐-Left

FIG. 86. *History:* 48-year-old male employed in a large mill with high noise levels. The noise spectrum is such that the speech frequencies are affected more than the higher frequencies. Fellow employees have similar hearing losses.

Otologic: normal

Audiologic: bilateral midfrequency dip with no air-bone gap. There is some evidence of recruitment but no abnormal tone decay.

Classification: bilateral sensory impairment

Diagnosis: noise-induced hearing loss

distinction from presbycusis, which progresses from the higher frequencies to the lower ones. This does not mean necessarily that all cases of dips are due to intense noise exposure, for they are not (Figs. 84, 85). Nor does it mean that the hearing loss is not due to noise exposure if the highest frequencies are damaged, for as exposure to intense noise continues, the frequencies on either side of 3,000 and 4,000 cycles also become affected. The classic course of progressive sensorineural deafness due to noise exposure is illustrated in Figure 83. This takes place generally over a period of many years. Susceptible subjects in rare instances may develop some hearing loss after a few months of exposure if the noise is exceptionally intense. There is no valid evidence that noises below 85 db are responsible for hearing losses.

The C-5 dip pattern is the most common but not the only early finding in noise-induced hearing loss. Exposure to certain types of noise produces the most damage, principally in the speech frequencies (Fig. 86). Communication handicaps manifest themselves much earlier in such a case.

Actually, the degree and the type of hearing loss depend on numerous factors, such as the intensity and the spectral characteristics of the noise and the time relation of the noise, that is, its suddenness, its intermittent or continuous character, the duration of exposure, and the little understood factor of individual susceptibility.

Extensive studies show conclusively that the early damage caused by intense noise takes place in the outer hair cells of the basilar coil of the cochlea. The site of pathology makes it a sensory hearing loss, and this diagnosis in a given patient is confirmed by showing the presence of marked recruitment. As the damage progresses, and the loss exceeds about 50 db, the inner hair cells also become involved, and then the supporting cells become damaged. Finally, the nerve fibers become affected, and clinical evidence of recruitment then becomes less marked.

In advanced cases of occupational hearing loss it often is difficult to distinguish the portion of the loss due to noise from the portion that is due to presbycusis. If in a specific case a reasonably good hearing level can be recorded in the frequencies above 8,000 cycles, the diagnosis in all likelihood is noise-induced hearing loss rather than presbycusis.

Because auditory fatigue can be a factor, it is advisable to evaluate the amount of occupational hearing loss present after the employee has been free of exposure to intense noise for at least several months.

The term "occupational deafness" is somewhat misleading. It implies the presence of obvious difficulties in hearing speech. Actually, the difficulty more often lies not so much in *hearing* speech as in *understanding* it. This trouble results from loss in the hearing of high frequencies, which is the characteristic finding in occupational deafness. Since many of the consonants that give meaning to words occur in the higher frequencies, it is natural that people who do not hear these frequencies or hear them feebly should be handicapped in understanding certain speech sounds, especially when they are poorly enunciated or masked by a noisy environment. Some of these speech sounds are s, f, z, ch and k. Therefore, unless one specifically looks for this lack of consonant discrimination, the presence of hearing loss is likely to be overlooked, since intense efforts generally are made by the employee to compensate for his handicap in reduced discrimination.

Ringing tinnitus is found commonly in acoustic trauma but rather infrequently in occupational hearing loss. A slight tinnitus may be present each night but disappears when the auditory fatigue subsides. Vertigo is never a real symptom accompanying occupational hearing loss. If vertigo is present, its true cause should be sought elsewhere.

Sudden deafness is not caused by continuous exposure to occupational noise. If deafness is sudden, and especially if it affects only one ear, the cause should be sought elsewhere. Military as well as civilian personnel on gunfiring duty, where the noise is intense, may experience much TTS after a day's exposure and perhaps some mild PTS, but more serious PTS involving the speech frequency range occurs only after many weeks of exposure even in the most susceptible people. When a person is removed from a noisy environment, his hearing improves. If after removal from noise his hearing continues to get worse over a period of months or years, another cause should be sought.

TEMPORARY HEARING LOSS

Although temporary hearing loss (auditory fatigue) or temporary threshold shift (TTS) is included in this section on sensory hearing loss, its true position is not certain. Animal experiments and even some observations in humans indicate that hair cells may not be involved in temporary threshold shift at nondamaging intensities, but that nerve fibers are involved. In human beings TTS differs in many respects from PTS.

There is as yet no proof that the relationship is quite so simple. For instance, the hearing of many workers who have sustained some degree of temporary shift daily for many years nevertheless returns to normal and remains normal. It is also known definitely that it is not possible to predict the sensitivity of an individual to intense noise by determining his temporary threshold shift characteristic, such as its degree or the rapidity of its return to normal. Until more definite and valid information is available, it is safer to consider the relation between TTS and PTS as still unresolved.

The degree of TTS depends to a great extent on the intensity and the duration of the stimulus in addition to the spectral configuration. The rate of recovery from TTS varies greatly in individuals but seems to be about

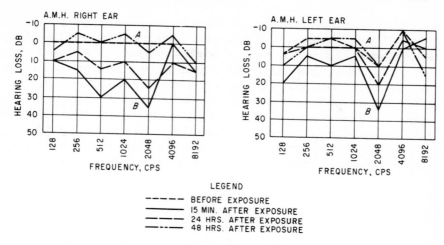

FIG. 87. Subject was exposed to intense noise of a certain type of jet engine for a long period. The hearing loss (B) returned to its original level (A) after 2 days of rest. During this period the subject experienced ringing tinnitus and much distortion with reduced discrimination.

the same in both ears in the same individual. There is some difference of opinion as to how long it takes for TTS to disappear after long exposure to intense noise. The estimates vary from several days to several months, but there is as yet no well-controlled study to establish the facts. Figure 87 describes the recovery studies in an interesting case of TTS occurring principally in the speech frequencies.

ACOUSTIC TRAUMA

In order to differentiate sudden hearing loss due to brief exposure to intense noise from the gradual loss caused by prolonged exposure over many months and years, the term "acoustic trauma" is restricted here to the former, and the latter is called noise-induced or occupational hearing loss.

In acoustic trauma the patient usually is exposed to a very intense noise of short duration like a rifle shot. This causes immediate hearing loss accompanied by fullness and ringing in the ear. If the cause is an explosion, there may be also a rupture of the eardrum and disruption of the ossicular chain. If this occurs, a conductive hearing loss is caused immediately without much serious sensory damage, because the middle ear defect now serves as a protection for the inner ear.

Following acoustic trauma to the inner ear the patient usually notes that the fullness and the ringing tinnitus subside, and his hearing improves. Generally, the hearing returns to normal. Most human beings have been exposed to gunfire at one time or another and have experienced some temporary hearing loss, only to have their hearing return to normal. In some cases, however, a degree of permanent hearing loss remains.

The amount of loss depends on the intensity and the duration of the noise and the sensitivity of the ear. Usually, the permanent loss is very mild and consists only of the high tone dip. If the noise is very intense, and the ear is particularly sensitive, the loss may be greater and involve a broader range of frequencies. The milder cases of hearing loss involve

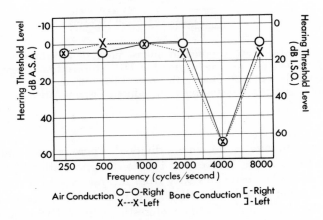

Air Conduction O–O-Right Bone Conduction [-Right
                    X---X-Left   ]-Left

Fig. 88. *History:* 9-year-old male with no clinical symptoms. The hearing defect was detected by the school nurse during routine screening. A year ago this child had been exposed to very loud cap pistol fire, immediately producing deafness and ringing tinnitus in both ears. Shortly thereafter the ringing and the deafness subsided.

Otologic: normal

Audiologic: The audiogram shows a typical bilateral C-5 dip, characteristic of acoustic trauma. There was no abnormal tone decay. Monaural loudness balance tests show almost complete recruitment:

Right		Left	
2,000 cps	4,000 cps	2,000 cps	4,000 cps
0	55	0	55
15	65	15	70
30	70	30	75
45	75	45	80
60	75	60	85
75	80	75	85

Classification: sensory impairment
Diagnosis: acoustic trauma

only one ear, usually the one closer to the gun or the source of the noise. If the noise is very intense, and the hearing loss is moderate, then usually both ears are affected to an almost identical degree, or perhaps one ear slightly more than the other. It is hardly possible (as a result of exposure to intense noise) to have a sensory hearing loss in one ear greater than about 40 decibels in all frequencies with normal hearing in the other ear. This has important medicolegal aspects.

Because there is practically always some degree of temporary hearing

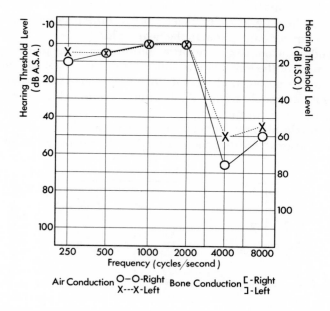

FIG. 89. *History:* 16-year-old male referred because of a slight ringing tinnitus and difficulty in understanding speech in a noisy environment. This difficulty, so typical with high tone loss, was aggravated when several people were speaking simultaneously. He also had difficulty hearing on the telephone. At the age of 6 he had experienced a severe exposure to cap pistol fire quite close to his ears. From that time he was aware of constant ringing tinnitus and hearing impairment. At the age of 10 his symptoms were aggravated by close exposure to the firing of a .22 caliber pistol.

Otologic: normal

Audiologic: bilateral C-5 dip with reduced thresholds at 8,000 cps also. This loss is sufficient to produce difficulty in discriminating certain consonants, particularly the sibilants. The difficulty is more pronounced in the presence of ambient noise or speech, due to the masking effect that these produce on the speech of nearby speakers.

Classification: sensory hearing loss

Diagnosis: acoustic trauma

loss or fatigue in acoustic trauma, the amount of permanent damage cannot be established until several months after the exposure. In the interim the individual must be free of other exposure to intense noise that might aggravate the hearing loss. The audiometric patterns in acoustic trauma are similar to those in noise-induced hearing loss, but the history is different, and probably the manner in which the permanent hearing loss is produced also is different. Figure 88 shows a typical case of acoustic trauma. Note that recruitment is present, is complete and continuous, and that there is no evidence of abnormal tone decay.

After the temporary hearing loss subsides, and only permanent loss remains, the hearing level stabilizes, and according to most investigators, there is no further progression in the hearing loss.

In Children. Comparatively little information is available concerning the sensitivity of the inner ears of children to loud noises. The infrequency of exposure to noises loud enough to produce acoustic trauma and the difficulty in accurately testing the hearing of young children may account for this paucity of information.

The example of three patients referred by a school nurse within several weeks dramatizes that more attention should be given to the effect

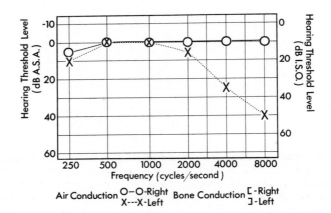

Air Conduction O–O-Right   Bone Conduction ⊏-Right
                X---X-Left   ⊐-Left

Fig. 90. *History:* 12-year-old male with no clinical symptoms referable to the ears. His hearing defect was detected during the school screening program. Several years ago he experienced sudden deafness and ringing tinnitus as a result of the loud report of a cap pistol fired close to his left ear. Both symptoms subsided the same day without recurrence.

Otologic: normal

Audiologic: right ear normal. Left ear has a high tone loss with recruitment.

Classification: sensory hearing loss

Diagnosis: acoustic trauma

of loud noises on the hearing acuity of children. In all three children permanent hearing defects were produced by inadvertent exposure to cap pistols or firecrackers. The hearing defects were of the inner ear and resembled those encountered among military personnel who have been exposed to gunfire. The loss was in the higher frequencies and occurred predominantly in one frequency, the so-called C-5 dip at 4,000 cycles. The hearing loss in such cases is not progressive, but once established, it is irreversible. Middle ear damage rarely accompanies this type of inner ear

			AIR CONDUCTION											
		RIGHT							LEFT					
DATE	LEFT MASK	250	500	1000	2000	4000	8000	RIGHT MASK	250	500	1000	2000	4000	8000
6/ 2/59	-5	-10	-5	0	-10	0	85	20	20	15	20	35	40
6/10/59							"	30	20	30	30	30	35
7/10/59							"	10	35	15	30	20	50
10/ 8/59							"	-5	10	10	-10	0	10

			BONE CONDUCTION									
		RIGHT							LEFT			
DATE	LEFT MASK	250	500	1000	2000	4000	TYPE	RIGHT MASK	250	500	1000	2000	4000
6/ 2/59								85	25	20	15	15	30
7/10/59								"	15	5	10	10	40
12/18/59								"	0	0	5	0	10

	DISCRIMINATION SCORE					
	RIGHT			LEFT		
% SCORE	TEST LEVEL	LEFT MASK	% SCORE	TEST LEVEL	RIGHT MASK	
			94	50	85	
			92	42	85	

Fig. 91. *History:* 30-year-old male. Fell and struck head 1 week previously. No unconsciousness or vertigo. Fullness and roaring in left ear.
Otologic: normal
Audiologic: temporary hearing loss with complete recruitment and no tone decay.

2,000 cps	
R	L
0	20
15	30
30	40
45	45

Classification: temporary sensory hearing loss
Diagnosis: direct trauma to head. It is difficult to predict if such a hearing loss will return to normal levels, as in this case, but it may do so if the damage is not severe.

involvement, unless the source of the noise is very close to the ear and is of a very intense low frequency. See Figures 88 to 90.

All three patients have been studied closely, and numerous audiograms have been recorded. Repeated hearing tests demonstrated that there was no evidence of progressive hearing loss in any of the youngsters. As might be expected, only the child with substantial bilateral hearing loss presented symptoms of clinical hearing impairment. It is not uncommon to find adults, as well as children, who are completely unaware of even profound unilateral hearing losses if the defects have been present since early childhood. The hearing defects in these three patients were found during the routine testing of 800 school children.

Direct Head Trauma

A direct blow to the head can produce hearing loss that may belong to almost any classification. To some extent the type as well as the degree of hearing impairment depends on the severity and the location of the head blow. In general, the harder the blow, and the more directly it hits the temporal bone, the more severe is the damage, and the more likely it is to involve the sensorineural mechanism. Hearing loss may be present with or without evidence of any fracture in the skull.

Longitudinal Temporal Bone Fracture. A moderate sensorineural type of hearing loss due to direct trauma can occur even without evidence of bone fracture. However, it usually accompanies a longitudinal temporal bone fracture. Interestingly enough, a sensory hearing impairment may be found in the ear on the side of the head opposite to the side that sustained the injury (contrecoup). The hearing loss has practically the same characteristics as that produced by exposure to intense noise. If the head injury is comparatively mild, only the hair cells of the basilar end of the cochlea are affected, and the effect on the hearing is like that shown in Figure 91. Note the complete recruitment, which localizes the principal site of the damage in the inner ear. If the injury is more severe, a greater area in the cochlea is affected, and even the nerve itself also may be damaged, with the classification then becoming sensorineural.

Transverse Fracture of the Temporal Bone. Another cause of sensorineural deafness is transverse fracture of the temporal bone. The fracture line on x-ray examination is perpendicular to the superior petrosal sinus and the long axis of the temporal bone. A severe blow to the back of the head can produce this type of fracture. The accompanying hearing loss generally is very severe, and often it is total. It is caused by fracture into the vestibule of the inner ear and destruction of the cochlea. Blood fills these areas and can be seen through an intact eardrum (in contrast with the torn eardrum caused by longitudinal fracture).

In many cases damage also to the facial nerve causes a complete facial paralysis, including the forehead on one side. Cerebrospinal fluid may fill the middle ear and drain out of the eustachian tube, especially if the eardrum is intact. Vertigo and nystagmus invariably are present after a transverse fracture of the temporal bone, and the hearing loss generally is permanent.

A purely neural type of hearing impairment can occur occasionally with transverse fracture of the temporal bone when the fracture includes the internal meatus and crushes the auditory nerve. Generally, facial paralysis also is present but may clear up. (See Fig. 92.)

Appraising Loss in Claims. The inner ear is so well protected that a blow to the head must be quite severe to produce hearing loss. When there is evidence of fracture, there is little question about the severity of the blow. However, when there is no visible fracture, and hearing loss is present, it may be difficult to determine in some cases that come to litigation whether the hearing loss was caused by the injury or was present previously. In such cases it is well to recall that if the patient did not exhibit any period of unconsciousness, the chances are that the blow was not severe enough to produce cochlear concussion with significant permanent hearing loss. Vertigo and tinnitus must be associated with such damage, and both are likely to persist for extended periods after the injury.

It also must be borne in mind that a portion of the conductive and the

				AIR CONDUCTION										
		RIGHT							LEFT					
DATE	LEFT MASK	250	500	1000	2000	4000	8000	RIGHT MASK	250	500	1000	2000	4000	8000
		0	0	−5	0	10	5	−	55	65	60	50	80	50
								85	NR	NR	NR	NR	NR	NR

				BONE CONDUCTION									
		RIGHT							LEFT				
DATE	LEFT MASK	250	500	1000	2000	4000	TYPE	RIGHT MASK	250	500	1000	2000	4000
		0	0	−5	0	5		−	5	10	0	5	15
								85	NR	NR	NR	NR	NR

SPEECH RECEPTION THRESHOLD					DISCRIMINATION SCORE					
					RIGHT			LEFT		
DATE	RIGHT	LEFT MASK	LEFT	RIGHT MASK	% SCORE	TEST LEVEL	LEFT MASK	% SCORE	TEST LEVEL	RIGHT MASK
			58	−				100	90	−
			NR	85				NR	100	85

Fig. 92. *History:* sudden onset of deafness in the left ear following a fractured skull with unconsciousness. Left facial paralysis. X-ray picture shows a fracture through the left internal auditory meatus.

Otologic: normal with absent caloric responses

Audiologic: Without masking the right ear there seems to be residual hearing in the left ear by air and bone as well as by speech. When masking is used, the absence of residual hearing in the left ear becomes apparent.

Classification: sensorineural deafness

Diagnosis: injury to the left auditory nerve

sensorineural hearing loss resulting from trauma may be reversible, and that it is necessary to wait at least several months before appraising the degree of permanent hearing loss.

A few cases have been reported in which patients did not become aware of their hearing difficulty until several weeks after the injury, and the impairment seemed to progress. This type of loss is unusual; although it is possible, there is no proof that the injury is the sole etiology.

AUDIOLOGIC FINDINGS. In the sensory type of hearing defect produced by trauma, audiologic findings reveal continuous and complete recruitment in the frequencies involved. If the speech frequencies also are involved, the discrimination score is reduced, and generally diplacusis is noted. If, in addition to the inner ear, the nerve endings become damaged, recruitment is not quite so prominent and may appear slightly above threshold.

There is no justification for assuming that merely because a patient sus-

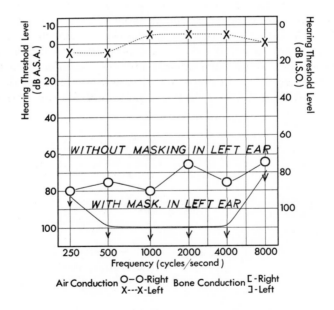

FIG. 93. *History:* 33-year-old male who claimed his right ear went deaf after he hit his head on a pole protruding from a building. There was no head wound or unconsciousness. He denied having vertigo or tinnitus.

Otologic: normal with normal caloric responses

Audiologic: no response in the right ear with the left ear masked

Classification: unilateral sensorineural deafness

Diagnosis: mumps deafness. Established by further detailed history.

Comment: So severe a unilateral deafness with normal labyrinthine responses is not produced by such a head injury.

tained a head injury, any hearing loss present was caused by the injury. If the deficit is conductive, either there must be evidence of a lesion of the eardrum, or the audiologic findings must indicate some ossicular chain damage. The latter can be confirmed very readily by elevating the eardrum and examining the ossicular chain. If the hearing defect is sensory or sensorineural, then the audiologic findings must fit the characteristic patterns that have been established for these types of hearing impairment.

Figure 93 shows a case in which an individual claimed a hearing loss as the result of a head injury. Because this was a total unilateral loss with normal hearing in the other side, every effort was made to try to explore this case very carefully. After much investigation it was found that the patient had had mumps many years ago, and that his hearing difficulty was due to mumps labyrinthitis rather than to the injury. On establishing a better understanding with the patient, he freely admitted the situation.

Schuknecht has crystallized the differential diagnosis of hearing loss due to head injuries (Table 1).

TABLE 1. DIFFERENTIAL CLINICAL FINDINGS IN HEARING LOSS*

	LABYRINTHINE CONCUSSION	LONGITUDINAL FRACTURE	TRANSVERSE FRACTURE
Bleeding from ear	Never	Very common	Rare
Injury to external auditory canal	Never	Occasional	Never
Rupture of drum	Never	Very common	Rare—commonly a hemotympanum
Presence of cerebrospinal fluid	Never	Occasional	Occasional
Hearing loss	All degrees—partial to complete recovery	All degrees—combined type, partial to complete recovery	Profound nerve type—no recovery
Vertigo	Occasional—mild and transient	Occasional—mild and transient	Severe—subsides; nystagmus to opposite side
Depressed vestibular function	Occasional—mild	Occasional—mild	No response
Facial nerve injury	Never	25%—usually temporary	60%—often permanent
X-ray signs	Negative	25%—in squamous and mastoid area	60%—in occiput in pyramid in vertex-mento films

* Schuknecht, H. F.: A clinical study of auditory damage following blows to the head, Ann. Otol. 59:331-359, 1950.

Drug Ototoxicity

Certain drugs can produce sensorineural hearing impairment when they are used over a long period of time. Among those drugs reported as ototoxic are dihydrostreptomycin, neomycin, quinine and kanamycin. It should be emphasized that the hearing damage occurs only after taking the drug systemically for a long period of time. There are exceptions to this in patients with renal disease. In such cases deafness can result after only a few doses of medication. Generally, however, the deafness is a gradual loss and can be followed audiometrically so that the drug can be stopped before it involves the speech frequency range. Ringing tinnitus is a frequent associated symptom and sometimes precedes the hearing loss.

The early impairment results from damage to the hair cells in the inner ear. A classic example and proof of this is described in Figure 94. Most of the time hearing loss due to drug ototoxicity is permanent, but it is not

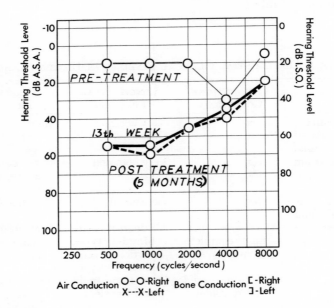

Fig. 94. *History:* Patient received daily injections of an ototoxic drug for 3 months. His hearing was followed weekly, and in the 13th week he developed a ringing tinnitus in the right ear, fullness and hearing loss. The drug was stopped immediately. No vertigo.

Otologic: normal

Audiologic: unilateral ascending hearing loss with recruitment and diplacusis.

Classification: sensory hearing loss

Diagnosis: cochlear deafness from ototoxic drug

AIR CONDUCTION														
RIGHT								LEFT						
DATE	LEFT MASK	250	500	1000	2000	4000	8000	RIGHT MASK	250	500	1000	2000	4000	8000
6/ /63		-10	-10	-10	-10	-5	-10							
6/ 7/63		-10	-10	-10	25	-5		Upper resp. infection.					Tinnitus	
6/11/63			-10	-10	20	-5							Tinnitus	
6/13/63			-10	-10	15	-5							Tinnitus	
6/14/63			-10	-10	-10	-5		Tinnitus subsided.						

FIG. 95. *History:* 2 days following the onset of an upper respiratory infection this 25-year-old male complained of a ringing tinnitus in his right ear.

Otologic: normal

Audiologic: all thresholds normal except for a dip at 2,000 cps in the right ear. Complete recruitment was present at 2,000 cps but not at 1,000 or 3,000 cps. The tinnitus matched the frequency of a 2,000-cps tone. No abnormal tone decay at 2,000 cps.

Classification: sensory impairment

Diagnosis: viral infection of the right inner ear

progressive. The hearing loss can occur without any vertigo, ringing tinnitus or other symptoms.

Virus Infections

Comparatively little proof is available to show that virus infections produce partial sensory or sensorineural hearing impairment. It is known that mumps and herpes zoster can produce severe sudden deafness by attacking the cochlea and the auditory nerve. However, the mechanism is not known with certainty, nor the reason for the loss being almost invariably in one ear. As far as partial sensory or sensorineural hearing loss is concerned, there is a strong feeling among clinicians that patients may sustain this type of damage after such typical viral infections as head colds, mouth ulcers and influenza (grippe). For this reason many clinicians in all sincerity tell patients that their hearing loss is probably due to some viral infection. There is no doubt that such a comment frequently is unwarranted, but it may very well be correct in some cases.

The author recently has seen a case which seems to provide reasonable clinical proof that viruses can cause certain types of sensory hearing deficiency. He was able to follow very closely an instance of sensory hearing loss associated with a viral upper respiratory infection in an audiologist. The case history is described in Figure 95. This is a most interesting example of a cause of hearing loss that is undoubtedly more common than generally is realized. The symptoms of ringing tinnitus, fullness in the ear

		AIR CONDUCTION												
	RIGHT							LEFT						
DATE	LEFT MASK	250	500	1000	2000	4000	8000	RIGHT MASK	250	500	1000	2000	4000	8000
		5	0	5	10	15	25	90	50	45	55	60	70	NR
Left stapes simply mobilized.														
One week post-op.								90	70	80	85	NR	NR	NR
One month post-op.								90	50	50	40	40	60	65

		BONE CONDUCTION											
	RIGHT							LEFT					
DATE	LEFT MASK	250	500	1000	2000	4000	TYPE	RIGHT MASK	250	500	1000	2000	4000
		0	-5	0	5	10		90	0	10	20	25	30
One week post-op.								90	35	40	50	NR	NR
One month post-op.								90	30	30	35	40	NR

	DISCRIMINATION SCORE					
	RIGHT			LEFT		
	% SCORE	TEST LEVEL	LEFT MASK	% SCORE	TEST LEVEL	RIGHT MASK
Pre-op.				82	90	90
1wk.post-op.				10	100	90
1mth.post-op.				42	85	90

Fig. 96. *History:* 26-year-old female with a diagnosis of otosclerosis. Operative notes indicate that the left stapes was mobilized merely by pressure on the end of the incus. No footplate manipulation was performed. Several days postoperatively the patient developed vertigo, roaring tinnitus, fullness and deafness in the left ear. Loud noises bothered her left ear.

Otologic: healed incision

Audiologic: Preoperative left ear thresholds revealed a moderate to severe air conduction loss. Bone thresholds were normal in the low frequencies and dropped off somewhat between 1,000 and 4,000 cps. The discrimination score was 82%. Postoperative thresholds revealed a great reduction in air and bone thresholds as well as reduced discrimination. For many months postoperatively there were hyperrecruitment, diplacusis, and lowered thresholds of discomfort. Some of these symptoms have gradually subsided.

1,000 cps	
R	L
5	35
20	65
35	70
50	75
65	80
80	80

Classification: conductive followed by sensorineural impairment

Diagnosis: postoperative labyrinthosis following stapes mobilization and the measurable hearing loss associated with recruitment and diplacusis seem to be related definitely to the typical upper respiratory viral infection that occurred in this patient. It appears that viruses can affect the inner ear and produce temporary partial hearing loss. The associated ringing tinnitus was found to match the frequency of the hearing loss and confirmed a common clinical impression that tinnitus can be produced by viral infections. The toxic mechanism of these phenomena undoubtedly will be investigated much more extensively in the future. There seems to be justification, however, for considering a viral infection as the possible etiologic factor in certain cases of partial sensory hearing impairment.

There also is evidence that viral infections during the first trimester of pregnancy can affect seriously the sensorineural mechanism of the fetus and result in congenital deafness.

			AIR	CONDUCTION									
			RIGHT						**LEFT**				
DATE	LEFT MASK	250	500	1000	2000	4000	8000	RIGHT MASK	250	500	1000	2000	4000	8000
Pre-op.	95	45	55	60	60	65	NR	-	10	20	35	45	55	NR
	95	75	85	NR	NR	NR	NR	Right stapedectomy						
	95	50	55	55	85	NR	NR							

			BONE	CONDUCTION								
			RIGHT						**LEFT**			
DATE	LEFT MASK	250	500	1000	2000	4000	TYPE	RIGHT MASK	250	500	1000	2000	4000
Pre-op.	100	0	15	25	NR	NR	←	-	10	10	25	45	55
	115	30	40	50	NR	NR	Right stapedectomy						
	100	NR	40	50	NR	NR							

SPEECH RECEPTION THRESHOLD				DISCRIMINATION SCORE						TUNING FORK TESTS (500 CPS.)		
				RIGHT			**LEFT**					
DATE	RIGHT	LEFT MASK	LEFT	RIGHT MASK	% SCORE	TEST LEVEL	LEFT MASK	% SCORE	TEST LEVEL	RIGHT MASK		R	L
Pre-op.	66	85	32	-	70	96	85	70	62	-	AIR-BONE COMPARISON		
	70	85			40	96	85	80	62	-	LATERALIZATION		
					20	104	85				B. C. COMPARISON TO NORMAL		

FIG. 97. *History:* 45-year-old female who several days postoperatively developed deafness, vertigo and nausea. There was a roaring tinnitus in the right ear.

Otologic: normal

Audiologic: Preoperative low frequency air-bone gap in the right ear with fair discrimination. Thresholds immediately postoperatively revealed a severe reduction in air and bone conduction thresholds. Three months later thresholds improved, but there were complete recruitment, diplacusis, distortion and reduced discrimination. There was a lowered threshold of discomfort (loud noises were very annoying).

Classification: sensory hearing loss

Diagnosis: postoperative labyrinthosis

SENSORY HEARING LOSS AFTER EAR SURGERY

The increase in stapedectomies for otosclerosis has focused attention on the sensorineural damage and hearing loss that may be associated with opening the vestibule of the labyrinth.

Mastoidectomy. Prior to the advent of the stapedectomy the oval window area and the vestibule of the inner ear were considered to be inviolable, and extreme caution was exercised to avoid disturbing the footplate during mastoid surgery. In spite of this caution surgical accidents did occur, and hearing often was lost totally in the operated ear during mastoidectomy procedures in which the oval window inadvertently was penetrated. Sometimes the deafness occurred long after surgery due to ear infection and cholesteatoma. Partial deafness from toxic labyrinthitis still is observed in chronic mastoiditis even when no surgery has been performed.

In simple stapes mobilization surgery sensorineural hearing loss is a rare complication, but such instances did and do occur (Fig. 96). The cause still is not established, but the symptoms associated with the deafness are highly suggestive of a viral labyrinthitis. Such complications are more common after stapedectomy, and they have occurred also after fenestration surgery.

Stapedectomy. With more frequent surgical entry into the vestibule during stapedectomy the incidence of sensory and sensorineural deafness has increased markedly as a complication. It has been estimated that after stapedectomy about 1 or 2 per cent of patients will experience either immediate or delayed severe sensorineural hearing loss in the operated ear. Some very cautious observers feel that practically every case in which the footplate is removed or fractured sustains some degree of temporary sensorineural damage. In most cases in which the surgeon is meticulous and avoids getting blood into the vestibule or sucking out perilymph, there is minimal sensorineural damage and few clinical symptoms. Yet even in some of these cases patients are known to complain of mild fullness in the ear and very slight imbalance along with a minimal ringing tinnitus.

Occasionally, after stapedectomy there is some measurable damage to the inner ear. Generally, the effect is temporary, but sometimes there is permanent high tone hearing loss associated with recruitment, impaired discrimination, and lowered threshold of discomfort for intense noise. Figure 97 shows these findings.

Another disturbing complication of stapedectomy is seen in patients who had had excellent results and then suddenly, many months after the original surgery, lost practically all their hearing in the operated ear. In most cases this loss is permanent. The causes for this and other sensorineural complications of stapedectomy surgery are not as yet entirely understood. Occasionally, there is a fibrous invasion filling the entire vestibule and completely blocking off the cochlea. In other cases of this type of delayed permanent severe deafness, the vestibule is found to have a normal appearance, and the perilymph also is normal. The cause for the cochlear damage in such cases still is unknown.

DISCRIMINATION. It is apparent, however, that one should not measure the success of stapes surgery solely by threshold hearing tests. Some patients have excellent pure tone thresholds, but their discrimination is reduced by the surgery, and their distortion can be distracting. With improving technics and better training for stapes surgery the incidence and the severity of sensorineural complications can be reduced steadily.

The dangers of surgery in **cases of tympanosclerosis** also are better recognized. When such cases are operated on to restore hearing, and the stapes footplate is removed in the presence of tympanosclerotic changes in the middle ear, the incidence of severe sensorineural deafness is very high. Many surgeons have resolved to complete this procedure in two stages or even to avoid doing it altogether because of the frequent complications that occur when the oval window is opened in the presence of this disease.

EARLY PRESBYCUSIS

For want of a better explanation, a high tone hearing loss occasionally encountered is called early or premature presbycusis if it occurs between the ages of about 30 to 50. Clinically, this condition is easy to overlook, but the audiogram shows a progressive hearing impairment in the high tones which may be associated with a high-pitched tinnitus and no other symptoms. The pathologic explanation generally subscribed to today is that the hair cells degenerate because of some hereditary tendency, and that the syndrome is not related to metabolism or infection. Little is known about this condition, but the picture occasionally is seen. In general, the loss is slowly progressive and eventually causes difficulty in discrimination as the speech frequencies are involved.

When the high frequency losses are accompanied by recurrent attacks of rotary vertigo, especially when there is tinnitus of some sort, the likely diagnosis is atypical Ménière's disease. Actually, it is not certain that this atypical picture truly is related to Ménière's disease. In some cases, especially if the hearing loss is bilateral, it may be due to so-called early presbycusis, whereas the accompanying vertigo is caused by labyrinthitis or some other labyrinthine disorder.

This type of case should be distinguished from hereditary progressive nerve deafness, which generally starts early, progresses faster, and does not exhibit marked recruitment.

CONGENITAL DEFECTS IN THE COCHLEA

Deafness present at birth can be caused in two ways: (1) malformation of the organ of Corti and (2) toxic effects on the inner ear in utero. More and more evidence is found that toxic degeneration is far more common than congenital malformation. Even some cases previously described as hereditary congenital nerve deafness now are being recognized as having been caused actually by toxic effects in the first trimester of pregnancy. German measles in the mother is one such cause, and probably Rh incompatibility may be another.

Usually, the organ of Corti is affected, and the result commonly is subtotal deafness or a moderately severe hearing loss that is greater in the higher than in the lower frequencies. In both instances the congenital defect is associated with a speech problem. If the hearing loss is severe, speech may not develop without much special training. When the hearing loss is partial, speech may be defective (see Chap. 27).

Although complete proof is not available, many otologists are convinced that viral infections during the first trimester of pregnancy do cause cochlear damage and deafness in the fetus. Anoxia shortly after birth also can cause damage to the cochlea, with resultant high tone hearing loss.

NEURAL HEARING IMPAIRMENT—ITS CAUSES

ACOUSTIC NEUROMA

The most urgent reason for distinguishing damage to the auditory nerve fibers from damage to the hair cells or the inner ear is that this distinction permits the physician to detect a tumor on the auditory nerve at the earliest possible moment. As the result of advances in hearing tests, it is now possible to diagnose most auditory nerve tumors long before other neurologic symptoms or signs become apparent. Figure 98 gives an example of such a case and emphasizes the need to perform discrimination, recruitment and tone decay studies in all cases of sensorineural deafness, especially if they are unilateral. A patient who comes in to have wax removed from an ear to correct a hearing loss sometimes actually has a neoplasm of the auditory nerve.

Early Symptoms. The earliest symptom of many acoustic neuromas is a mild unilateral neural hearing impairment. Tinnitus is common, and vertigo may or may not be present. Vertigo occurs early if the neoplasm involves or presses on the vestibular portion of the 8th nerve. The vertigo is more of a constant imbalance in contrast with Ménière's disease, in which vertigo imbalance usually is intermittent and accompanied by a seashell-like tinnitus.

The important diagnostic criteria of acoustic neuroma are: (1) progressive unilateral neural hearing impairment, (2) abnormal tone decay, (3) absence of marked recruitment, (4) reduced discrimination more marked than that to be expected from an estimate of the pure tone hearing threshold, (5) abnormal results from caloric studies such as absent responses on the involved side and perverted responses on the other ear, (6) persistent or spontaneous nystagmus, and (7) corneal anesthesia on the involved side and anesthesia of the upper posterior external auditory canal skin.

Other Diagnostic Criteria. When other neurologic symptoms such as facial paralysis become apparent, the neoplasm already has extended beyond the 8th nerve.

Although an auditory nerve tumor usually occurs on one side, its presence must not be ruled out merely because a patient has bilateral sensori-

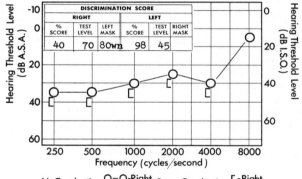

Air Conduction O—O-Right Bone Conduction ⌐-Right
X---X-Left ⌐-Left

Fig. 98. *History:* 36-year-old male complained of having wax in his right ear, causing stuffiness for several weeks. No tinnitus or vertigo.

Otologic: normal ear canals and eardrums and no excess wax. No spontaneous nystagmus.

Audiologic: mild ascending hearing loss in the right ear with reduced bone conduction. Tuning fork lateralized to the good ear, and air was better than bone conduction on the bad ear. No diplacusis and no recruitment were present. Discrimination was remarkably poor in the right ear, especially in view of the mild hearing loss. Abnormal tone decay was present with the threshold going to 75 db at 1,000 cps after 1 minute.

Classification: neural hearing loss

Diagnosis: acoustic neuroma

Aids to classification: The presence of unilateral nerve deafness with absent recruitment but abnormal tone decay and reduced discrimination indicates some pressure on the auditory nerve. In addition, there were corneal anesthesia, absent caloric responses in the right ear and perverted responses in the left ear. An acoustic neuroma was removed at surgery.

		AIR CONDUCTION												
		RIGHT							LEFT					
DATE	LEFT MASK	250	500	1000	2000	4000	8000	RIGHT MASK	250	500	1000	2000	4000	8000
1/55		0	-5	0	0	-5	-5	85	25	30	35	40	40	45
3/55								"	25	45	55	60	60	55
6/55								"	65	60	65	65	NR	NR
10/55								"	75	NR	NR	NR	NR	NR

		BONE CONDUCTION											
		RIGHT							LEFT				
DATE	LEFT MASK	250	500	1000	2000	4000	TYPE	RIGHT MASK	250	500	1000	2000	4000
1/55								85	20	30	35	40	NR
6/55								85	NR	NR	NR	NR	NR

SPEECH RECEPTION THRESHOLD					DISCRIMINATION SCORE						TUNING FORK TESTS (500 CPS.)		
					RIGHT			LEFT					
DATE	RIGHT	LEFT MASK	LEFT	RIGHT MASK	% SCORE	TEST LEVEL	LEFT MASK	% SCORE	TEST LEVEL	RIGHT MASK		R	L
1/55								55	75	85	AIR-BONE COMPARISON		
6/55								22	100	85	LATERALIZATION		
											B. C. COMPARISON TO NORMAL		

FIG. 99. *History:* 24-year-old male complaining of deafness, occasional buzzing and slight vertigo.

Otologic: normal. No spontaneous nystagmus

Audiologic: unilateral hearing loss with reduced bone conduction. Tuning fork tests showed lateralization to the right; A > B on left. No recruitment. Marked tone decay and poor discrimination.

1,000 cps

L	R
35	5
45	15
50	25
65	35

Classification: neural deafness

Diagnosis: acoustic neuroma

Aids to diagnosis: corneal anesthesia on left, absent caloric responses on left and perverted responses on right side. The patient refused surgery initially because of the mildness of the symptoms. Later his deafness increased, and he developed much vertigo. A large neuroma was removed, leaving a left facial paralysis.

neural deafness. In multiple neurofibromatosis tumors can occur on both auditory nerves and may affect only the cochlear or only the vestibular portions. An instance of an auditory nerve tumor causing a comparatively mild hearing loss and a very marked reduction in discrimination threshold, using phonetically balanced word lists, is cited in Figure 98. The patient in such instances may volunteer that he simply cannot understand anything in that ear even though he hears voices. This complaint should always be followed through, and if recruitment is absent, and tone decay is pathologic, caloric studies should be done to confirm or to rule out the presence of a neoplasm.

It is essential to bear in mind that the mere presence of abnormal tone decay does not mean necessarily that the patient has a tumor of the auditory nerve. It indicates merely that nerve fibers have been damaged. Other causes also can produce damage to auditory nerve fibers.

Testing for corneal anesthesia is easy to do and often supplies important information. Merely brushing a wisp of absorbent cotton over both corneas and comparing the reflex closing of the eyelids can show a marked difference when one side is anesthetic. The same technic applies to testing sensitivity in the external canal.

The simple tuning fork test for recruitment always should be done, especially when facilities for more accurate quantitative measurement are

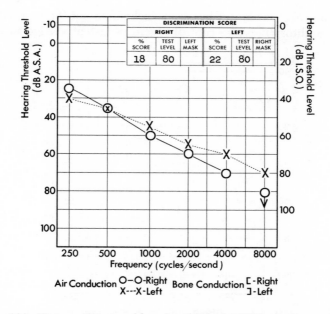

Fig. 100. *History:* 52-year-old male who had Ménière's disease in both ears and had undergone a bilateral vestibular nerve section. According to the patient, discrimination was sharply reduced postoperatively.

Otologic: normal

Audiologic: bilateral mild to moderate hearing loss with no air-bone gap. Very poor discrimination ability which worsened in the presence of environmental noise.

Classification: neural hearing loss

Diagnosis: surgical lesion of auditory nerves resulting from section of vestibular nerves.

not available. The audiometric pattern in acoustic nerve tumors varies. Figure 99 shows the progress of a patient with an acoustic neuroma.

Fractured Skull and Auditory Nerve Injury

A transverse fracture of the temporal bone can go through the internal auditory meatus and compress or sever the auditory nerve. Occasionally, the 7th nerve also is damaged with the result of facial paralysis. Since the deafness usually is total, findings such as abnormal tone decay and disproportionately poor discrimination cannot be detected, but x-ray pictures and absent caloric responses on the involved side with normal responses on the other side help to establish the diagnosis.

Section of the Auditory Nerve

Some neurosurgeons in the past were inclined to cut the vestibular portion of the auditory nerve to control severe persistent vertigo in patients

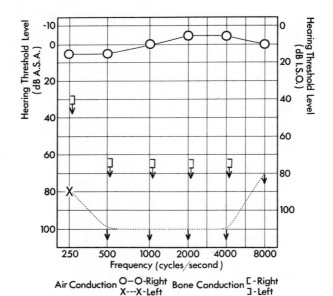

Fig. 101. *History:* 58-year-old male who developed severe herpes with pain in left ear. He had a left facial palsy for several weeks, and this resolved. He also had a buzzing tinnitus that cleared up. No vertigo.

Otologic: normal at time of examination. Caloric tests normal
Audiologic: total deafness left ear
Classification: neural deafness
Diagnosis: herpetic auditory neuritis

with Ménière's disease. During the operation it was difficult for the surgeon to avoid severing at least some portion of the adjacent hearing fibers. Although the vertigo was controlled in most instances, many of the patients were left with additional hearing loss due to section of the auditory nerve fibers. Almost invariably, the high tones were chiefly affected by the surgery. Figure 100 describes a case in which both vestibular nerves were sectioned by a neurosurgeon. In this case the low frequencies likewise were affected, but part or all of this may have been attributable to the preexisting Ménière's disease. Some of the high frequency loss was present preoperatively, but this was greatly aggravated by the surgery. In addition to the change in threshold, this patient's ability to understand speech was reduced seriously after the nerve section. A hearing aid was practically useless for this individual.

VIRUS INFECTION

Certain viral infections, notably herpes, are supposed to cause deafness by affecting the auditory nerve proper. In this instance the site of injury is supposed to be in the ganglion. The hearing loss produced often is quite severe. Figure 101 shows an interesting case.

CONGENITAL NERVE DEAFNESS

It is common practice to call all cases of deafness present at birth "congenital nerve deafness" or "hereditary nerve deafness," especially if it is present in other members of the family. It is not certain that the congenital defect always is in the nerve itself, but in many cases it does appear to be in this site, especially if the deafness is severe. Since some cases of congenital deafness have their sites of damage in the cochlea, a more nearly accurate term would be cochlear deafness, but the distinction is at present only of academic interest. When therapeutic measures become available that offer more hope for either sensory or neural deafness, the distinction, of course, may become more important.

Chapter 15

Mixed, Central and Functional Hearing Impairments

MIXED HEARING IMPAIRMENT

Whenever the hearing loss of a patient includes a mixture of both conductive and sensorineural characteristics, he is said to have a mixed hearing impairment. The hearing deficiency may have started originally as a conductive failure, such as otosclerosis, and later developed a superimposed sensorineural component; or the difficulty may have been sensorineural in the beginning, such as presbycusis, and a conductive defect, perhaps resulting from middle ear infection, may have developed subsequently. In some cases the conductive and the sensorineural elements may have started simultaneously as, for example, in a severe head injury affecting both the inner ear and the middle ear.

In clinical practice most cases with an original sensorineural etiology remain in that classification without an added conductive element. In contrast, most cases that start as conductive hearing impairment later develop some sensorineural complication. Familiar examples are otosclerosis with presbycusis and chronic otitis media with labyrinthitis.

Sensorineural Involvement

Otosclerosis was at one time thought to retain its purely conductive character for years; today it is recognized that this condition develops sensorineural complications, if judgment is based on criteria that at present are considered to be valid. Of a series of 75 patients on whom we operated for unilateral otosclerosis, over 70 per cent showed evidence of reduced bone conduction, high tone hearing loss, and occasionally even recruitment—all of them suggestive of sensorineural deafness. However,

200

AIR CONDUCTION													
	RIGHT							LEFT					
DATE	LEFT MASK	250	500	1000	2000	4000	8000	RIGHT MASK	250	500	1000	2000	4000	8000
		70	80	70	75	90	NR	Pre-op.					
		30	35	45	45	65	70	Post-op.					

BONE CONDUCTION												
	RIGHT							LEFT				
DATE	LEFT MASK	250	500	1000	2000	4000	TYPE	RIGHT MASK	250	500	1000	2000	4000
		NR	50	50	60	NR		Pre-op.				
		30	30	35	40	NR		Post-op.				

Fig. 102. *History:* 67-year-old male with insidious deafness for 25 years. No tinnitus or vertigo. Wears a hearing aid on the right ear.

Otologic: normal. Complete stapes fixation confirmed at surgery.

Audiologic: bilateral reduced air and bone conduction thresholds with some air-bone gap in the right ear. The left ear was not as severely involved as the right but did not exhibit any air-bone gap. Tuning fork tests showed bone conduction better than air in the right, with lateralization to the right ear. The tuning fork sounded louder on the teeth than on the mastoid.

Classification: mixed hearing loss

Diagnosis: otosclerosis with secondary sensorineural involvement

Aids to diagnosis: The presence of an air-bone gap, good tuning fork responses, especially by teeth, and satisfactory hearing aid usage in conjunction with negative otoscopic findings are important in making the diagnosis. In this case the air-bone gap was closed. The apparent improvement in postoperative bone conduction is seen commonly, but it does not mean that the sensorineural deafness has been improved.

one should avoid hasty conclusions, for perhaps some mechanical impairment in the ossicular chain may account partly for these findings. Figures 51 and 102 show examples of sensorineural features in otosclerosis.

Similar evidence of sensorineural involvement often is seen in chronic otitis media. According to one hypothesis, some toxic inflammatory metabolite produces a cochleitis or labyrinthitis (Fig. 103).

Mixed hearing loss is becoming more common also in otosclerosis after stapedectomy. The sensorineural deficit may be caused by penetration of the oval window with exposure of the perilymph. Despite meticulous surgical care, the inner ear can be traumatized readily and made more susceptible to infection by this procedure. In surgical trauma to the inner ear, high tone hearing loss often falls below the preoperative level, and the patient may complain of reduced discrimination though his pure tone threshold is improved. Other symptoms suggestive of sensory damage, such as recruitment, distortion and a lower threshold of discomfort, may be noted.

Figure 104 shows an important aspect of mixed deafness. The patient attributed his hearing loss to wax in his ears, but when the wax was removed, we noted an underlying sensorineural deafness of which the patient had not been aware. This example serves as a warning to physicians to avoid assuring any patient that his hearing loss can be corrected merely by removing cerumen, since mixed deafness subsequently may be found.

EVALUATING CONDUCTIVE AND SENSORINEURAL COMPONENTS

On the other hand, pure conductive hearing loss may on occasion be

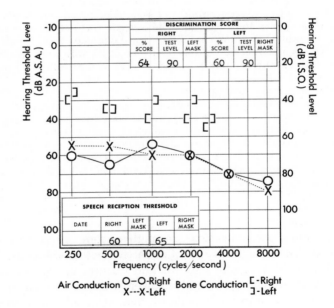

FIG. 103. *History:* 60-year-old male with bilateral chronic otorrhea for 40 years. Insidious hearing loss for many years, which is now stationary. No tinnitus or vertigo.

Otologic: putrid discharge with evidence of cholesteatoma

Audiologic: moderate to severe bilateral flat loss. Bone conduction is reduced at all frequencies but a 20- to 30-db air-bone gap remains. Discrimination is reduced bilaterally.

Classification: mixed hearing loss

Diagnosis: chronic otitis media and neuritis or cochleitis

		AIR CONDUCTION												
		RIGHT							LEFT					
DATE	LEFT MASK	250	500	1000	2000	4000	8000	RIGHT MASK	250	500	1000	2000	4000	8000
		Impacted Cerumen							Impacted Cerumen					
		25	30	35	45	50	50		25	30	35	45	55	55
		Cerumen Removed							Cerumen Removed					
		5	10	15	30	50	50		5	10	15	30	50	55

		BONE CONDUCTION										
		RIGHT							LEFT			
DATE	LEFT MASK	250	500	1000	2000	4000	TYPE	RIGHT MASK	250	500	1000	2000	4000
		5	5	10	25	30			5	10	15	30	50

FIG. 104. *History:* 45-year-old male with fullness in both ears and hearing loss for 1 week. No tinnitus or vertigo. No history of ear infections. Wants the wax removed to restore his hearing.

Otologic: bilateral impacted cerumen. Removed, and eardrums normal.

Audiologic: bilateral reduced air conduction thresholds with greater loss in high frequencies. No bone thresholds obtained before removal of cerumen, but tuning fork tests showed bone better than air, bilaterally. After cerumen was removed, air conduction thresholds improved, but a high frequency loss remained. Bone conduction thresholds approximated the air conduction thresholds. Tuning fork tests showed air better than bone after removal of wax.

Classification: mixed hearing loss before removal of cerumen. Sensorineural loss after removal of cerumen.

Diagnosis: impacted cerumen with progressive nerve deafness

Aids to diagnosis: It is always advisable to do audiometric studies before and after removing impacted cerumen and before reaching a diagnosis.

misdiagnosed as mixed deafness because the high tones and the bone conduction are somewhat reduced. (See Fig. 24.) In the case cited, hearing returned to normal when the fluid was removed from the middle ear; actually, there was no sensorineural damage. Whenever there is any possibility of fluid in the middle ear, a diagnostic myringotomy is indicated to avoid an erroneous diagnosis of sensorineural deafness. A high tone hearing loss with reduced bone conduction may create a mistaken impression of sensorineural damage.

The bone conduction test as now performed is not a completely reliable measure of sensorineural efficiency. Excessive reliance on this test may mislead the physician. Figure 105 illustrates a case in which the bone conduction was almost undetectable with a vibrating tuning fork on the patient's mastoid bone or forehead. Yet when the instrument was placed directly on the patient's teeth, a good bone conduction response was obtained. This was a case of mixed deafness followed by a satisfactory surgical result.

		AIR CONDUCTION												
		RIGHT							LEFT					
DATE	LEFT MASK	250	500	1000	2000	4000	8000	RIGHT MASK	250	500	1000	2000	4000	8000
3/60		80	95	NR	NR	NR	NR		75	75	85	95	95	NR
5/60		40	45	65	70	75	NR							
4/61									45	55	65	65	75	NR

		BONE CONDUCTION											
		RIGHT							LEFT				
DATE	LEFT MASK	250	500	1000	2000	4000	TYPE	RIGHT MASK	250	500	1000	2000	4000
3/60		40	50	50	NR	NR			45	45	50	NR	NR

	DISCRIMINATION SCORE					
	RIGHT			LEFT		
	% SCORE	TEST LEVEL	LEFT MASK	% SCORE	TEST LEVEL	RIGHT MASK
4/61	62	95		60	95	

Fig. 105. *History:* 62-year-old female with severe deafness. Using a powerful aid for many years. Voice is normal. No tinnitus or vertigo. Several aunts also use hearing aids.

Otologic: normal

Audiologic: Bone conduction is better than air, but patient denied hearing the tuning fork on the mastoid or the forehead but heard it fairly well on the teeth.

Classification: mixed hearing loss

Diagnosis: otosclerosis with sensorineural deafness

Comment: Both oval windows were overgrown with otosclerosis which required drilling. Note the good hearing improvement in spite of poor response to tuning fork. Surgery was done only because she did well with a hearing aid and had a good air-bone gap. A 1-year interval was allowed between operations on the two ears.

In every case of mixed hearing loss one should determine how much of the deficit is conductive and how much is sensorineural. The prognosis depends largely on this estimate. For instance, a patient's chronic otitis media may be resolved and leave a 55-db hearing loss. The tentative conclusion that a tympanoplasty is likely to restore the patient's hearing must be revised when bone conduction and discrimination studies show a severe sensorineural involvement, so that the chances of restoring hearing are poor. On the other hand, in some cases of otosclerosis with bone and air conduction levels almost below the measurable limits of the audiometer, the prognosis for restoring hearing to the bone conduction hearing level by stapes surgery may be surprisingly good.

The best way to approximate the conductive and the sensorineural components of a hearing loss is to perform all possible tests for estimating the patient's sensorineural potential or "cochlear reserve." In addition to routine bone conduction, speech discrimination scores are essential. A good rule to follow is this: If the patient hears and discriminates well when speech is made louder, then the conductive element probably is a major cause of the hearing difficulty, and surgery has a good chance of improving the hearing. If, on the other hand, the patient understands no better with a hearing aid or when the voice is raised, then the outlook for improved hearing is not favorable even if the conductive portion of the mixed hearing loss is corrected. (Compare Fig. 105.) Note that in this case the patient heard reasonably well with a hearing aid in the right ear, though there seemed to be no useful residual hearing. Successful stapes surgery confirmed the preoperative evaluation. Because of the severe hearing loss in the right ear, it was not possible under office conditions to amplify speech sufficiently to test the patient's discrimination. However, the results with a hearing aid indicated fairly good discrimination. In another patient with mixed hearing impairment and almost as much neural involvement the discrimination was not good. Consequently, after a successful stapes mobilization the hearing level was improved, but the discrimination was not helped, and so the patient was not nearly so pleased with the results.

Mixed hearing loss usually includes the following **range of conditions:** (1) visible pathology in the external ear canal or in the middle ear, associated with reduced bone conduction and other findings of sensorineural deafness; (2) normal otologic observations, somewhat reduced bone conduction, but a significant air-bone gap; (3) reduced speech discrimination, though usually of a mild degree, with improved discrimination as the intensity of speech is raised; and (4) unilateral hearing loss with the conductive element predominating, and the tuning fork lateralizing to the more severely impaired ear. In such cases there is always an air-bone gap.

The prognosis of mixed hearing impairment depends on the relative proportion of conductive and sensorineural pathology. If the sensorineural component is slight, the surgical prognosis is good, and under favorable circumstances the hearing may approximate the level of the bone conduction. However, the discrimination is not improved much, even after correcting the conductive defect.

CENTRAL DEAFNESS

For the purposes of this book a hearing impairment is classified as "central" if it is caused by a lesion that affects primarily the central nervous system between the auditory nuclei and the cortex. The process of verbal communication is complex. The entire auditory pathway consists of a series of transducers that repeatedly change the speech stimulus so that it can be handled effectively by the cortex. The eardrum and the ossicular chain modify the amplitude of the sound waves, and the cochlea analyzes these waves into fundamentals that then are reflected as impulses to the cortex. The chief function of the auditory cortex is to interpret and to integrate these impulses, and to provide the listener with the exact meaningful information intended by the speaker, or to permit the listener to react appropriately to the actual implication of the sound.

REACTION TO TESTS IN DIAGNOSIS

It would appear, then, that interference with the neural impulse pattern traveling up the central pathways to the cortex would manifest itself not so much by a lowering of the hearing threshold for pure tones as by reduced ability to interpret information. On the strength of this reasoning otological authorities have suggested various technics to diagnose central deafness. Since damage to the central auditory pathway causes little or no change in the pure tone threshold, the tests are designed to measure a more complex function. For example, one test involves filtering out the higher frequencies of certain speech samples, and then comparing the ability of normal-hearing persons to understand such speech sequences with that of patients with central deafness. It has been found that when this test is given to patients with unilateral central deafness (due to a brain tumor, for example), the *opposite* ear, which presumably hears normally, has much poorer discrimination than the ear of a normal-hearing person. This means that in unilateral central deafness the contralateral ear seems to be affected. A similar adverse effect is noted in the ear opposite to the tumor when certain words periodically are interrupted or accelerated. Interestingly enough, the patient with central deafness has no difficulty in perceiving high frequency sounds such as the letters *s* and *f* that are affected so characteristically in peripheral sensorineural lesions, but he has difficulty in interpreting what he hears.

PRINCIPAL CHARACTERISTICS

The following are the principal characteristics of central hearing impairment: (1) hearing tests do not indicate peripheral hearing impairment, (2) the pure tone threshold is relatively good compared with the ability of the patient to discriminate, and especially to interpret, what he hears, (3) the patient has difficulty in interpreting complex information, (4) there is usually an accompanying shortened attention span and other

		AIR CONDUCTION												
		RIGHT							LEFT					
DATE	LEFT MASK	250	500	1000	2000	4000	8000	RIGHT MASK	250	500	1000	2000	4000	8000
5/60		55	55	50	35	25	25		45	45	40	30	20	20
9/62		60	45	50	20	20			20	25	0	15	15	
3/63		50	40	45	15	20			35	30	10	10	15	
3/65		35	25	45	15	15	15		15	15	0	10	10	15

		BONE CONDUCTION											
		RIGHT							LEFT				
DATE	LEFT MASK	250	500	1000	2000	4000	TYPE	RIGHT MASK	250	500	1000	2000	4000
5/60		NR	50	40	30	20			NR	45	20	20	15
9/62		NR	45	55	25	20			25	40	15	30	30

	DISCRIMINATION SCORE					
	RIGHT			LEFT		
	% SCORE	TEST LEVEL	LEFT MASK	% SCORE	TEST LEVEL	RIGHT MASK
5/60	18	95	80	56	80	-
3/63	56	65		60	40	-

Fig. 106. *History:* In 1960 this patient was 8 and had to be helped to walk because of muscular incoordination and vestibular imbalance resulting from varicella encephalitis at age 18 months. Her eyesight and walking were affected, and deafness started 3 days after the encephalitis was diagnosed. The hearing gradually improved, and her speech is very good with only a slight voice defect. In 1960 she had another encephalitis attack, and hearing was depressed but gradually improved.

Otologic: normal, and caloric test was normal.

Audiologic: The very poor discrimination score in the right ear in 1960 was confirmed on several subsequent studies. The improvement in discrimination scores is not uncommon in such cases. There was no tone decay, and recruitment was not significant.

Classification: central deafness

Diagnosis: encephalitis

neurologic findings, and (5) apart from unusual cases with unilateral vascular lesions or neoplasms, deafness of this type resembles a bilateral perceptive disorder without any evidence of recruitment.

Some authors include sensory aphasia in the classification of central deafness, but most otologists consider this condition to be beyond the scope of their specialty.

The prognosis for central hearing impairment is poor, but re-education seems to offer a useful approach. There is no characteristic audiometric pattern except that the disparity between the hearing level and the speech interpretation is quite marked.

Present knowledge of central deafness is obviously rather meager. There can be extensive brain damage without apparent hearing abnormality. When symptoms do occur, they usually are associated with some general disease such as encephalitis (Fig. 106), vascular accident or neoplasm. Other causes include brain tumors and infections.

FUNCTIONAL HEARING IMPAIRMENT

Functional or psychogenic hearing impairment is the customary diagnosis when there is no organic basis for the patient's apparent deafness. His inability to hear results entirely or mainly from psychological or emotional factors, and his peripheral hearing mechanism may be essentially normal. If there is some slight damage to the peripheral end-organ, the observed hearing loss is disproportionate to the organic lesion.

Cause and Characteristic Features

The basis for functional deafness in most patients is neurotic anxiety, the product of emotional conflict. Anxiety is to the emotions what pain is in the physical realm. *Normal* anxiety is the natural reaction to an actual threat to one's welfare; it is recognized as such and recedes when the cause is removed or with the passage of time. In contrast, *neurotic* anxiety is an excessive reaction and may exist even in the absence of an external threat. Seldom is the true cause recognized consciously by the patient, and the anxiety persists beyond any recognizable need.

When anxiety is converted in part to a somatic symptom such as deafness, there are always other evidences of emotional disturbance, such as insomnia. Tinnitus is a characteristic feature of "hysterical deafness," and patients often claim that the noise is unbearable. Hearing acuity usually varies, depending on the patient's emotional state at the time of testing. Patients may appear to be overly concerned about their auditory symptoms when in reality some or all of the tinnitus and the deafness is caused by anxiety, the origin of which lies elsewhere.

When all or nearly all of the anxiety is transferred to the ear, the case is one of true conversion or hysteria. The patient then usually is indifferent to his symptoms despite their apparent severity, and he may delay seeking medical advice until persuaded to do so by his associates. He underreacts emotionally and appears to be calm and indifferent. The reason is that he has partially solved an emotional conflict by permitting it to assume a somatic form. This illusion generally is incomplete, and careful scrutiny will show residual emotional symptoms.

Psychogenic deafness often has a sudden onset and follows some emotional disturbance. Because of his anxiety the patient adapts his life to his symptoms, rather than adjusting to life. Indeed, he tends to make a "way of life" out of his symptoms. He becomes so obsessed with them and mentions them so often that everyone who knows him thinks of him as "the deaf man."

A Product of Both Military and Civilian Life. Functional hearing loss, then, is an unconscious device by which the patient seeks to escape from an intolerable problem that he cannot face consciously. Hysterical blindness or paralysis are other examples of the same type of somatization or "conversion reaction." More often seen in military life during wartime, such situations occur also in civilian life. For example, the patient may come with his wife to consult the physician. The physician asks the patient about his problem, but before he can answer, his wife says, "He just doesn't hear me, doctor." When hearing tests indicate no hearing impairment, the physician talks to the patient alone. It then may become apparent (though the process of interrogation may take considerable time) that the patient subconsciously does not want to listen to his wife and therefore has developed a psychogenic hearing loss as a defense mechanism.

Probably the classic example of psychogenic deafness is the young soldier in battle, too frightened to charge and yet ashamed of retreating while his buddies bravely go forward. In the absence of a rational way out, his unconscious mind conjures up the concept of deafness or blindness.

The chief statistics of functional deafness originate in the Armed Forces and the Veterans Administration hearing centers. Here some 25 per cent of hard-of-hearing patients are reported to have significant functional hearing losses. Strangely enough, a large percentage of such cases during World War II had little or no combat service. Disruption of family life and subjection to military discipline produced sufficient trauma to bring on psychogenic hearing loss.

The complexities of civilian society also have produced an abundance of emotional conflict and insecurity—sufficient to account for a complete spectrum of emotional disturbance, including psychogenic hearing loss. Often such cases escape medical attention or diagnosis.

FUNCTIONAL OVERLAY

It is, of course, entirely possible for hearing loss of functional origin to be superimposed on true organic deafness, in which case the term "functional overlay" is used. The problem then is to recognize the two components in the patient's hearing impairment.

The history and the otologic examination often provide important clues, such as the unrealistic attempts of a patient to account for his difficulty. For example, he may claim that his hearing was excellent until a physician cleaned out his ears with such force that he suddenly went stone deaf. Another patient may carry on a perfectly normal conversation with his physician and hear everything he says, while repeated hearing tests consistently suggest a severe deafness quite inconsistent with the patient's conversational accomplishments.

DIAGNOSIS BY SPECIFIC FEATURES

The diagnosis of functional hearing impairment should not be made solely by exclusion or merely because tests performed reveal no organic evidence. There are specific features that characterize functional hearing impairment, and upon these a positive diagnosis must depend.

A critical appraisal of routine hearing tests usually will justify a diagnosis of functional deafness if this is present. In an organic lesion all tests must not only give fairly consistent results when they are repeated, but they must also correlate with one another. It is a mistake to attribute well-marked discrepancies to individual variations. Several authors have suggested critical observations that should alert physicians to the possible presence of a functional hearing loss. These leads have been found to be useful:

1. A medical history that experience indicates could not possibly explain the patient's condition, such as the sudden onset of profound deafness following instillation of drops into the ears. Care must be taken to exclude all organic causes and not simply to disprove the patient's explanation.

2. Too spectacular an improvement with a hearing aid, especially when the patient has set the controls at minimal amplification, or a sudden disproportionate improvement in hearing after a simple procedure such as drum massage or blowing out the eustachian tube. In such cases the power of suggestion probably should receive the credit rather than the mechanical procedure.

3. Decided fluctuations in hearing acuity as determined by any single test. The importance of repeated tests cannot be overemphasized. They are needed especially to establish basic hearing against which to evaluate the results of any treatment to be undertaken.

4. Inconsistency in the results of two or more tests. For example, the patient may hear everything when spoken to, and yet his audiogram may show a very severe hearing loss, such as 70 db or even greater. In functional deafness of the neurotic type these inconsistencies usually are constant and repeatable, whereas in malingering they usually are inconstant, and the results of the tests vary considerably when they are repeated.

5. In alleged complete deafness the presence of cochlear nerve reflexes with loud noise indicates either malingering or hysteria. Psychogalvanic

skin resistance tests also are used to establish true hearing when subjective responses are unreliable.

In psychogenically induced hearing loss there is usually a uniform flat tone loss in all frequencies, suggestive of a well-marked conductive deafness. However, in these patients the bone conduction is practically absent. In a patient with unilateral functional deafness there may be complete absence of bone conduction on the side of the bad ear, though the good ear has normal acuity. Such a patient may even disclaim hearing shouts directed at the bad ear in spite of the good hearing in the opposite ear.

AUDIOMETRIC PATTERNS IN FUNCTIONAL HEARING IMPAIRMENT

There is no characteristic audiometric pattern in functional deafness,

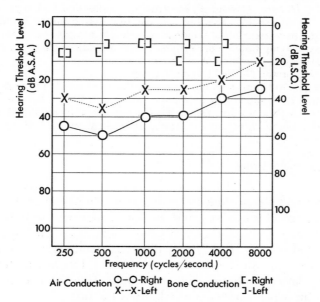

FIG. 107. *History:* 34-year-old female with otosclerosis and hearing loss for over 10 years. Mother and aunt have same difficulty, but all refuse to use hearing aids. Patient reluctantly admits having some hearing loss. She often says, "What?" even when addressed loudly and habitually asks for repetition even though she evidently hears. She often repeats a question before answering and obviously has much better hearing than her responses indicate. The patient appears to be frustrated and emotionally disturbed and does not use her residual hearing effectively. Her associates have been led to believe that her hearing loss is worse than it actually is. This is a functional overlay on an organic otosclerosis. After positive suggestion this patient acquired a hearing aid and is doing much better. She refuses ear surgery.

		AIR CONDUCTION												
		RIGHT							LEFT					
DATE	LEFT MASK	250	500	1000	2000	4000	8000	RIGHT MASK	250	500	1000	2000	4000	8000
5/11/61	-	25	15	15	20	30	35	-	45	50	55	55	60	75
								80	65	70	75	70	70	NR
								-	70	75	75	80	85	NR
Rudmose Audiometry		15	15	25	15	15	15	-	40	40	40	40	50	60
PGSR								-	10	15	15	20	25	35

		BONE CONDUCTION											
		RIGHT						LEFT					
DATE	LEFT MASK	250	500	1000	2000	4000	TYPE	RIGHT MASK	250	500	1000	2000	4000
5/11/61	-	15	20	25	25	25		-	45	55	55	45	45
								80	NR	55	NR	NR	NR

Fig. 108. *History:* 37-year-old construction worker knocked to ground by a beam. No unconsciousness, but left ear required sutures. Noted some hearing loss in left ear after accident, which has progressively worsened. Denies ever having tinnitus or vertigo. This is a medicolegal problem, and he is suing for compensation of deafness.

Otologic: normal. Normal caloric findings

Audiologic: Note varying and inconsistent hearing levels during repeated audiograms. It is difficult to determine how much of the hearing loss is organic and how much functional. Psychogalvanic skin resistance testing confirmed a marked functional overlay, with only about a 15-db loss in all frequencies.

Classification: functional hearing loss

Etiology: malingering

but the consistent inconsistencies serve to alert the physician. Usually, the hearing impairment is bilateral, and the bone conduction level is the same as the air conduction level. Figure 107 shows a functional hearing loss due to a functional overlay. Here the patient has some organic hearing loss due to otosclerosis, but she does not use her residual hearing effectively and actually hears much less than she should. This is not uncommon in otosclerosis, in which emotional instability is the rule.

SHOULD THE PHYSICIAN UNDERTAKE PSYCHOTHERAPY?

The general practitioner or otologist must decide for himself whether psychiatric involvement in patients with functional deafness is or is not too profound and complex for him to handle personally. The physician is more likely to assume the responsibility of psychotherapy if any of the following favorable factors are present: (1) the patient is young, (2) the duration of the functional disturbance is short, and there is a history of previous stability, (3) the history shows that an important emotional crisis

AIR CONDUCTION

DATE	Exam.	LEFT MASK	250	500	1000	2000	4000	8000	RIGHT MASK	250	500	1000	2000	4000	8000	
			RIGHT							**LEFT**						
2/2/59			60	60	70	80	75	60		60	·55	75	75	75	60	
2/2/59			60	55	70	80	70	65		55	60	75	75	70	70	
2/6/59			55	60	70	75	70	65		60	60	75	70	75	70	
2/9/59			65	60	65	75	75	65		60	60	70	75	70	70	
2/9/59			10	10	20	← PGSR →				10	5	10				
2/9/59			0	0	5	5	10	20	After ← PGSR → 0	0	10	20	25	20		

BONE CONDUCTION

DATE	Exam.	LEFT MASK	250	500	1000	2000	4000	RIGHT MASK	250	500	1000	2000	4000	
			RIGHT						**LEFT**					
2/2/59			NR	NR	NR	NR	NR		NR	NR	NR	NR	NR	
2/2/59			NR	NR	NR	NR	NR		NR	NR	NR	NR	NR	

SPEECH RECEPTION

DATE	RIGHT	LEFT MASK	LEFT	RIGHT MASK	FREE FIELD
	Inconsistent	Results			

Fig. 109. *History:* 21-year-old female with a series of emotional conflicts including breakup with her boy friend, flunking out of college and a pending divorce of her parents. She now claims she cannot hear what goes on around her and for that reason flunked out of school. Her responses are generally delayed, and she seems to be "distant."

Otologic: normal

Audiologic: Even though she gave consistent pure tone thresholds which showed a severe hearing loss, she often seemed able to hear soft voices behind her back. She denied hearing by bone conduction with a tuning fork. PGSR showed normal hearing.

Classification: functional

Etiology: emotional disturbance. Her hearing returned to normal after psychotherapy.

is now past, and (4) the physician is reasonably sure of his ability to win the patient's confidence.

On the other hand, if the patient shows evidence of chronic or repeated emotional disturbances, psychiatric attention may be advisable.

MALINGERING

Malingering is the deliberate fabrication of symptoms that the patient knows do not exist. He is motivated by the desire to seek some advantage: financial compensation, escape from military service or evasion of responsibility for failure. Malingering is becoming increasingly common in school children. Characteristically, the malingerer abandons his symptoms when he thinks he is no longer being observed. In contrast, a neurotic patient with a functional hearing loss believes in his symptoms, and they interfere with his pleasures as well as his work.

A minor form of malingering, pleading a headache to forego a dull social affair, generally is tolerated as a "white lie." However, to sham a disability as severe as deafness transcends normal behavior and denotes a defective personality. Such a person may have antisocial tendencies.

Unlike the neurotic individual who believes his symptoms are real, the malingerer who pretends deafness has no "pattern" in his alleged disability. His hearing tests are a crazy quilt of inconsistencies. When he is subjected to tests that he does not understand, he suspects he may be tripped up by the doctor and his testing machine. He wishes to preserve the fiction

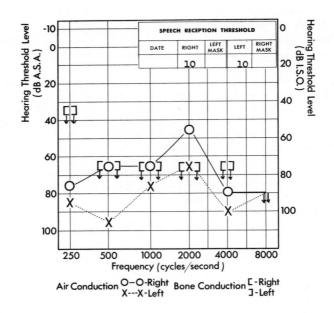

FIG. 110. *History:* 11-year-old female who is doing poorly at school, and parents are concerned because she does not seem to hear them. No history of otologic disturbance, but an aunt uses a hearing aid.

Otologic: normal

Audiologic: In spite of an apparent severe bilateral hearing loss the girl responded to speech at 10 db.

Classification: functional

Diagnosis: emotional conflict. This child was using a hearing loss (on the basis of her aunt's handicap) to solve her school and home difficulties. She was aided by several discussions in the office and came along well.

that he is deaf, but when he is asked whether he can hear a signal of a given strength, he does not know when to say, "Yes," and when to say, "No." He falters in his answers. Yesterday's audiogram may have shown a 70-db hearing level, and today's, a 35-db. The record may indicate a 60-db hearing loss for pure tone but a loss of only 10 db for speech reception. When the tests are repeated, his answers may vary by as much as 30 to 40 db.

If the patient claims he has one "good" and one "bad" ear, and the examiner obstructs his "good ear" with a finger, then shouts into it loudly enough to be heard easily by bone conduction alone, the malingerer claims he hears nothing.

When a patient malingers to the extent of exaggerating a true organic hearing loss, the task of learning the truth becomes more difficult. Such a problem may assume considerable importance in medicolegal cases, particularly if they involve compensation claims for occupational deafness. For a more detailed discussion of this subject see Chapter 26. Figures 108 to 110 show audiograms of several patients with functional hearing impairments; the captions explain the motivating factors.

Chapter 16

Tinnitus and Vertigo

TINNITUS

Tinnitus, or noise in the ear, is one of the most challenging symptoms in otology and medicine. It usually indicates some damage to the auditory pathway. It has been speculated that tinnitus may be the result of a continuous stream of discharges along the auditory nerve to the brain due to abnormal irritation in the sensorineural pathway. Though no sound is reaching the ear, the spontaneous nerve discharge may cause the patient to experience a false sensation of sound. Although this theory sounds logical, there is as yet no scientific proof of its validity.

Various efforts to stop the tinnitus, even by the desperate expedient of cutting the auditory nerve, have only beclouded the theory, for an occasional patient continues to hear the tinnitus though his auditory nerve is severed completely, and all hearing apparently is gone. The bilateral innervation of the auditory pathway and other difficult aspects complicate a thorough understanding of this phenomenon.

One of the surprising features about tinnitus is that not everybody has it. After all, the cochlea is exquisitely sensitive to sounds, and relatively loud sounds are being produced inside each human head: the rushing of blood through the cranial arteries, the noises made by muscles in the head during chewing. That an individual rarely hears these body noises may be explained by the way that the temporal bone is situated in the skull and by the depth at which the cochlea is imbedded in the temporal bone. The architecture and the acoustics of the head ordinarily prevent the transmission of these noises through the bones of the skull to the cochlea, and thus to consciousness; yet the cochlea is so built and situated that normally it can respond to very weak sounds carried by the air from outside the head. Only when there are certain changes in the vascular walls—perhaps caused by arteriosclerosis—or in the temporal bone structure, does the ear pick up these internal noises. The patient may say that he hears his own pulsebeat as a result of a vascular disorder, and it may seem to be louder when the room is quiet, or at night when he is trying to go to sleep. Pressing on various blood vessels in the neck rarely stops this type of tinnitus, unassociated with hearing loss.

Although it is always troublesome, tinnitus may serve as an early warning of auditory injury. For example, a high-pitched ringing or hissing may be the first indication of impending cochlear damage from ototoxic drugs—a clear signal that the drug should be stopped or its dosage reduced. Generally, the tinnitus disappears, and no hearing loss may result, though in some instances the head noises may persist for months or even years.

Among the common drugs capable of producing tinnitus are aspirin and quinine in large doses, and especially the antibiotics, kanamycin, neomycin and dihydrostreptomycin. These drugs should be used with extreme caution, especially when kidney function is deficient.

Except for tinnitus associated with certain vascular disorders and soft palate abnormalities, when an observer can hear independently or feel the cause of the head noises that bother the patient, the vast majority of cases of tinnitus are subjective, i.e., heard by the patient alone. Objective tinnitus is comparatively easy to detect and to localize, because either it can be heard with a stethoscope or it can be determined by special studies such as x-ray studies and angiography.

Diagnostic Significance of Description of Tinnitus

Because tinnitus, like pain, is subjective, it can be described by the patient only by comparing it with some familiar noise. The patient may say it sounds like the hissing of steam, the ringing of bells, the roar of the ocean, a running motor, buzzing or a machine shop. Very often it is difficult for the patient to localize the noise in the ears; he even may not be able to tell from which ear it is coming, for it may sound as though it were in the center of his head. Some people declare that the noises are not in their ears at all but inside the head. Quite frequently, a patient claims that the noise is in one ear and not in the other; yet when by some surgical or medical procedure the noise is stopped in the ear in question, the patient notices the noise in the opposite ear. This means that the patient heard the tinnitus in the ear in which it was loudest but did not realize that it was present also in the opposite ear.

How the patient describes his tinnitus is often of diagnostic significance. For example, a low-pitched type of tinnitus is more common in otosclerosis and other forms of conductive deafness. Sounds like ringing bells and hissing are more usual in sensorineural deafness. The ocean-roaring type of noise or a noise like a hollow seashell held to the ear is complained of most often in Ménière's disease.

Patients sometimes say that their ear noises are so loud that they are unable to hear what is going on around them. They claim also that if only the head noises would stop, they would be able to hear better. Unfortunately, this is not the case. It is possible to measure how loud these noises actually are. These measurements show that tinnitus is rarely louder than a very soft whisper, and it is actually the concomitant hearing loss that prevents patients from hearing; or else a psychological disturbance, rather than the masking effect of the tinnitus, is at fault.

TINNITUS IN OTOSCLEROSIS

In otosclerosis tinnitus is usually low-pitched and described as a buzzing or, occasionally, a roaring sound. Sometimes the patient may say he hears a pumping noise or a pulsation timed to his heart beat. To some patients with otosclerosis the tinnitus is even more disturbing than the hearing loss. However, not all victims of otosclerosis have tinnitus, and some with very severe otosclerotic deafness deny ever having had head noises. In most instances tinnitus disappears in the course of many years of hearing impairment. Tinnitus rarely is found in older patients who have had long-standing otosclerosis.

In view of all that has been learned about the pathology of otosclerosis, it might be thought that it would be possible to clear up the tinnitus by correcting the fixation of the stapedial footplate. This is not borne out necessarily by experience. Many patients who have had successful stapes surgery and a return to almost normal hearing have found that the tinnitus seems to persist, although it may not be as loud as it was prior to surgery. Yet in other patients tinnitus seems to subside completely when hearing is restored surgically. It would appear, then, that there are other factors beside stapes fixation in the etiology of tinnitus and otosclerosis. Possibly, the ototoxic effects of otosclerosis eventually produce a sensorineural deafness and tinnitus.

TINNITUS IN MÉNIÈRE'S DISEASE

One of the most disturbing and persistent types of tinnitus is found in Ménière's disease. It generally is described as an ocean roar or a hollow seashell sound. In the early stages of Ménière's disease tinnitus may appear or become accentuated only during the attack, but afterwards the tinnitus often persists all the time and becomes the most distracting symptom.

Many patients would even sacrifice their hearing to get rid of the tinnitus, but unfortunately there is no positive therapy, not even by surgery, that will guarantee the disappearance of the tinnitus. Fortunately, the tinnitus and the inner ear involvement are restricted usually to one ear, but when they invade both ears, the psychological impact on the patient becomes a serious challenge to both the patient and the physician.

TINNITUS AFTER BLOW TO HEAD, EXPOSURE TO NOISE

Ringing tinnitus is experienced almost invariably after a slap across the ear or close exposure to a sudden very loud noise such as the explosion of a firecracker or the firing of a gun. In most instances the tinnitus is accompanied by a high tone hearing loss. If the loss is temporary, the noise usually subsides in a few hours or days. If permanent hearing loss has occurred from damage to the inner ear, a ringing tinnitus may persist for many years.

The close relationship of head injury and tinnitus is clearly evident in the classic cartoon that portrays an individual knocked out by a punch on the jaw or a blow on the head, complete with stars circling his eyes and bells ringing in his ears. The bells dramatize the tinnitus that the patient hears after a severe blow, especially on the chin or on the side of the head. The noise is due probably to a concussion in the cochlea. The damage seems to be reversible most of the time, for the ringing gradually subsides.

AUDITORY NEURITIS AND MISCELLANEOUS CAUSES

For want of a more specific etiology, tinnitus often is attributed to neuritis of the auditory nerve, especially if a high tone deafness accompanies it. It is not known precisely whether the irritation actually injures the nerve itself, but there seems to be good reason to believe that the damage occurs in the cochlea. Diseases such as hepatitis, influenza and other viral diseases frequently result in high-pitched tinnitus, tentatively attributed to cochleitis or auditory neuritis. Tinnitus occasionally is associated with presbycusis, impacted cerumen on the eardrum and with a number of unknown causes. It rarely is found in infections of the middle ear.

TINNITUS WITH A NORMAL AUDIOGRAM

It is standard procedure in otologic practice to perform an audiogram on every patient who complains of tinnitus. If the otoscopic findings are normal, and the audiogram shows normal hearing from the lowest frequencies to 8,000 cycles, and yet the patient complains of tinnitus, several causes should be considered: (1) temporomandibular joint disparity; (2) functional causes; (3) vascular and neurologic disorders; and (4) hearing defect above the 8,000-cycle frequency.

Temporomandibular Joint Problems

Just how an overbite or other temporomandibular joint disparity can cause tinnitus is not yet known, but there are some patients whose tinnitus has been cleared up completely by adequate dental correction. The evidence conflicts with the assumption that all of these cases are of emotional origin. Only a few patients with overbite ever complain of tinnitus, and even when overbite and tinnitus are present in the same patient, it does not follow necessarily that the overbite causes the tinnitus. Since dental correction is sometimes a formidable undertaking, one might consider a tentative procedure to indicate whether a complete corrective program would stop the tinnitus. Such a procedure may consist of placing a plastic prosthesis over the lower molars at night. If there is a noticeable improvement in the tinnitus after a satisfactory trial period, then more permanent measures may be indicated. Indiscriminate or radical efforts to remove tinnitus by correcting the overbite without a valid therapeutic test to establish the causal relationship should be avoided. Many otologists question the reality of any true relationship between overbite or temporomandibular joint disparity and hearing loss.

Tinnitus due to an overbite is rare and usually unilateral. When it is present, it generally is a high-pitched ring or a low roar and accompanied by fullness in the ear. It has been postulated that pressure on the eustachian tube is responsible, but experimental efforts to produce tinnitus by putting artificial pressure on the eustachian tubes generally fail to prove the point. However, a ringing tinnitus can be produced in many normal persons when they clench their teeth tightly together and tense their jaw muscles. A sharp blow to the jaw with the bite closed often produces a ringing tinnitus, not necessarily originating in a concussion of the inner ear. Tinnitus due to an overbite is heard best when it is quiet at night, especially with the opposite ear pressed against the pillow to shut out masking noise. The precise mechanism is controversial.

An abnormally large space between the upper and the lower front teeth when the patient closes his jaw suggests overbite. Placing the index fingers over the temporomandibular joint and asking the patient to open his mouth widely, then close it, may make a clicking or grinding noise. Sometimes the lower jaw extends an abnormal distance beyond the upper jaw (prognathism). Muscle spasm over the jaw joint (of the masseter and the

AIR CONDUCTION

	RIGHT									LEFT							
250	500	1000	2000	4000	8000	10000	12000	14000	250	500	1000	2000	4000	8000	10000	12000	14000
5	0	-5	-10	5	5	35	30	35	5	5	-5	-10	-10	-5	15	10	5

FIG. 111. *History:* 38-year-old female with fullness in right ear and high-pitched constant tinnitus for several months. No obvious cause. She had had eustachian tube inflations, allergic desensitization, bite correction and nose treatments without help. Patient was referred as a marked neurotic.

Otologic: normal

Audiologic: normal hearing with high tone hearing loss above 8,000 cps.

Classification: high tone sensory hearing loss

Diagnosis: After further questioning the patient subsequently associated the onset of tinnitus with a bad cold. Loss probably due to a viral cochleitis.

AIR CONDUCTION

	RIGHT									LEFT							
250	500	1000	2000	4000	8000	10000	12000	14000	250	500	1000	2000	4000	8000	10000	12000	14000
-10	-5	-5	-10	-5	45	30	35	60	0	-5	-5	-5	0	-10	-5	-5	0

FIG. 112. *History:* 18-year-old female with ringing tinnitus 8 weeks after fall on right side of head, with unconsciousness. Skull was fractured, and she had vertigo and bleeding from right ear. For 6 weeks she had light-headedness. A persistent ringing tinnitus is present.

Otologic: normal

Audiologic: Note the loss in the very high frequencies in the right ear.

Classification: sensorineural deafness

Diagnosis: direct trauma to inner ear

temporalis muscles) and head pain in the temporal area are symptoms in temporomandibular joint disparity.

TINNITUS WITH HIDDEN HIGH FREQUENCY HEARING LOSSES

Tinnitus and hearing loss are associated so frequently with each other that some physicians attribute tinnitus to a psychological disturbance if the audiogram shows normal hearing. Such a diagnosis hardly is justified. A diagnosis of psychological disturbance should be made on positive findings rather than on the fact that the audiogram is normal. Studies now being published by the author and his associates show that many patients who complain of ringing or hissing tinnitus may have perfectly normal hearing in the frequencies that all audiometers test, that is, up to 8,000 cycles. However, when the hearing is tested at higher frequencies up to

14,000 cycles, it is not uncommon to find a hearing deficit in the ear in which the patient claims he has tinnitus.

Continuous audiometry up to 10,000 cycles performed with a Bekesy audiometer is of tremendous help in cases of this special type. Figures 111 and 112 relate cases of tinnitus that were diagnosed as functional because no hearing loss was found during routine audiometry. However, more detailed hearing tests revealed the presence of auditory damage which could well account for the patient's tinnitus.

In addition, the standard audiogram shows thresholds only at a few fixed octave frequencies. The hearing damage may well be at a point intermediate between these major frequencies. For example, a 40-db loss at 3,500 cycles would not be seen on the ordinary audiogram, because hearing is measured at 2,000 and 4,000 cycles.

FUNCTIONAL CAUSES

For all the reasons enumerated, a diagnosis of functional or psychological tinnitus should be made with great caution. Nevertheless, in a large number of cases in which a patient with normal hearing complains of head noises, a tentative diagnosis of functional tinnitus may have to be considered. Most such patients become so preoccupied with their tinnitus they continue to talk about it to their friends and go the rounds of numerous doctors and nonprofessional persons for relief that is not forthcoming. Unfortunately, the otologist can do little to cure such patients of their tinnitus, since the cause is not known. However, the general practitioner can help the patient to adjust more sensibly to the mild auditory disorder by practical psychotherapy. It is helpful in such cases to bear in mind that tinnitus itself is really not very loud, but many patients overreact to their symptoms and allow their problem to assume distressing proportions.

MANAGING THE PATIENT WITH TINNITUS

Some patients become so obsessed with the noises in their ears that they become emotionally disturbed and are unable to sleep at night, for they maintain the noise keeps them awake. This happens mainly in highly nervous individuals, but the problem requires much patience and understanding on the part of the physician. Reassurance and encouragement are very helpful. Whatever symptomatic therapy may be available for the tinnitus should be provided. One practical suggestion is for the patient to put an automatic timer on his radio and play it when he goes to sleep. After an hour or two the automatic timer shuts off the radio, and by then the patient is fast asleep. Music from the radio may mask out the patient's tinnitus by distracting his attention from endogenous noises.

In managing the patient with tinnitus it is advisable to have a forthright talk with the patient and to explain to him the most likely cause of the tinnitus, and the fact that as yet there is no specific cure for it. Nevertheless, it is possible in most instances to mitigate the problem and particularly to alleviate the patient's excessive concern about his symptoms. If a hearing aid is indicated, its daily use usually makes the patient less aware of the tinnitus by focusing attention on other matters. Everyday noises definitely help to mask out tinnitus. However, when the patient takes off the hearing aid at night, the tinnitus may become more noticeable. Periods of tension and stress also tend to make tinnitus more troublesome. People with tinnitus who keep occupied, especially at work, are almost never aware of their noises.

The use of tranquilizers, constructive suggestions and specific cures for such conditions as otosclerosis and Ménière's disease are important therapeutic regimens in managing the patient with tinnitus. In many cases the tinnitus subsides gradually or even suddenly for no obvious reason. Medical attention to related vascular abnormalities, such as hypertension, Buerger's disease and atherosclerosis, is recommended. Psychotherapy and encouragement are of tremendous value.

AUDIOMETRY IN PRESENCE OF TINNITUS

Occasionally, when an audiogram is being performed on a patient with marked tinnitus, he complains that he cannot detect the tone produced by the audiometer because of his tinnitus. This is a real problem, and it can be handled best by modifying the technic of audiometry. Instead of sounding a tone on the audiometer for a second or less, it is best to present quickly interrupted tones, so that the patient can distinguish the discontinuous audiometer tone from his constant tinnitus. In this way the tester will get a much more accurate threshold than by using the routine method of tone presentation.

The character of a patient's tinnitus can be determined by asking him to match it with sounds applied to his good ear. For example, a 1,000-cycle tone may be applied to the good ear and gradually amplified until the patient matches it with the tinnitus in his bad ear both as to intensity and frequency. Another method is to apply a masking noise to the ear with tinnitus and then to determine the amount of noise needed just to mask out the patient's tinnitus and make it disappear. Both of these methods provide reasonably good measures of the intensity and the type of a patient's head noise.

VERTIGO

In addition to deafness and tinnitus, vertigo is an important symptom associated with disorders of the ear. The intimate relationship of the vestibular portion of the labyrinth to the cochlea makes it easy to understand the reason that many diseases and lesions affect both balance and hearing, such as Ménière's disease, head trauma and vascular accidents. Some diseases, like mumps, classically affect only the cochlea. Certain toxins and viruses affect only the vestibular portion without affecting the hearing. Intense noise affects only the cochlea.

Vertigo, like deafness and tinnitus, is a subjective experience and is a symptom, not a disease. Its cause must be sought in each case. The term "dizziness" or "vertigo" is used by patients to describe a variety of subjective sensations, many of which actually are not related to the vestibular system. Vertigo of labyrinthine origin is basically a disturbance of the patient in relation to his environment. It is a feeling of motion, either subjectively, in which the patient feels himself moving, or objectively, in which the room moves about the patient. There may be also a sensation of imbalance, of falling or being pushed, but in all instances it is related to motion. If, on careful questioning of a patient who complains of vertigo, it is found that the sensation is rather one of faintness, spots before the eyes, body weakness, tightness in the head, or general lightheadedness, involvement of the vestibular pathway generally can be ruled out. "Cloudiness" or dullness in the head also may be described as vertigo by the patient, but these sensations do not have their origin in the ear. In many patients it is difficult to get an accurate description of the subjective experience. If, however, the symptoms are not accompanied by deafness and tinnitus or fullness in the ear, a disorder of the auditory and vestibular mechanism must be ruled out.

The vestibular system is complex and connects with the muscles of the eyes, the vagus nerve, the temporal lobe cortex, the cerebellum, and the muscles of the neck, the trunk and the limbs. Under normal conditions this bilateral system is constantly in operation to receive impulses, to regulate body movements and to maintain position. All this occurs without the individual's being aware of it. When the labyrinth is subjected to exceptional stress, the resultant experience can produce a sensation of vertigo. Such a situation may arise in motion sickness or disease of the vestibular apparatus. As the result the patient can experience a feeling of imbalance or falling, which causes him to make a reflex effort to counteract the sudden subjective sensation. If the abnormal stimulus is severe enough, nystagmus, nausea, vomiting and sweating may occur.

Two Important Questions

When a patient complains of "dizziness" that may originate in the inner ear, two important questions must be settled. (1) Is the symptom the result of a vestibular pathway disturbance? (2) If so, is the etiology in the central nervous system or in the peripheral vestibular apparatus? The first point can be verified readily by taking a careful history and determining that the vertigo consists of a disturbance of motion, probably associated with tinnitus, deafness or ear fullness.

Nervous System Involvement and Other Causes

Vertigo involving the central nervous system is an urgent problem and must be ruled out in every case, especially in those cases in which it is associated with unilateral fullness in the ear or hearing loss.

Certain symptoms strongly suggest that the cause of the vertigo must be sought in the central nervous system. If spontaneous nystagmus is present and persists, the physician immediately should look for associated neurologic signs, such as falling and papilledema. If the rotational vertigo is associated with loss of consciousness, the physician should suspect also that the vertigo originates in the central nervous system. The association of intense vertigo with localized headache makes it mandatory to rule out a central lesion.

Among the common causes of vertigo caused by central nervous system involvement are: (1) vascular crises, (2) tumors of the posterior fossa, (3) multiple sclerosis, (4) epilepsy, (5) encephalitis and (6) concussion.

The vertigo in a vascular crisis is of sudden onset and generally is accompanied by nausea and vomiting as well as tinnitus and deafness. In many instances there is involvement of other cranial nerves. In a special type of vascular crisis, such as Wallenberg's syndrome, there is thrombosis of the postero-inferior cerebellar artery, resulting in sudden overwhelming vertigo, dysphagia, dysphonia and Horner's syndrome, as well as other neurologic findings. The episode often is so severe that death is not uncommon.

It is also possible to have a much more discrete vascular defect in the vestibular labyrinth without an involvement of the cochlea. This usually results in an acute onset of severe vertigo. Recovery is rather slow, and the vertigo may persist as postural imbalance. The nystagmus may subside, but unsteadiness and difficulty in walking may continue much longer.

A still milder form of vascular problem related to vertigo occurs in hypotension and vasomotor instability. These people have recurrent brief episodes of imbalance and instability, particularly after a sudden change of position, such as suddenly arising from tying their shoelaces or turning quickly. Investigators are convinced that histamine sensitivity plays an important role in this type of vertigo, especially when migraine attacks also are present. Histamine desensitization by subcutaneous injections over a long period of time has been reported to be of great help in this type of vertigo, particularly in cases in which the patient shows a marked sensitivity on intradermal testing.

In multiple sclerosis vertigo is occasionally a symptom, but it is rarely severe enough to confuse the picture with other involvement of the vestibular pathways. In epilepsy vertigo occasionally may be a premonitory sensation before an epileptic attack, but unconsciousness usually accompanies the attack and helps to distinguish the condition.

A complaint of vertigo in postconcussion syndrome is extremely common. The vertigo usually is associated with movement of the head or the body, severe headache and marked hypersensitivity to noise and vibration. The patients usually are jittery, tense and very touchy.

Carotid sinus syndrome and psychic disturbances frequently produce vertigo that may be confused with vertigo of vestibular origin. Taking a careful history and testing the carotid sinus make it possible to distinguish these conditions.

Of special interest to the otologist is the vertigo that sometimes is associated with a lesion of the posterior cranial fossa and particularly with an acoustic neuroma. It is a standing rule in otology that when a patient complains of true vertigo, an acoustic neuroma must be ruled out. This is especially true when the vertigo is accompanied by a hearing loss or tinnitus in one ear. Vertigo is not always a symptom in all posterior fossa lesions, but when it occurs, a number of simple tests help to establish the possibility that a tumor is present. One such test is to use a piece of absorbent cotton to test the corneal reflex. In many early cases of acoustic neuroma the cornea becomes somewhat less sensitive to touch on the side of the lesion. If a hearing loss is present in one ear, and the bone conduction is poor, the following three findings point to an acoustic neuroma: (1) discrimination for speech is reduced markedly, (2) pathologic fatigue of the nerve is present, and (3) recruitment is absent.

Other occasional causes of vertigo are encephalitis, meningitis, direct head injuries and toxic reactions to alcohol, tobacco or other toxic drugs, such as streptomycin.

A most common cause of peripheral vertigo, Ménière's disease, is described in detail in Chapter 14. The vertigo is classically of sudden onset, comparatively brief in duration and recurs in paroxysmal attacks. During the attack it generally is accompanied by an ocean-roaring tinnitus, fullness in the ear and hearing loss. Occasionally, there may be some residual imbalance between attacks, but this does not happen often.

Another type of vertigo associated with some abnormality in the vestibule is being recognized more frequently. In positional vertigo the attack occurs briefly with sudden movements of the head. It generally is not associated with deafness or tinnitus. Depending on the position of the head, the posterior semicircular canal may be the source of the difficulty, or one of the other canals may be involved. Therapy for this condition is still in the symptomatic stage, and usually the symptoms resolve spontaneously.

Certain viruses such as herpes classically produce vertigo by involving the peripheral end-organ. The attack is usually of sudden onset associated with tinnitus and deafness, and it subsides spontaneously. Certain toxins readily produce vertigo.

Whenever a patient complains of vertigo, and there is evidence of a chronic otitis media, it is essential to determine whether a cholesteatoma is present that is eroding into the semicircular canal and causing the vertigo. Vertigo can be present also with certain types of otosclerosis that involves the inner ear. In all such cases the specific cause of the vertigo should be determined, and whenever possible, proper therapy based on the specific cause should be instituted.

In every case of vertigo of an undetermined origin it is essential to do vestibular tests as well as hearing studies. Vestibular tests include rotational tests, caloric studies, and more complicated examinations within the realm of the otologist and the neurologist.

NYSTAGMUS

Every examination of the head and the neck must include a search for spontaneous nystagmus, especially if vertigo is a complaint. A brief test can be done by first asking the patient to look straight ahead and then to hold his head straight but move his eyes from side to side. Normally, no nystagmus is present in an individual who is gazing straight ahead, but over 50 per cent of people have a slight unsustained nystagmus when they are looking to the right or the left. This is a normal reaction, probably due to tension in the eye muscles. It generally lasts only a few seconds. In pathologic nystagmus of vestibular pathway origin there is generally a slow and a fast component. The nystagmus is aggravated by looking in the direction of the fast component, and the nystagmus is so named, that is, to the right or to the left, depending on the direction of the fast component. The nystagmus persists for some time when it is pathologic. In central nervous system disorders it may persist for months. In acute attacks of Ménière's disease it may last for several days or as long as the attack continues. In positional vertigo the episode may be fleeting and last only as long as the head is held in a certain position. When marked nystagmus occurs spontaneously, and the patient does not complain of vertigo, it is highly suggestive of damage to the central nervous system. Vertigo that accompanies spontaneous nystagmus also may suggest a central nervous system defect, but other conditions may produce the same symptoms, such as acute episodes of Ménière's disease, toxic labyrinthitis and positional vertigo. Whenever pathologic nystagmus is present, comprehensive otologic and neurologic studies are indicated.

Chapter 17

Charts Summarizing Differential Diagnoses

CHART 1. AUDIOLOGIC CRITERIA FOR

	AIR CONDUCTION PATTERN	BONE CONDUCTION PATTERN	AIR-BONE-GAP	LATERALIZATION OF 500 cps FORK	RE-CRUIT-MENT
Conductive	Greater low tone loss except when fluid is in the ear. Maximum loss is 60 db.	Normal or almost normal	At least 15 db	To worse ear	Absent
Sensory	Greater low tone loss or high tone dip	Bone conduction equals air conduction (BC = AC).	No gap	To better ear with low intensity To worse ear with high intensity	Marked and continuous
Neural	Greater high tone loss	BC = AC, or BC worse than AC	No gap	To better ear	Absent
Sensorineural	Greater high tone loss or flat loss	BC = AC	No gap	To better ear	Absent or slight
Functional	Flat	Usually no BC	No gap	Vague	Absent
Central	Variable or even normal threshold	BC = AC, or absent BC	No gap	None	None

* These criteria are the usual ones, but many variations and exceptions are encountered.

Classifying Hearing Impairment*

Abnormal Tone Decay	Discrimination	Audiometric Responses	Tinnitus	Bekesy Tracings	Patient's Voice	Other Findings
Absent	Good	Vague and slow	Absent or low buzz	Overlap of pulsed and continuous tracings	Soft or normal	No diplacusis Hears better in noisy environment
Absent	Poor	Sharp	Low roar or seashell	Pulsed tracings slightly wider at higher frequencies Little or no separation	Normal	Diplacusis Hears worse in noisy environment Lowered threshold of discomfort
Marked tone decay in acoustic neuroma and nerve injuries	Reduced	Sharp	Hissing or ringing	Separation of tracings in acoustic neuroma	Louder	No diplacusis Hears worse in noisy environment
Absent	Reduced	Sharp	Hissing or ringing	Slight separation of tracing	Louder	No diplacusis Hears worse in noisy environment
Variable	Usually good or no response	Inconsistent	Absent	Separation of tracing with poorer threshold for pulsed tone	Normal	No diplacusis Hears worse in noisy environment
Undetermined	Reduced	Slow	None	Undetermined	Normal	No diplacusis Hears poorly in noise

CHART 2. CAUSES OF CONDUCTIVE HEARING LOSS WITH ABNORMAL FINDINGS ORIGINATING IN EXTERNAL CANAL

DIAGNOSIS	HISTORY	ONSET OF HEARING LOSS	OTOSCOPIC FINDINGS	TINNITUS	AUDIOLOGIC	SPECIAL FINDINGS
Congenital aplasia	Ear deformed at birth with hearing-impairment Unilateral or bilateral	Congenital	Auricular deformity and canal closed	None	Flat hearing loss, about 50-60 db	If deformity is bilateral, speech development is slow.
Treacher-Collins syndrome	Abnormal findings present at birth bilaterally	Congenital	Auricular deformity and canal closed	None	Flat hearing loss, about 50-60 db	Bilateral deformity: slanted eyes, receding jaw and malar bones
Stenosis	Ear blocked either since birth or following infection, trauma, or surgery to the ear	Congenital or slowly developing	Eardrum not visible due to closure of canal	None	Flat hearing loss, about 50 db	Auricle is normal, but canal is closed uniformly. Usually no inflammation is present.
Cerumen	Ear blocked after attempting to clean canal or after chewing	Slow or sudden after attempting to clean ear canal	Wax blocking canal and drum not visible	Rarely	Flat loss, about 35 db	Wax is visible, and hearing returns after wax is removed.
Fluid in canal	After swimming or bathing or	Sudden	Fluid in canal	Occasionally	Mild loss with greater loss in	Ear drum normal after fluid is re-

	applying medication in ear				higher frequencies Bone conduction normal	moved with cotton
External otitis	Pain and itching in canal, aggravated by chewing or moving auricle Tenderness No pain on nose blowing	Insidious	Canal wall inflamed and debris present Eardrum intact	None	Flat loss, about 35 db	Tender canal walls and surrounding areas Hearing improves with removal of debris
Exostosis	Either constant blockage or intermittent if small opening opens and closes with wax or debris	Sudden or intermittent	Hillocks of bony projections from canal wall	None	Flat loss, about 35 db	Canal closed by hillocks or mounds of bone from canal wall X-ray pictures: normal middle ears and external bony projections
Granuloma	Fullness in ears— often painless	Slow	Firm granulation with or without excessive bleeding	None	Flat loss, about 35 db	Often no pain or inflammation Middle ear normal

CHART 2. CAUSES OF CONDUCTIVE HEARING LOSS WITH ABNORMAL FINDINGS
ORIGINATING IN EXTERNAL CANAL (*Concluded*)

DIAGNOSIS	HISTORY	ONSET OF HEARING LOSS	OTOSCOPIC FINDINGS	TINNITUS	AUDIOLOGIC	SPECIAL FINDINGS
			Ear drum normal if visible Often no inflammation			Occasional palpable bony defect in canal Positive biopsy
Cysts	Little or no discomfort but fullness	Slow	Soft mass in canal covered with skin	None	Flat loss, about 35 db	Drum normal if visualized
Collapse of canal	Hearing loss only during testing	Only with earphones	Relaxed opening to external canal	None	Mild low tone loss	Patient says he hears worse with earphones
Foreign body	Foreign body in ear In children, no clear history	Sudden	Foreign body in ear	None, except live insect in ear	Mild flat loss	Mass in ear not attached to canal wall and not covered with skin

Etiology and Principal Findings	History	Onset of Hearing Loss	Tinnitus	Audiologic	Otoscopic	Special
1. Myringitis bullosa (blebs on drum)	Mild discomfort, fullness in ear, not aggravated by swallowing or chewing and not associated with general malaise	Slow	Slight	Very mild hearing loss of about 15 or 20 db	Clear or hemorrhagic blebs on drum involving only outer layer	Drum is intact and moves with air pressure through canal or nose.
2. Ruptured ear drum	Severe explosion, slap on ear, or foreign body poked into ear, with sudden pain, hearing loss, and possible bleeding and fullness	Sudden	Sometimes ringing	Flat loss from 30 to 50 db	Jagged central perforation of drum with no inflammation if seen early	Perforation in drum is jagged and not associated with infection.
3. Perforated drum due to burns	Spark in ear from welding or exposure to fire	Sudden	None	Flat loss of about 50 db	Usually complete destruction of drum with little infection	Marked destruction of drum with history of severe pain due to burn
4. Dry perforation in drum A. Anterior or central	Previous otitis media due to adenoid hypertrophy, allergy,	Slow	None	Usually less than 30 db and worse in lower frequencies	Central or anterior perforation. No infection and	Discharge usually recurs intermittently with colds or water

[235]

CHART 3. CONDUCTIVE DEAFNESS WITH ABNORMAL FINDINGS VISIBLE IN TYMPANIC MEMBRANE AND MIDDLE EAR (Continued)

Etiology and Principal Findings	History	Onset of Hearing Loss	Tinnitus	Audiologic	Otoscopic	Special
	or eustachian tube pathology, or following secretory otitis media.				normal middle ear mucosa. Edge of perforation usually smooth and regular.	in ears.
B. Superior (Shrapnell's area) or posterior perforation on large portion of drum	Previous otitis media with chronic otorrhea or mastoid infection	Slow	None	Variable from 5 to 50 db	Perforation in Shrapnell's area	The amount of hearing loss depends on damage to ossicular chain and other pathology in the middle ear.
5. Healed perforation	Previous ear infections	Gradual	None	From minimal to 60-db flat loss	Thick scars on transparent closure in drum that looks like perforations	Drum moves with gentle air pressure in canal or through nose; hearing loss depends on damage in middle ear.
6. Hypertrophied adenoids	Intermittent ear blocking and fullness	Gradual	None	Maximum loss about 30 db and often	Clear fluid level in middle ear or thickened or	Large lymph tissue masses in lateral recesses

				worse at higher frequencies	retracted drum	of nasopharynx
	Some mouth breathing					
7. Cleft palate	Recurrent otitis in childhood	Gradual	None	As above	Opaque, thickened, or retracted drum	Inability to close nasopharynx leads to occasional ear infections.
8. Retracted drum	Stuffiness in ears	Gradual	None	As above	Abnormalities in nasopharynx or eustachian tubes, such as allergy, adenoids or neoplasm	Pressure disparity in middle ears and poor eustachian tube function
9. Serous otitis media	Stuffiness in ears, feeling of fluid	Gradual	None	As above	Fluid level in middle ear with evidence of inflammation and associated with upper respiratory infection	Blocked eustachian tube and abnormal findings in nasopharynx or tubes
10. Acute otitis media	Stuffiness, pain, and fullness in	In several hours	None	Maximum loss about 30 db	Inflamed or bulging drum with	Associated with inflammation in

CHART 3. CONDUCTIVE DEAFNESS WITH ABNORMAL FINDINGS VISIBLE IN TYMPANIC MEMBRANE AND MIDDLE EAR (Continued)

ETIOLOGY AND PRINCIPAL FINDINGS	HISTORY	ONSET OF HEARING LOSS	TINNITUS	AUDIOLOGIC	OTOSCOPIC	SPECIAL
	ear; sometimes fever			and often worse at higher frequencies	prominent vessels; absent landmarks	nasopharynx and upper respiratory infection
11. Secretory otitis media	Generally without upper respiratory infection but may follow it; recurrent fullness; no pain or systemic symptoms	Slowly	None	As above Bone conduction may be slightly reduced.	Fluid level or bubbles and straw-colored fluid or even gellike mass	Eustachian tube is patent, and condition recurs. Nasal mucosa also is secretory.
12. Aerotitis media	Sudden pain and fullness on descending in airplane or elevator	Sudden	None	Mild and usually mostly in higher frequencies	Retracted drum with possible fluid level Hearing returns with politzerization or myringotomy.	Resolution often is spontaneous, but early myringotomy resolves hearing loss.
13. Chronic otitis media	Previous otitis media with	Gradual	None	Flat loss, 50-60 db	Large marginal perforation in	Usually, end of incus or crura

A. Dry with ossicular damage	prolonged otorrhea for many months before cessation; no pain				drum and disruption of ossicular chain by erosion	are eroded. X-ray pictures show sclerosis but no active infection in mastoid.
B. Mucoid discharge	Intermittent otorrhea, especially following upper respiratory infection, but dry in between; no pain	Gradual	None	Mild with maximum of 30 db and mostly in lower frequency	Usually anterior perforation	Associated with eustachian tube and nasopharyngeal infections. Ossicular chain intact. X-ray pictures: no mastoid involvement
C. Putrid and purulent discharge	Persistent otorrhea with evidence of mastoid bone destruction; occasional discomfort	Gradual	None	Flat loss up to 60 db	Marginal perforation or no drum	Degree of hearing loss depends on damage to ossicles. X-ray pictures show chronic mastoiditis.
D. Putrid and purulent discharge with cholesteatoma	As above Usually discharge	Gradual	None	Flat loss up to 60 db	Marginal perforation or no drum; white cholesteatoma; debris in canal	As above, and cholesteatoma

CHART 3. CONDUCTIVE DEAFNESS WITH ABNORMAL FINDINGS VISIBLE IN TYMPANIC
MEMBRANE AND MIDDLE EAR (*Continued*)

ETIOLOGY AND PRINCIPAL FINDINGS	HISTORY	ONSET OF HEARING LOSS	TINNITUS	AUDIOLOGIC	OTOSCOPIC	SPECIAL
E. Putrid and purulent discharge with cholesteatoma and erosion into semicircular canal	As above Vertigo	Gradual	Occasional tinnitus	Flat loss up to 60 db	As above; vertigo and nystagmus with pressure of air in ear canal	As above; positive fistula test
14. Glomus jugulare tumor	Gradual stuffiness in one ear or persistent discharge	Gradual	Often hears own heartbeat	Very mild hearing loss at first and later up to 60 db	Red appearance of drum and middle ear or hemorrhage; granulomatous tissue	Much bleeding in ear on manipulation; x-ray pictures show erosion.
15. Tuberculosis	Mild hearing loss with chronic ear infection; may be associated with tuberculosis elsewhere	Gradual	None	Minimal to 60-db flat loss	Granulation tissue that resists treatment; later, cervical adenopathy	Biopsy and culture show TB.

16. Granuloma	Chronic otorrhea with fullness in ear and little pain	Gradual	None	Minimal to 60-db flat loss.	Firm granulations that regrow after removal	Biopsy shows specific etiology.
17. Carcinoma	As above, and sometimes some pain and nodes	Gradual	None	As above	As above	As above
18. Letterer-Siwe's disease	Generalized skin rash; chronic otorrhea	Gradual	None	As above	Bleeding and erosive granulations causing stenosis of canal	X-ray pictures show bone erosion and punched-out areas in skull.
19. Tympano-sclerosis	Chronic otitis media in the past	Gradual	None	Usually flat and about 50-60 db.	Eardrum eroded or scarred and thick; deformed appearance in middle ear	Sclerosis in mastoid bone
20. Aquaphor in round window	Previous ear infection or ruptured drum and ointment instilled in middle ear	Gradual	None	20-60 db flat loss	Either drum is absent, or there is large posterior perforation, with mass of ointment in round window niche.	To correct phase difference, ointment such as Aquaphor is instilled in round window niche, and hearing improves.

CHART 3. CONDUCTIVE DEAFNESS WITH ABNORMAL FINDINGS VISIBLE IN TYMPANIC MEMBRANE AND MIDDLE EAR (*Continued*)

ETIOLOGY AND PRINCIPAL FINDINGS	HISTORY	ONSET OF HEARING LOSS	TINNITUS	AUDIOLOGIC	OTOSCOPIC	SPECIAL
21. Hemotympanum	Blow to head or ear, with pain and fullness	Sudden	Roaring	30-60 db with greater loss at higher frequencies	Bloody fluid in middle ear	No infection is present, and eardrum does not move with pressure.
22. Systemic diseases: measles, scarlet fever	Acute otitis media, often followed by chronic otitis and hearing loss	Sudden	None	20-60-db flat loss	Perforated drum with or without chronic otitis	Chronic ear infection since childhood disease
23. Adhesion in middle ear	Slight hearing loss and fullness in ear with colds	Gradual and fluctuating	None	Up to about 25 db, or worse in lower frequencies	Drum retracted or scarred, reflecting previous otitis media	Hearing loss not corrected by inflation
24. Flaccid tympanic membrane	Feeling of flutter in eardrum corrected by self-politzerization and nose blowing	Gradual and fluctuating	None	As above	Wrinkled and loose eardrum	Drum is easily blown out and seems to be loose and redundant.
25. Blue eardrum	Fullness in ear	Fluctuates	None	Up to about 35 db and worse in higher frequencies	Drum seems to be blue or purple and does not move.	Drum is dark blue and does not politzerize easily.

						Normal x-ray findings in mastoid. No infection
26. Simple mastoidectomy	Ear infection followed by surgery—usually postauricularly; no subsequent ear discharge	None	After infection	Often little or no hearing loss, but sometimes up to 60 db if ossicular chain is disrupted	Eardrum often almost normal, or only small perforation and normal auditory canal	Usually postauricular scar and no progressive hearing loss
27. Modified radical mastoidectomy	Ear infection and surgery without removal of ossicles	None	After infection	About 30-db flat loss	Eardrum slightly deformed and posterior canal wall taken down	Postaurical or endaural scar and malleus are visible.
28. Radical mastoidectomy	Ear infection and surgery with removal of eardrum remnants and ossicles	None	After infection	60-db flat loss	No eardrum or ossicles visible and mastoid cavity seen through canal wall	X-ray picture shows surgical defect in mastoid.
29. Fenestration	Hearing loss and surgical correction	May be low-pitched.	Insidious hearing loss over years	Variable hearing loss from 20 to 60 db, depending on success of surgery	Partially exenterated mastoid cavity with displaced eardrum	Positive fistula test

CHART 3. CONDUCTIVE DEAFNESS WITH ABNORMAL FINDINGS VISIBLE IN TYMPANIC MEMBRANE AND MIDDLE EAR (*Concluded*)

ETIOLOGY AND PRINCIPAL FINDINGS	HISTORY	ONSET OF HEARING LOSS	TINNITUS	AUDIOLOGIC	OTOSCOPIC	SPECIAL
30. Myringoplasty	Hearing loss and hole in drum with surgical repair; often vein or skin was used.	Mild and gradual	None	Flat loss up to 60 db.	Healed perforation or large thick drum repair; landmarks may be missing.	Drum is in good position, and patient has scar at donor site.
31. Tympanoplasty	Chronic otitis and hearing loss followed by surgery for hearing and infection	Gradual	None	About 40-60 db	Large middle ear often is covered with skin; ossicles are absent, and cavity resembles radical mastoidectomy.	Varying findings, depending on type of surgery done
32. Artificial prosthesis	Ear infection with large defect in eardrum	Gradual	None	40-60 db flat loss	Much of drum is absent, and patient uses artificial prosthesis that is inserted into canal to middle ear.	Patient improves hearing with prosthesis.
33. X-radiation to nasopharynx or thyroid	Clear fluid in ear following irradiation	Gradual	None	20-30 db, with greater loss in higher frequencies	Fluid level and pressure disparity	X-ray treatment

CHART 4. SENSORY HEARING LOSS

HISTORY	ONSET OF HEARING LOSS	OTOSCOPIC	TINNITUS	AUDIOLOGIC AND/OR SPECIAL	DIAGNOSIS
1. Recurrent intermittent vertigo, nausea Ear feels full Voices sound tinny and hollow Difficulty understanding speech	Intermittent and then permanent	Normal	Ocean roar or hollow sea-shell	Recruitment complete, continuous, and hyperrecruitment Diplacusis Poor discrimination compared with hearing loss Discrimination worse with increase in intensity Small amplitude Bekesy tracings Recruitment is complete and often hyperrecruitment Diplacusis Patient distraught Usually unilateral	Ménière's disease with vertigo
2. Hears but cannot understand	Insidious	Normal	Hollow or absent	Same, except no hyperrecruitment Same Often bilateral	Ménière's disease without vertigo
3. Occasional mild imbalance Some ear fullness No noise exposure	Insidious or sudden	Normal	Absent or high-pitched	Marked recruitment Loss only in high frequencies Complete recruitment Usually unilateral No noise exposure	Virus disease

CHART 4. SENSORY HEARING LOSS (*Continued*)

	HISTORY	ONSET OF HEARING LOSS	OTOSCOPIC	TINNITUS	AUDIOLOGIC AND/OR SPECIAL	AUDIOLOGIC AND/OR SPECIAL	DIAGNOSIS
4.	Exposure to sudden noise, such as gunfire or explosion	Sudden deafness with tinnitus and then improves	Normal	Ringing	Starts with 4,000-cps dip and widens if severe Sometimes permanent	Highest frequency normal unless advanced age and severe damage; nonprogressive	Acoustic trauma
5.	Direct blow to head	Sudden, with ringing tinnitus; may be some improvement	Normal	Some ringing tinnitus	4,000-cps dip, loss in high frequencies or dead ear. Labyrinth also may be affected.	X-ray picture may reveal fracture of temporal bone. Vertigo may be present.	Head trauma
6.	Surgery for otosclerosis Sound distortion and some imbalance	Following surgery for stapes mobilization or stapedectomy	Normal	Usually present with buzz or roar	High tone hearing loss—worse postoperative; discrimination reduced	Discrimination worse postoperatively than preoperatively, even if hearing loss is improved.	Poststapedectomy
7.	Daily exposure to intense noise for many	Insidious	Normal	Uncommon	Early 4,000-cps dip or slightly broader dip	Marked and continuous recruitment	Occupational deafness (early)

months No vertigo					Only a little discrimination change because only high tones involved	Presbycusis
8. Slight difficulty in understanding speech	Insidious	Normal	Occasional hissing	High tone drop at 8,000, 6,000 and 4,000 cps Mild recruitment but continuous Discrimination slightly reduced Bilateral usually	Age group about 50 to 60 Bilateral hearing loss. This type of presbycusis is not clearly established.	Presbycusis
9. Taking ototoxic drugs, especially in presence of kidney infection	Insidious or sudden	Normal	Generally high-pitched	High tone loss bilaterally, but may progress to all frequencies	Recruitment present Deafness usually associated with prolonged administration of drug	Drug ototoxicity

CHART 5. NEURAL HEARING LOSS

HISTORY	ONSET OF HEARING LOSS	OTOSCOPIC	TINNITUS	AUDIOLOGIC	SPECIAL	DIAGNOSIS
Early unilateral high tone hearing loss Later, persistent vertigo	Insidious	Normal	Uncommon	Abnormal tone decay. Wide separation on continuous and interrupted Bekesy tracings. Poor discrimination compared with hearing loss	Unilateral. Marked tone decay. No response to caloric test. Spontaneous nystagmus. Erosion visible by x-ray picture late in disease. Corneal reflex absent	Acoustic neuroma
Trouble understanding some people with soft voices	Insidious	Early atrophic eardrum; more white than normal	Occasional hissing	Gradual high tone hearing loss. Reduced discrimination. No abnormal tone decay. Bone conduction often worse than air conduction	Age range roughly includes 60-75. Bilateral progressive deterioration of hearing. No abnormal tone decay	Presbycusis
Severe head injury with loss of consciousness	Sudden	Normal, or blood in canal if fracture involves middle ear.	Ringing or none	Total, usually unilateral loss of hearing from injury to auditory nerve	X-ray picture shows fracture around internal auditory meatus.	Skull fracture
Sudden hearing loss, occasionally with vertigo or pain in ear	Sudden	Normal	High-pitched	Severe unilateral hearing loss	Other symptoms of herpes may be present.	Virus infection

CHART 6. SENSORINEURAL HEARING LOSS

	History	Onset of Hearing Loss	Otoscopic	Tinnitus	Audiologic	Special	Diagnosis
1.	Difficulty in hearing and understanding speech	Insidious	Normal	Occasional	Usually reduced hearing in all frequencies, especially in higher range. Reduced discrimination	Usually over age 50. Bilateral progressive hearing loss. No abnormal tone decay. Starts at 3,000 to 6,000 cps	Presbycusis
2.	Exposure to intense noise over many months or years	Insidious	Normal	Rare	Early high tone loss (C-5 dip), later involving lower frequencies. Reduced discrimination. Bekesy tracings depend on stage.	In working age group. Bilateral. Starts with higher frequencies and progresses downwards. Usually no abnormal tone decay	Noise-induced hearing loss (Occupational hearing loss)
3.	Severe head injury, often with unconsciousness; subjective vertigo	Sudden	Normal or some middle ear pathology due to fracture	Hissing	Deafness is usually severe but may be only high tone dip or high tone loss.	Fractured temporal bone with absent caloric responses. Eardrum often appears to be normal. No	Head trauma

CHART 6. SENSORINEURAL HEARING LOSS (*Continued*)

History	Onset of Hearing Loss	Otoscopic	Tinnitus	Audiologic	Special	Diagnosis
4. Ototoxic drug, usually in large doses, or a small dose in presence of kidney disease	Sudden	Normal	High-pitched	Rapid, severe bilateral deafness	Rapid and severe bilateral deafness; spontaneous nystagmus, except early	Ototoxicity (neomycin, dihydrostreptomycin, kanamycin or other ototoxic drugs)
5. Exposure to intense noise	Sudden hearing loss and tinnitus, followed by gradual recovery	Normal	Temporary ringing	High tone dip or more severe losses, mostly in high frequencies	Except in unusual cases, recovery occurs within several days.	Auditory fatigue Temporary threshold shift (TTS)
6. Rh incompatibility in parents; kernicterus and speech defect in child	Congenital	Normal	None	Descending audiogram; nonprogressive hearing loss	Speech defect; usually athetoid cerebral palsy	Rh factor
7. Sudden unilateral deafness during or following mumps	Sudden	Normal	None	Total unilateral deafness	Normal vestibular reaction	Mumps

8. Severe deafness after meningitis with high fever	Sudden	Normal	None	Generally subtotal bilateral deafness	Labyrinth also is involved in many cases.	Meningitis
9. Sudden unilateral hearing loss with or without dizziness	Sudden	Normal	High-pitched or motor-like	Subtotal high tone loss, usually unilateral	Occasionally associated with hypotension but generally no specific vascular disease	Vascular disorders
10. Child has retarded or defective speech.	Congenital	Normal	None	High tone loss bilaterally	Often follows maternal rubella in first trimester of pregnancy, or anoxia, trauma or jaundice at birth	In utero and birth lesions
11. Disturbing unilateral tinnitus and deafness	Sudden and sometimes progressive	Normal	May be hissing	High tone loss or subtotal loss of hearing, usually unilateral	Often follows a viral infection	Auditory neuritis

CHART 7. DISTINGUISHING EXTERNAL OTITIS FROM OTITIS MEDIA

	EXTERNAL OTITIS	OTITIS MEDIA
History	Onset after getting water in ear or irritating auditory canal	After rhinitis or blowing nose hard or sneezing
Pain	In auditory canal and around meatus; aggravated by moving auricle and chewing	Deep in ear; aggravated by sneezing and blowing nose
Tenderness	Around auricle	No tenderness
Otoscopic	Skin of canal infected and absence of normal cerumen; eardrum not inflamed	Skin of canal not infected but eardrum injected or bulging
Discharge	Debris from skin of canal	Often mucoid or mucopurulent through tympanic perforation
With air pressure in canal	Eardrum moves with positive pressure.	Eardrum does not move well, especially if perforation is present.
Hearing	Hearing loss disappears when canal is cleared.	Hearing loss is present even with clear canal.
With politzerization	Eardrum moves.	Eardrum does not move well.
	If the external canal is infected, and there is a mucoid discharge, it is a combination of external otitis and otitis media, since the mucus comes from the middle ear through a perforated ear drum.	
Fever	Comparatively little	Often general malaise and fever
X-rays	Normal mastoids and middle ears	Congestion in mastoid and middle ears

Chapter 18

The Otologic History

The first thought of a physician who is consulted by a patient with a hearing difficulty should be to put him at ease. The patient's nerves are likely to be on edge, because he already has suffered much embarrassment from failure to understand other people, who have not always been patient with his handicap. The first thing to do is to face the patient and to speak to him in a distinct and moderate tone. If the patient is wearing a hearing aid, there is usually no need to address him in a loud voice, but it helps to speak slowly and distinctly.

A hearing difficulty is quite a different problem from the usual complaints examined in a physician's practice. Other patients may be concerned about discomfort, itching or pain. Perhaps they are worried that they have cancer. In contrast, the patient with a hearing loss is likely to be in good health.

What drives the hard-of-hearing patient to the physician is not so much the hearing loss itself as the social and the vocational difficulties he has been encountering because of his inability to hold his own in communication. Therefore, when he first tells the doctor about his problem, he probably will have a great deal to unburden about his psychological, social and business problems.

ESSENTIAL QUESTIONS

The physician often can save much time and be more helpful to his patient by asking certain meaningful questions that have a direct bearing on the nature of the patient's problem. The answers to these questions may help him to make a differential diagnosis of the hearing impairment.

These are among the essential questions:

How long have you been aware of your hearing trouble?

Did it come on suddenly or slowly?

Has it been getting worse?

What makes it worse?

Did your hearing trouble start with pregnancy? (Ask in appropriate cases.)

Is there deafness in your family?

Do you hear better in a quiet or noisy room?

Are there noises in your ears, and what do they sound like?

Have you ever had dizziness? If so, describe in detail.

Does your hearing fluctuate noticeably?

Have you ever had ear infections? If so, do you know what medicine was prescribed for it?

Did you ever have a speech defect as a child?

What kind of work do you do?

What sort of medicines have you been taking?

In the case of children, parents should be asked to supply information on any possible history of difficulties at birth and of early childhood diseases, such as anoxia, severe jaundice, blood dyscrasias or a hemorrhagic tendency. A history of convulsions and high fevers with their causes also is important.

THE IMPORTANCE OF GETTING ACCURATE ANSWERS

Very frequently, the patient without realizing it gives inaccurate answers to some of the questions in the history. This is particularly true of the length of time the hearing loss has been present. Usually, the patient underestimates the duration of the handicap.

Quite often it is an advantage to have the patient's husband or wife present at the taking of the history, as he or she often is able to supply more accurate information. One reason is that many hearing losses develop so insidiously that the patient is quite unaware of having any hearing trouble until it is quite pronounced, long after the hearing loss has become obvious to everyone else. Mild suggestions that perhaps his hearing is less keen may have been made to him for a long time, but the patient laughed them off and forgot about them.

In some instances patients refuse to recognize or to admit that their hearing is defective even after the trouble has become extremely apparent to all their associates. This common observation illustrates the psychological overtones that frequently complicate certain forms of hearing impairment.

The exact time of onset of deafness may be critical, particularly when it is rather sudden. Hearing may be lost suddenly after a patient puts his finger in his ears and thereby blocks the ear canal with a plug of wax. Or the sudden onset may be due to Ménière's disease, mumps, rupture of a blood vessel, allergy, or undetermined diseases affecting the inner ear or the auditory nerve. In practically all such cases only one of the ears is involved. When the cause is meningitis or a severe head injury, both ears may be affected. Most frequently, a hearing loss develops slowly over a long term of years, especially in presbycusis, otosclerosis, deafness following exposure to intense noise, and hereditary nerve deafness.

Since otosclerosis, presbycusis and hereditary nerve deafness are determined genetically, or at least have a tendency to recur in families, the question of familial occurrence is of some importance. Quite frequently, the patient is certain there is no history of deafness in his family, and yet at the completion of the studies the diagnosis may point to a hereditary or familial condition. On further questioning the patient sometimes does recall that one or several members of his family were afflicted with a hearing impairment. More often the patient keeps insisting that there has been no deafness in his family. This statement can be true, for in many cases of hereditary deafness the hearing loss may not manifest itself for many generations. In otosclerosis, for example, there may be no recent evidence of deafness in any living member of the family, and yet it is known that otosclerosis has a heritable tendency.

PROGNOSIS AND DIAGNOSIS

A vital question in the minds of both the physician and the patient is: "Will the hearing loss get worse?" The answer depends on the diagnosis. For example, hereditary nerve deafness is likely to get worse and may become quite profound. On the other hand, otosclerosis may progress but level off and not become very severe. Some otosclerotics, however, have a tendency to develop nerve deafness, and the hearing of the patients deteriorates early in life. Congenital deafness infrequently progresses.

The patient often can help the otologist arrive at a more definite diagnosis, even on his first visit, by indicating with some certainty whether the hearing loss has remained constant or has been getting worse over a period of months or years. It helps the otologist to distinguish deafness due to noise from that due to heredity or advancing age. A diagnosis that reveals an inherently nonprogressive condition is a source of great comfort and satisfaction to both the otologist and the patient.

DIFFERENTIATING SYMPTOMS

SENSORINEURAL OR CONDUCTIVE HEARING LOSS

Asking a patient whether he hears better in a quiet or a noisy environment usually provokes an expression of bewilderment. "I wonder what he means by that?" seems to be written on the patient's face. Actually, the answer to this question provides a valuable preliminary clue as to whether the patient has a sensorineural or a conductive hearing loss. In many cases of conductive deafness, especially in otosclerosis, there is a tendency to hear better in noisy places, whereas in perceptive hearing loss there often is a tendency to hear much more poorly in a noisy environment. The ability to hear better in the presence of noise is called paracusis Willisiana and is named after Thomas Willis, the physician who first described this phenomenon.

TINNITUS

One of the least understood and therefore most frustrating conditions encountered by the otologist is tinnitus. Various types of tinnitus are associated so often with specific types of hearing handicaps that a complaint of tinnitus and a description of its characteristics can be helpful.

VERTIGO

Along with tinnitus, dizziness (vertigo) is a frequent companion of deafness. Because the hearing and the balance mechanisms are related so intimately and bathed in the same labyrinthine fluid, vertigo often complicates hearing difficulties. Some disturbances in the labyrinthine fluid produce not only hearing loss but also disturbance of balance. To the otologist vertigo does not mean lightheadedness, fainting or seeing spots before the eyes. It does not mean even a slight sensation of loss of balance. It generally portrays a sensation of turning, a feeling as if the room or the objects in it were revolving around the subject. Quite often, a sick feeling in the stomach, or nausea, accompanies the sensation of rotary vertigo, which is similar to that felt by an inexperienced sailor on a storm-tossed ship. Labyrinthine vertigo can produce a loss of balance during walking; the patient may find it difficult to walk in a straight line because of a sensation of swaying from side to side. A full discussion of tinnitus and vertigo is found in Chapter 16.

FLUCTUATION IN HEARING

Practically all people with hearing trouble are aware of fluctuation in their hearing. Most patients seem to hear better in the morning and worse at night. Some claim they hear better after they inflate their ears (by pinching the nose, closing the lips and blowing—the so-called Valsalva maneuver). Many factors are involved in a fluctuating hearing level. For instance, most people seem to hear much better when they are rested and relaxed than when they are tired and upset, as at the end of a hard day. Alertness may sharpen, whereas inattention may dull, auditory efficiency. Some types of deafness, such as Ménière's disease, are inherently subject to sharp fluctuations in hearing.

Self-inflation. Although it is true that some people actually can improve their hearing by inflating their ears, the vast majority experience only a clear feeling of air in their ears, which leads them to feel subjectively better without actually hearing better. This subjective improvement is usually short-lived and provides little benefit. On the other hand, indiscreet self-inflation can lead to ear infections and abnormal eardrums.

Ototoxic Drugs

Since large doses of certain drugs are known to cause hearing loss, questions concerning the use of dihydrostreptomycin, neomycin and kanamycin may have an important bearing on the diagnosis. A history of previous ear infections, as well as systemic infections, also may yield important clues.

Speech

Because the development of speech is dependent on hearing, it is not surprising that deafness or defective hearing in infancy or early childhood can result in speech problems. This is the reason that for centuries people who were deaf from birth also were considered to be dumb. One of the important clues the otologist uses in his diagnosis is the patient's speech. Features such as loudness, strain and poor articulation all help him to establish the type and the prognosis of a hearing loss.

For example, a hard-of-hearing patient who speaks in a loud and strained voice in all probability has a sensorineural type of hearing loss. If his voice is unusually soft, he probably has otosclerosis. If a child has a speech defect, particularly with the letters *s* and *x*, in all likelihood he has a high tone nerve defect.

Noise-induced Loss

Questions to determine the patient's line of work help to bring out whether he has been exposed to very intense noise. A history of military service or other exposure to gunfire also is important. The increasing number of people who lose their hearing because of exposure to intense industrial noise is a subject of serious concern to many elements of society. This problem is considered in Chapter 26.

The history is of such pertinence in an otologic examination that quite often it suggests a diagnosis which then may require only a few special tests for confirmation. In such instances many needless studies can be eliminated, and much time and energy can be saved.

PREVIOUS EAR SURGERY

Another question of increasing importance concerns previous ear surgery. At one time it could be readily established that the patient had had a mastoidectomy by looking for the postauricular scar. Nowadays modern otologic surgery leaves little or no scar. Surgery for correction of otosclerosis and ossicular defects leaves no detectable scar, and even the most observant otologist cannot know whether a patient has had previous surgery. Not uncommonly, a patient who has had stapes surgery is embarrassed or unwilling to admit it to his new otologist, and so the otologist may reoperate without realizing that he is performing a revision rather than an initial procedure. Therefore, it is always helpful to ask directly whether a patient has had any surgery to correct his deafness.

Chapter 19

The Otologic Examination

Every patient complaining of a hearing loss, tinnitus, vertigo or any other aural symptom requires a complete examination of the head and the neck. Simply examining the ears is not sufficient, since the cause of some otologic symptoms lies in the nasopharynx, the posterior choanal fossa, the temporomandibular joint or even the throat.

A STANDARD PATTERN FOR A COMPLETE EXAMINATION

It is advisable to develop a standard pattern for a complete examination so that nothing is overlooked. If this pattern is followed persistently, it becomes routine to examine the opposite ear and the nasopharynx even though the presumptive cause of the patient's symptoms is located immediately and cleared up, as by removing impacted cerumen from one ear.

Some physicians begin their examinations by first inspecting the ear to which complaints are directed. The author finds it preferable to examine first the nose, then the neck and the throat, then the presumably normal ear, and finally the so-called "bad ear." The chief reason for this is that too frequently he has overlooked the opposite ear and the nasopharynx after becoming completely engrossed in an examination of the ear that produced the symptoms. Occasionally, the patient asks pointedly, "Doctor, aren't you going to look at my other ear or my throat?"

Passing Probes

The time required to perform a complete examination can be shortened by first inspecting the nose with a nasal speculum and at the same time spraying the nasal cavities with 1 per cent cocaine or Pontocaine to prepare them to receive the nasopharyngoscope. After examining the condition of the turbinates and looking for discharge and obstruction by polyps, a small amount of 4 per cent cocaine then is applied to the floor of the nose with a fine probe tipped with cotton. It takes very little of this medication and only a few minutes to anesthetize the floor sufficiently to pass the nasopharyngoscope. It may seem presumptuous to point out the sensitivity of the nasal passages, but so many complaints from patients are heard about the discomfort in their noses after examinations that it warrants comment. Extreme gentleness is indicated in passing probes, and especially a nasoscope, into the nasal passage. If after shrinking the mucosa a direct passage still is not clearly visible, the other nares should be used. Many times the passage is blocked by spurs or a deviated septum, and it is unwise to try to force a rigid instrument past a bony obstruction. With care and patience it is possible to pass instruments through the vast majority of nasal passages without causing pain or irritating the nasal mucosa.

If pus is found in the nose, its source should be determined, if possible. Is it from the middle meatus or from further back toward the nasopharynx? The discharge should be sucked out with a fine nasal tip before passing the nasoscope. The appearance and the consistency of the mucosa over the turbinates also should be noted. Is it pale and boggy, or red and tense? Does it shrink markedly after being cocainized? How about the nasal airway? Is it adequate before shrinkage, and what happens after shrinking? The author avoids passing the nasopharyngoscope until the last part of the examination. This gives time for the cocaine to take effect and reserves the most frightening part of the examination until last, the more so since by then the patient already has gained confidence in the examination. When the nasoscope is passed, it should be slid along the floor of the nose with utmost gentleness. During the passage of the instrument the roof of the nose and the posterior turbinates can be seen. Finally, the nasopharynx, the eustachian tubes and Rosenmüller's fossae are scrutinized carefully on both sides.

THE EUSTACHIAN TUBES

The functional efficiency of the eustachian tubes can be estimated in part by having the patient swallow while the physician looks at the prominent cartilaginous lips (tori) of the tubal orifices through the nasoscope. The tori should move freely. If a bubble covers the tubal orifice, and the tube is normal, the bubble should break during swallowing. It is most important to look for thick bands of adhesions or growths of adenoid tissue in the fossae of Rosenmüller behind the tubal openings. Sometimes these can be seen best by placing a good-sized mirror on the depressed tongue and looking up into the nasopharynx.

Neck, Throat, Mouth

Before inspecting the throat it is wise to palpate the thyroid area and the cervical and the posterior areas for glands and neoplasms. Temporomandibular joints also should be felt while the patient opens his mouth very wide. If crackling, dislocation or tenderness is detected, it should be brought to the patient's attention, especially if a defective bite is observed. The teeth and the mouth should be examined routinely, as well as the larynx, with the aid of a laryngeal mirror. The epiglottis and the base of the tongue should not be overlooked.

EARS

Before the nasopharyngoscope is passed, the ears are examined, attention being given first to the "better" one. The auricle and the entrance to the external canal are seen better with a head mirror than with the otoscope. Sometimes a small cyst or furuncle situated just at the entrance to the canal otherwise may be overlooked and cause pain when the otoscope is inserted. Choose an otoscope with as large a tip as will fit comfortably. A large tip not only affords broader vision but also fits more snugly in the canal, so that alternate positive and negative pressure can be applied to the eardrum with a small rubber bulb to test the mobility of the eardrum. This procedure is useful also to discover whether there is a perforation in the eardrum.

Eardrum

Removal of Wax or Debris. If wax or debris is present, it should be removed carefully, so that the entire drum can be seen. Whenever possible, the wax should be picked out gently in one piece with a dull ear curette. Irrigation should be reserved for those cases in which there is no likelihood of a perforation, and the wax is impacted and difficult to pick or wipe out. When the drum has a perforation, irrigation may result in middle ear infection. Any debris, such as that due to external otitis or otitis media, should be wiped out carefully with a thin cotton-tipped applicator or removed with a fine suction tip. If bony protrusions (exostoses) are noted in the canal, care should be taken to avoid injuring the thin skin covering them, so as to prevent bleeding and infection. If a large tip on the otoscope makes it difficult to see the drum for any reason, a smaller tip is used, but care is essential in inserting it deeply.

Cone of Light. A great deal of information can be derived from a discerning scrutiny of the eardrum. In a normal eardrum a cone of light classically is seen coming from the end of the umbo or handle of the malleus, because of the manner in which the sloping drum reflects the otoscopic light. In some eardrums the cone of light may not be seen, but this does not mean necessarily that an important abnormality exists. Absence of the cone of light may be due to the abnormal slope of the drum, or the angle of the external canal, or a thickening of the eardrum or senile changes that perhaps do not allow the light to be reflected.

Intact or Perforated Eardrum. An essential point to look for in the drum is whether it is intact. Most of the time a hole in the eardrum is readily visible. Sometimes, however, it is difficult to see a perforation, and occasionally what appears to be one is really an old perforation that now is healed over completely with a thin transparent film of epithelium. If a patient has a discharge that does not come from the external canal, or if the discharge seen is found to be mucoid, then the physician must always look carefully for the perforation through which the discharge issues. It is important to look for the pinpoint perforation likely to be present when a patient complains that he hears air whistling in his ear whenever he blows his nose or sneezes.

There are several ways to detect a perforation in the eardrum. One is to move the drum back and forth with air pressure in the external canal. This is done with a special otoscope or the rubber bulb attached to some otoscopes. If the drum freely moves back and forth, it is in all likelihood intact. If it does not move, or moves only slightly, the perforation may become visible, since the perforated area moves more sluggishly than the rest of the drum. If a perforation is high in the area of Shrapnell's membrane, the drum still may move fairly well. Another technic (politzerization) to detect a perforation is to have the patient swallow while a camphorated mist is forced into one nostril, and the other nostril is pinched shut. If the eustachian tube is patent, and there is a perforation in the drum the examiner, looking into the external auditory canal, will see the mist coming out through the small perforation. Sometimes spraying a film of powder, such as boric acid powder, on the drum delineates the edges of the perforation. All these procedures can be used also to see whether there is a transparent film over a healed perforation, but gentleness and care are essential to avoid breaking the film.

Shadow Formations. Another important thing to look for is the shadow formations behind the drum, particularly those caused by fluid in the middle ear. To accomplish this the otologist should try to look through the drum rather than merely at it. In this way what seemed to be a simple surface becomes a map with a dark shadow for the round window niche and a lighter area for the promontory, a pink area for the incus, and many other features.

REVELATION OF FLUID IN THE MIDDLE EAR. Fluid in the middle ear often eludes detection, even though it causes hearing loss. This failure easily may result in a wrong diagnosis. For instance, a patient may have a 30-db conductive hearing loss with an eardrum that to all intents and purposes appears to be practically normal. The diagnosis then would naturally be otosclerosis, and stapes surgery would be indicated. When the eardrum is reflected during surgery, however, a thick mucoid gelatinous mass is encountered, especially around the oval and the round windows, and the correct diagnosis is not otosclerosis but secretory otitis media. The fluid was simply not detected preoperatively.

A diligent search should be made for fluid in the middle ear if bone conduction is reduced slightly in an otherwise classic picture of conductive hearing loss. There are several ways to detect fluid in the middle ear. If a well-defined fluid level is seen through the eardrum, the diagnosis is simple. It should be borne in mind, however, that strands of scar tissue in the drum and bands in the middle ear can simulate a fluid level. It helps to see if the apparent fluid level stays in position while the patient's head is bent forward and backward. With air pressure in the external canal, it is difficult to get free to-and-fro motion of the drum if there is much fluid behind it in the middle ear. This is in contrast with a normal drum, which is moved easily. Occasionally, bubbles can be seen in the fluid. This assures the diagnosis.

Politzerization is of great help in detecting fluid but should not be performed in the presence of an upper respiratory infection, particularly one affecting the nose. During the politzerization the fluid and the bubbles can be seen briefly through the drum; then they usually disappear. The patient may profess to hear better suddenly.

Whenever there is any doubt about the presence of middle ear fluid, a *myringotomy* should be performed for diagnostic and therapeutic reasons. In adults this is done best without local or general anesthesia by using a sharp knife to puncture the posterior portion of the drum. If fluid is present, some usually will ooze out spontaneously, or it can be forced out by politzerization or suction in the myringotomy, if it is done deftly. Manipulation in an attempt to produce some local anesthesia often prolongs the procedure and causes discomfort.

Scars and Plaques; Color; Tumor. The eardrum may reveal still other findings, such as scars and plaques. These reflect previous infections and tissue changes in the eardrum. They rarely in themselves cause any significant degree of hearing loss. Occasionally, an eardrum appears to be blue or purple. This may be due to a block in the middle ear, or to entrapped fluid, or it may be merely a peculiar type of retracted eardrum. A reddish color occasionally is due to a tumor (glomus jugulare) extending into the middle ear. If there is any possibility that such a tumor might be present, exploration should be done with great circumspection.

Retracted Eardrum. This is another abnormal finding. It is easy to understand why one physician will look at a drum and say it is normal, whereas another observer will say it is retracted. Eardrums vary in their appearance, and the concept of retraction is subject to comparable variations. Be this as it may, it should make little difference in otology, for even a moderate amount of retraction per se may not cause any significant hearing loss. Only when the drum is retracted markedly, and especially when it is pulled into the promontory, is there a correlation between retraction and hearing. In such instances politzerization can restore hearing by returning the drum to its original position. Occasionally, the drum is overdistended during politzerization, and then it appears to be flaccid and relaxed.

In all cases of retracted eardrum the cause should be sought in the nasopharynx, the sinuses and the eustachian tubes. Allergies and adenoids are the most common causes, but neoplasms also must be excluded, especially in unilateral cases. Aerotitis media may be another cause of a retracted eardrum. In some patients politzerization is not possible, and a small eustachian catheter has to be introduced gently into the mouth of the eustachian tube, generally guided by a nasopharyngoscope positioned through the other naris. The air can be forced in carefully until the tube is opened. By placing a listening tube in the patient's ear and the other end in the physician's ear the sound of air can be heard as it enters the middle ear.

Erosion; Previous Surgery; Drainage. Perhaps the most confusing otologic picture presents itself when the eardrum is largely eroded, and the middle ear is discharging; a similar problem arises when some kind of mastoid surgery has deformed the normal landmarks. It is necessary in such cases to appraise the condition of the middle ear in order to decide on the proper treatment and to evaluate the chances of restoring hearing. In view of the extensive amount of otologic surgery that has been performed in recent years, it is always wise to look at scars of previous operations, both postauricular and endaural, the latter being situated just above the tragus. A postauricular scar usually indicates mastoid surgery. If the eardrum is practically normal, it was in all likelihood a simple mastoidectomy, and the hearing very well may be within normal limits. If the eardrum is gone, and the malleus and the incus also are absent, there was a radical mastoidectomy, and the hearing level should be about 50 to 60 db. Intermediate between the simple and the radical mastoidectomies are various surgical procedures aimed at both preserving as much hearing as possible and eradicating the infection. These procedures usually are called modified radical mastoidectomies or tympanoplasties. Usually, the drum or part of it is visible, and some form of ossicular chain is present. In modern technics a polyethylene or Teflon tube may have been inserted to restore ossicular continuity; also a vein graft or skin graft may have been applied to replace the eardrum that had been removed previously. The endaural scar could indicate also a fenestration operation, in which case an eardrum will be visible, but it will seem to be out of place, and at least some part of the mastoid bone will have been exenterated. Quite often these cavities are covered with debris and require gentle cleaning to permit a clear view. Caution is necessary in cleaning such a cavity around a fenestrated area to avoid inducing vertigo and nystagmus.

A large amount of stapes surgery is being performed, but usually this leaves no evident scar, and so previous stapes surgery must be uncovered in the history. In stapes surgery the incision is made inside the external auditory canal on its posterior wall, and the drum is reflected forward upon itself, so that the surgeon can work in the middle ear. Healing is almost free of visible scars in the canal.

It is becoming increasingly common to see eardrums of a very peculiar appearance, in which infection has played no part. In most cases the unusual features are the result of myringoplasties with skin, fascia or vein grafts. The drum may appear to be thick and flaccid or whitish, and it may show few landmarks. The patient best can supply the pertinent information in such instances. Another strange experience with an eardrum is to see something sticking out of it that looks like a small tube; and that is precisely what it is, a tiny piece of polyethylene or Teflon tubing that has been inserted through a small perforation to prevent closure and to allow drainage from the middle ear. This is usually done in cases of persistent secretory otitis media.

OTHER CONDITIONS

Chickenpox occasionally leaves a small pockmark on the eardrum that may persist for many years. Blood in the middle ear following head injury has an important connotation. It generally indicates a fracture in the middle cranial fossa. Hearing tests help to determine the extent of involvement, especially if the inner ear is damaged.

Objective Tinnitis. Two other rare conditions are mentioned here. In one the patient insists that the physician, too, should be able to hear the whistling or gurgling that he himself hears in his ears. In these cases the physician should by all means put his ear to the patient's ear or use a listening tube to find out if there is a bruit indicating some vascular disorder or a click from the nasopharynx or the middle ear. The other phenomenon is an intermittent spasm of the soft palate. This produces a clicking sensation heard in the ear. The cause is unknown, but the condition easily is recognized when it is encountered. Both these rare conditions are called objective tinnitus, because they can be heard by an examiner.

Whenever there is a possibility of an **acoustic neuroma** being present, vestibular tests are essential. The interpretation of these tests is not included in this book. However, it is essential to point out that whenever a patient has spontaneous nystagmus of the labyrinthine type, i.e., when the nystagmus has a fast and a slow component, vestibular and hearing tests are of utmost importance.

Chapter 20

The Physics of Sound

One need not be a physicist to record or to interpret an audiogram, but a brief review of the basic notions underlying the perception and the measurement of sound will increase understanding of what physicians do in the service of patients with a hearing loss.

Why does an audiologist or an otologist use a different base line for his decibels in his office from that used by an engineer or an industrial physician who measures the noise level in a factory? Why is it that when hearing at high sound frequencies is tested, the patient may hear nothing and then suddenly hear a tone loud? Yet all the examiner did was to move the earphone a fraction of an inch. Why is it that when two machines are placed close together, each making 60 decibels of noise, the total noise is not 120 db?

The conscientious physician, interested in the problems of his hard-of-hearing patient, should know the ABC's of the physics of sound as they relate to these and other practical problems.

WHAT ARE SOUND WAVES?

When a sound wave is generated by striking a tuning fork, by exercising the vocal cords or by other means, a vibrating object imparts its vibrations to air molecules, causing them alternately to be compressed and rarefied in a rhythmic pattern. This pattern communicates itself, more or less in a straight line, to adjacent air molecules at a very rapid rate (1,100 feet per second). Air-borne sound is therefore a rapid alternation in atmospheric pressure.

CHARACTERISTICS OF SOUND WAVES

Sound waves will travel through air and more rapidly through water.

They are conducted also by solids. An ear placed close to the iron rail of a train track will detect the approach of the train before the air-borne sounds can reach the observer. Thus sounds travel through different media at different speeds; the speed also varies when the medium is not uniform. However, sound waves are not transmitted through a vacuum. This can be demonstrated by the classic experiment of placing a ringing alarm clock inside a bell jar and then exhausting the air through an outlet. The ringing will no longer be heard when the air is exhausted, but it will be heard again immediately when air is readmitted. This experiment emphasizes the importance of the medium through which sound waves travel.

The bones of the head also conduct sounds, but ordinarily the ear is much more sensitive to sounds that are air-borne. Under certain abnormal conditions, as in cases of conductive deafness, a patient may hear better by bone conduction than by air conduction. Such an individual can hear the vibrations of a tuning fork much better when it is held directly touching the skull than when it is held next to the ear but without touching the head.

Sound waves travel in straight lines in all directions from the source, decreasing in intensity at a rate inversely proportional to the square of the distance from their source. This means that if a person shortens his distance from the source of a sound and moves from a position 4 feet away to only 2 feet from the source, the sound will be 4 times as loud rather than merely twice as loud. In practical application this inverse square law applies only in instances in which there are no walls or ceiling. It is not strictly valid in a room where sound waves encounter obstruction or reflection, and this is one very important reason that voice tests commonly performed by increasing the distance of a whisper or a watch tick from the subject rarely can be truly accurate or reliable.

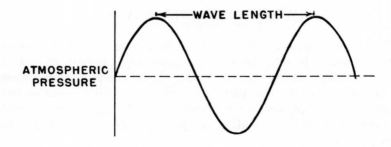

Fig. 113. Diagram of a pure tone (sine wave).
(Figures 113 to 115, 117, 118, 121 and 136 are from Sataloff, Joseph: Industrial Deafness, New York, Blakiston Division, McGraw-Hill, 1957)

When sound travels through air and encounters an obstruction such as a wall, the sound waves can bend around the obstacle almost like water passing around a rock in a stream. Distortion of sound waves by wind is a common occurrence, as, for instance, when sounds travel with or against the wind. The effect also varies according to whether the wind blows faster near the ground or above it.

Frequency, Amplitude, Pitch and Loudness. A simple type of sound wave, called a *pure tone*, is pictured in Figure 113. This is a graphic representation of one complete vibration, with the area of compression represented by the top curve and the area of rarefaction by the bottom curve.

A pure tone has two important characteristics: (1) *frequency*, which is the number of times per second that a complete vibration occurs; and (2) *intensity*, which is a measure of the maximum swing of vibration of an air particle. When a pure tone is represented graphically, its intensity is indicated by the height of the wave from the base line.

A tuning fork of a specified frequency is so constructed that it vibrates the required number of times per second to produce the tone of that frequency. No matter how hard or how gently the tuning fork is struck, its prongs always will vibrate back and forth the same number of times each second. If it is struck hard, it will not vibrate faster, but it will vibrate more intensely: that is, its prongs will cover a greater distance or amplitude from their starting place (Fig. 114).

The *pitch* that the ear hears from a vibrating tuning fork is related intimately to its frequency. Similarly, the *loudness* of the tone is related intimately to its intensity or amplitude. In general, the greater the frequency, the higher is the pitch, and the greater the intensity, the louder is the sound. We say these terms are related intimately rather than inter-

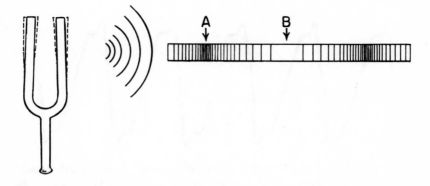

FIG. 114. Areas of compression (A) and rarefaction (B) produced by a vibrating tuning fork.

changeable, because the relationships are somewhat more complicated than may appear at first glance, though no purpose would be served by attempting a formal explanation. Suffice it to say that frequency and intensity are terms used in physics to denote exact physical measurements. Their correlates of pitch and loudness are terms used in psychology or psychoacoustics to describe sensations perceived by the brain through the ear. For example, a tuning fork may vibrate at a frequency of 1,000 cycles per second, but it is heard as a certain pitch or musical note, as on a violin or a piano.

THE OCTAVE. When two frequencies have a relationship of 2 to 1, they constitute an octave. For example, the 500-cycle tone on the audiometer is one octave above the 250-cycle tone, and one octave below the 1,000-cycle tone. When frequencies have this kind of whole-number relationship, the higher frequency is said to be a *harmonic* of the lower, and the lower frequency is called the *fundamental*.

COMPLEX SOUNDS. The pure tone is in contrast to more complex sounds, such as speech, music and noise. Rarely are pure tones encountered in daily life. Most sounds are very complex with many different wave forms superimposed on each other. Noise usually is composed of unrelated random frequencies, whereas musical tones usually are related to one another (Fig. 115).

It is somewhat difficult to define noise accurately, because so much of its meaning depends on its effect at any specific time and place rather

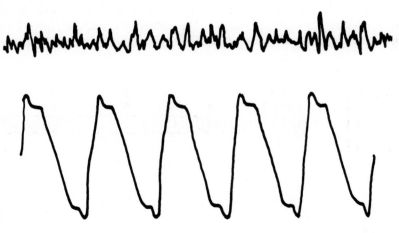

FIG. 115. Upper graph depicts typical street noise. Lower graph depicts C on a piano. (Fletcher, Harvey: Speech and Hearing in Communication, Bell Telephone Laboratories Series, New York, Van Nostrand, 1953; Sataloff, Joseph: Industrial Deafness, p. 9, New York, Blakiston Division, McGraw-Hill, 1957)

than on its physical characteristics. Sound can in one instance or by one individual be considered as most annoying noise, whereas on another occasion or to another observer the same sound may seem to be pleasant and undeserving of being stigmatized as "noise." For the purpose of this book, the term *noise* is used broadly to designate any unwanted sound.

The Standing Wave. An interesting aspect of sound waves related to hearing testing is a phenomenon called the "standing wave." Without delving too deeply into this subject, it is sufficient to say that under certain circumstances two wave trains of equal amplitude and frequency traveling in opposite directions can cancel out at certain points called "nodes." Figure 116 is a diagram of such a situation. It will be noted that when a violin string is plucked in a certain manner, at point "n" (node) there is no displacement. If this point falls at the eardrum or some other sensitive spot receiving the sound in the ear, the listener will not be aware of any sound, because the point has no amplitude and cannot excite the ear. This phenomenon occasionally occurs in hearing tests, particularly in testing at 8,000 cycles and above. These higher frequencies are likely to be involved, because the ear canal is only about 1⅛ inches long, and the wavelength of sound at such high frequencies is of the same order of magnitude.

Furthermore, when sound waves are produced within small enclosures, as when a receiver is placed over the air, the sound waves encounter many reflections, and much of the sound at high frequencies is likely to be in the form of standing waves. Hardly any sound energy is transmitted by these standing waves, and so the intensity is almost zero or at best very low, even though the pressures in each wave may be quite large. Such waves often do not serve as exciting stimuli to the inner ear, and no sensation of hearing is produced because of the absence of transmission of sound energy.

Sometimes, by simply holding the earphone a little more tightly or loosely to the ear in testing the higher frequencies, suddenly no sound may be produced at all when it should be loud, or a loud sound may be heard when a moment before there seemed to be no sound. This phenomenon occurs because of the presence of standing waves.

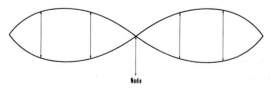

Node

Fig 116. Diagram of a standing wave showing the nodal point at which there is no amplitude.

Wavelength. It is comparatively easy to estimate the length of a wave if its frequency is known. If it is recalled that sound waves travel about 1,100 feet per second, it is possible, for example, to determine the wavelength of a 1,000-cycle per second frequency by simple division. This will result in 1.1 feet per cycle, since the "seconds" cancel themselves out. The wavelength of a frequency of 8,000 cycles per second thus would be 1,100 divided by 8,000, which equals .13 feet or about 1 inch.

The long wavelength of the low frequencies makes these sounds very difficult to attenuate or to absorb and explains the reason that they are so imperfectly attenuated by ear protectors or reduced by simple noise abatement measures.

MEASURING SOUND

In the kind of noise measurement done in industry the chief concern is with very intense noise, whereas in the testing of hearing the primary concern is with very weak sounds, because the purpose is to determine the individual's threshold of hearing. How, then, is it possible to compare and to measure the intensity of sound that is described as low, weak, loud, etc.?

Sound, a Form of Energy

Since sound is a form of energy, it can be measured in various ways. The measurement of its power can be expressed in units called watts or horsepower; the measurement of its pressure can be expressed in microbars, 1 million microbars being equal to a standard atmospheric pressure of 14.7 pounds per square inch. Since the human ear responds not to the power but to the pressure fluctuation in the sound wave, in calculations the pressure units must be used rather than the power units. The unit of measurement, then, is the *microbar*, with 1 microbar being one millionth of the normal atmospheric pressure, or, as it often is expressed, one dyne per square centimeter ($dyne/cm^2$).

Range of Sound Detectable by the Human Ear

The weakest sound pressure that the keen, young human ear can detect under very quiet conditions is about .0002 microbar, and this very small amount of pressure is used as the basis or the reference level for *noise* measurements. This basis usually is determined by using a 1,000-cycle tone (a frequency in the range of the maximum sensitivity of the ear) and reducing the pressure to the weakest measurable sound pressure to which the young ear will respond. In some instances the keen ear under ideal conditions will respond to a pressure even weaker than .0002 microbar, but it is the .0002 microbar pressure that is used as a base.

Of course, sound pressures can be increased tremendously above this weakest tone. The usual range of audible sound pressures extends upward to about 2,000 microbars, a point at which the pressure causes discomfort and pain in the ears. This range is equivalent to an energy increase of over a trillion times the basic pressure. Higher pressures can damage or even destroy the inner ear. This is such a very great range (.0002 microbar to 2,000 microbars) that the use of the microbar as a measurement of sound is too cumbersome.

DECIBEL

From the field of communication engineering the term "decibel" has been borrowed, and it is this term that most generally is used to describe sound intensity. The detailed manner in which this unit was derived and the manner in which it is converted to other units is somewhat complicated and not within the scope of this book. However, a very clear understanding of the nature of the decibel and the proper use of the term is most valuable in understanding how hearing is tested, and noise is measured.

The decibel is simply a **unit of comparison**—a ratio—between two sound pressures. In general, it is not a unit of measurement with an absolute value, such as an inch or a pound. The concept of the decibel is based on the pressure of one sound or reference level, with which the pressure of another sound is compared. Thus, a sound of 60 decibels is a sound that is 60 decibels more intense than a sound that has been standardized as the reference level. The reference level must be either implied or specifically stated in all sound measurements, for without the reference level the expression of intensity in terms of decibels is meaningless. It would be the same as saying that something is "twice," without either implying or referring specifically to the other object with which it is being compared.

Two Reference Levels. For the purposes of this book two important reference levels are used. In making physical noise measurements, as in a noisy industry, the base used is the sound pressure of .0002 microbar, which is known as *acoustical zero* decibels. Sound measuring instruments such as sound-level meters and noise analyzers are calibrated with this reference level. When a reading is made in a room, and the meter reads so many decibels, the reading means that the sound pressure level in that room is so many decibels greater than acoustical zero.

The other important reference level is used in audiometry and is known

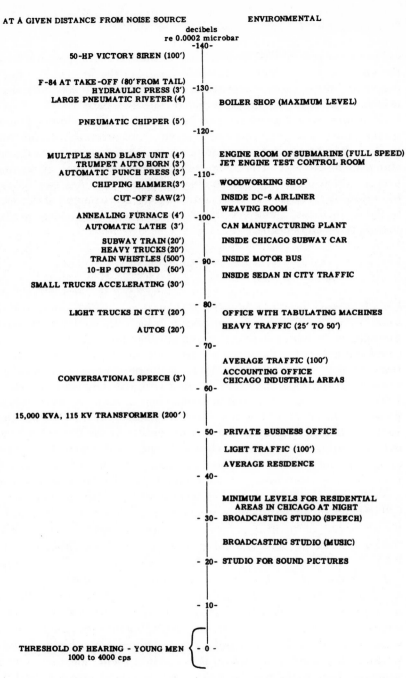

AT A GIVEN DISTANCE FROM NOISE SOURCE	decibels re 0.0002 microbar	ENVIRONMENTAL
	-140-	
50-HP VICTORY SIREN (100')		
F-84 AT TAKE-OFF (80' FROM TAIL) HYDRAULIC PRESS (3') LARGE PNEUMATIC RIVETER (4')	-130-	BOILER SHOP (MAXIMUM LEVEL)
PNEUMATIC CHIPPER (5')	-120-	
MULTIPLE SAND BLAST UNIT (4') TRUMPET AUTO HORN (3') AUTOMATIC PUNCH PRESS (3')	-110-	ENGINE ROOM OF SUBMARINE (FULL SPEED) JET ENGINE TEST CONTROL ROOM
CHIPPING HAMMER (3')		WOODWORKING SHOP
CUT-OFF SAW (2')		INSIDE DC-6 AIRLINER WEAVING ROOM
ANNEALING FURNACE (4') AUTOMATIC LATHE (3')	-100-	CAN MANUFACTURING PLANT
SUBWAY TRAIN (20') HEAVY TRUCKS (20') TRAIN WHISTLES (500') 10-HP OUTBOARD (50')	-90-	INSIDE CHICAGO SUBWAY CAR INSIDE MOTOR BUS
SMALL TRUCKS ACCELERATING (30')		INSIDE SEDAN IN CITY TRAFFIC
	-80-	
LIGHT TRUCKS IN CITY (20') AUTOS (20')		OFFICE WITH TABULATING MACHINES HEAVY TRAFFIC (25' TO 50')
	-70-	
CONVERSATIONAL SPEECH (3')		AVERAGE TRAFFIC (100') ACCOUNTING OFFICE CHICAGO INDUSTRIAL AREAS
	-60-	
15,000 KVA, 115 KV TRANSFORMER (200')		
	-50-	PRIVATE BUSINESS OFFICE
		LIGHT TRAFFIC (100') AVERAGE RESIDENCE
	-40-	
	-30-	MINIMUM LEVELS FOR RESIDENTIAL AREAS IN CHICAGO AT NIGHT BROADCASTING STUDIO (SPEECH)
		BROADCASTING STUDIO (MUSIC)
	-20-	STUDIO FOR SOUND PICTURES
	-10-	
THRESHOLD OF HEARING - YOUNG MEN 1000 to 4000 cps	-0-	

FIG. 117. Typical over-all sound levels measured with a sound-level meter. (General Radio Co.; Sataloff, Joseph: Industrial Deafness, p. 16, New York, Blakiston Division, McGraw-Hill, 1957)

as *zero decibels of hearing loss* or *average normal hearing*. This level is not the same as that used as a base for noise measurement. In the middle frequency range (around 3,000 cycles per second) it is about 15 or 16 decibels above the reference level known as acoustical zero. In testing hearing with an audiometer, 40-decibel loss in hearing on the audiogram means that the individual requires 40 decibels more of sound pressure than the average normal person to be able to hear the tone presented.

Since the base line or reference level is different for the audiometer than it is for noise measuring devices, it should be clear now that a noise of, say, 60 decibels in a room is not the same intensity as the 60-decibel tone on the audiometer. The noise will sound less loud, for it is measured from a weaker reference level.

Formula for the Decibel. With these reference levels established, the formula for the decibel is worked out. To compare the two pressures, we have designated them as Pressure 1 and Pressure 2, with Pressure 2 being the reference level. This ratio can be expressed as $\frac{P_1}{P_2}$. Another factor that must be taken into account is that in computing this ratio in terms of decibels, the computation must be logarithmic.

A logarithm is the exponent or the power to which a fixed number or base (usually 10) must be raised in order to produce a given number. For instance, if the base is 10, the log of 100 is 2, because 10×10 equals 100. In such a case 10 is written with the exponent 2 as 10^2. Similarly, if 10 is raised to the 4th power and written as 10^4, the result is $10 \times 10 \times 10 \times 10$, or 10,000; the logarithm of 10,000 is, therefore, 4. If only this logarithmic function is considered, the formula has evolved as far as $db = \log \frac{P_1}{P_2}$. But it is not yet complete.

When the decibel was borrowed from the engineering field, it was a comparison of sound powers and not pressures, and it was expressed in bels and not decibels. The decibel is 1/10 of a bel, and the sound pressure is proportional to the square root of the corresponding sound power. It is necessary, therefore, to multiply the logarithm of the ratio of pressures by 2 (for the square root relationship) and by 10 (for the bel-decibel relationship). When this is done, the decibel formula is complete, and the decibel in terms of sound pressure level is defined thus:

$$db = 20 \log \frac{P_1}{P_2}$$

For instance, if the pressure designated as P_1 is 100 times greater than the reference level of P_2, substitution in the formula gives $db = 20 \times \log \frac{100}{1}$. Since it is known that the log of 100 is 2 (as $10^2 = 100$), it can be seen that the formula reduces to $db = 20 \times 2$, or 40 decibels. Therefore, whenever the pressure of one sound is 100 times greater than that of the reference level, the first sound can be referred to as 40 decibels. Likewise, if P_1 is 1,000 times greater, then the number of decibels would be 60, and if 10,000 times greater, the number of decibels is 80.

In actual sound measurement, if P_1 is 1 microbar—being a pressure of 1 dyne per square centimeter—then the ratio is $\dfrac{1}{.0002}$ or 5,000. By the use of a logarithmic table or a special table prepared to convert pressure ratios to decibels, the pressure level in such a case is found to be 74 db, based on a reference level of .0002 microbar. Figure 117 shows where a number of common sounds fall on this decibel scale in relation to a .0002 microbar reference level. This base level is used for calibrating standard sound measuring instruments.

IN AUDIOMETRIC TESTING, which uses a higher reference level than that for noise measurement, the tester does not need to concern himself with additional mathematical formulas, because the audiometer used in testing is calibrated to take into account the 15- to 16-decibel increase above acoustical zero to provide the necessary reference level for audiometry of average normal hearing (zero decibels of hearing loss).

Important Points. The important thing to be remembered is that the decibel is a logarithmic ratio. It is a convenient unit, because 1 decibel approaches the smallest change in intensity between two sounds that the human ear can distinguish.

An important aspect of the logarithmic ratio is that as the ratio of the pressures becomes larger, because the sound becomes more intense, the rate of increase in decibels becomes smaller. Even if the ratio of the pressures is enormous, such as one pressure being 10,000,000 times that of another, the number of decibels by which this ratio is expressed does not become inordinately large, being only 140 db. This is the principal reason for using the decibel scale. From the psychoacoustic aspect, it takes comparatively little increase in sound pressure to go from zero to 1 decibel, and the normal ear can detect this. However, when an attempt is made to increase the sound pressure from 140 to 141 decibels—also an increase of 1 decibel, which the ear can barely detect—it takes an increase of about 10,000,000 times as much in absolute pressure.

A point to be remembered is that the effect of adding decibels together is quite different from that of adding ordinary numbers. For example, if one machine whose noise has been measured as 60 decibels is placed near another machine also producing 60 decibels of noise, the resulting level is 63 decibels and not 120 decibels.

Figure 118 is a chart showing the results obtained from adding noise levels. On this chart it will be seen that if 70 and 76 decibels are being added, the difference of 6 decibels is located on the graph, and this difference is found to produce an increase of 1 decibel, which is added to the

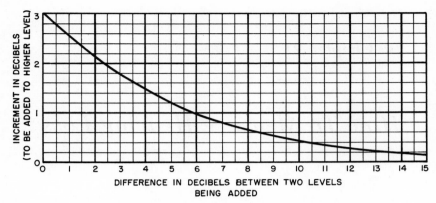

FIG. 118. Results obtained from adding noise levels.

higher number. Therefore, the combined level of noise produced by the two machines is 77 decibels above the reference level.

There are other important and interesting aspects of the physics of sound that might be discussed; the subject is a complex and fascinating one. The average physician concerned with the problems of deafness will find that a reasonable comprehension of the material thus far presented will be helpful—especially the fact that the term "decibel" expresses a *logarithmic ratio to an established reference level.*

Chapter 21

How To Measure Hearing Loss

ASPECTS OF TESTING

COOPERATION OF THE PATIENT

To obtain an accurate measure of the hearing level of a patient, it is necessary to have his cooperation. At present physicians do not have at their disposal a reliable objective method of measuring hearing in all individuals. Some response of the patient is necessary as an indication that he hears the sound used to test his hearing. The sound may be a word, a sentence, a pure tone, a noise or even the blast of a loud horn. The response of the patient may consist of raising his finger or his hand, pressing a button, answering a question or repeating a sentence, merely blinking his eyes, or turning in the direction of the sound. The test sound may be reduced in intensity until the patient hears it only 50 per cent of the times it is presented. In such an instance the intensity level at which he just hears the sound is called his *threshold of hearing*. Or speech may be used at a reasonably loud level, and the patient is asked to repeat words or combinations of words to determine how well he distinguishes certain speech sounds. This is called *discrimination testing*.

DEVELOPMENT OF THE AUDIOMETER

The ideal method of testing hearing would be to measure and to control everyday speech accurately, and to present it to the patient in such a manner that without the patient's giving any voluntary response, the physician could determine whether the patient had received and understood it clearly through either ear and with the participation of his brain. Unfortunately, such a method has not yet been developed, and the problems that would have to be solved to realize that ambition are inconceivably complex. Even the very first step of controlling and measuring the intensity of speech itself has not yet reached a satisfactory degree of perfection.

The old method of testing hearing—one that many physicians still use—is to stand 15 feet away and to whisper numbers or words to the patient, who is plugging his distal ear with a finger. The examiner gradually reduces his distance from the patient until the latter just begins to repeat the whispered words correctly. If the patient responds correctly to every word at 15 feet, the examiner gives him a score of 15/15 or normal hearing, but if the physician has to approach to within 5 feet to obtain a correct response from the patient, the latter receives a 5/15 score for his hearing impairment. Then the patient is turned to face the other way, with a finger plugging the other ear, and the procedure is repeated.

It is extremely difficult to duplicate the test under identical conditions, and it is virtually impossible to compare results in different patients or to maintain an absolute sound intensity level. The acoustics of the test room, the choice of words, the examiner's accent, enunciation and ability to control and to project his voice, as well as the degree of hearing loss in either or both of the patient's ears—not to mention still other factors—all conspire to render this testing procedure highly inaccurate.

The Pure Tone Audiometer. These shortcomings and the impossibility of controlling and reproducing speech sounds accurately with the early forms of electronic equipment led to the development of the pure tone audiometer. Its developers recognized that their chief objective was to determine to what degree speech must be amplified to be barely heard by the patient. They therefore analyzed speech and found that it encompassed frequencies from about 128 to 8,192 cycles per second.

At that time electronic equipment was readily available to measure pure tones with a great deal of accuracy, though no equipment was available to measure speech. Since it was not practical to test all frequencies from 128 to 8,192 cycles, the developers of the audiometer decided to sample certain pure tone frequencies within the speech range, and they selected a series of doubles: 128, 256, 512 and so on to 8,192. Frequencies bearing this double relationship to each other represent octaves on the musical scale.

FREQUENCY RANGE. Later the numbers were rounded off, so that today some audiometers are calibrated for frequencies 250, 500, 1,000, 2,000, 4,000, and 8,000 cycles. The newest audiometers also include three other frequencies, 1,500, 3,000 and 6,000 cps. This frequency range does not cover the entire gamut of normal hearing but merely the speech range. The human ear is sensitive to sound waves from frequencies as low as 16 cycles per second to as high as 16,000 or even 20,000 cycles per second, especially in young children. Its most sensitive area is in the range be-

tween 1,000 and 3,000 cycles. In this so-called middle frequency range it
takes less sound energy for tones to reach the threshold of hearing than it
does for tones above 3,000 cycles and below 1,000 cycles. The diagram in
Fig. 119 shows that at the higher and the lower frequencies the ear is not
as sensitive as in the middle frequencies, and so it is necessary to make
higher and lower tones louder to permit the normal ear to hear them.

When it is recalled that the audiogram has a 0 decibel reference level
for normal hearing, and that it is depicted as a straight line across the

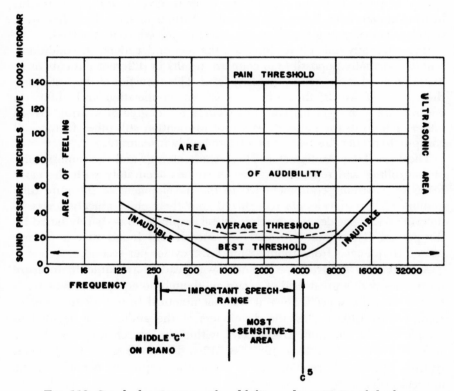

FIG. 119. Graph showing area of audibility and sensitivity of the human
ear. The best threshold (solid line) separates the audible from the inaudible sounds. This level generally is the reference level for sound-level
meters. The average threshold of hearing (dashed line) lies considerably
above the best threshold and is the reference level used in audiometers.
The ear is most sensitive between 1,000 and 3,000 cycles. The sound pressures are measured in the ear under the receiver of an audiometer. (With
modifications from Davis, H., and Silverman, S. R. [eds.]: Hearing and
Deafness, rev. ed., New York, Holt, 1960)

audiogram, it is apparent that it was necessary to introduce a *correction factor* to the lower and the higher frequencies to adjust the reference level and to make it a straight rather than a curved line, as shown in the figure. The straight line reference level makes it easier to read and to interpret an audiogram.

Above the range of normal human hearing, as at 16,000 cycles, is the ultrasonic domain, which is inaudible to the human ear. However, dogs and bats can hear frequencies far in excess of 16,000 cycles, and the ears of the bats are so sensitive that they use these frequencies to guide their flight in a manner closely paralleling the principle of the modern radar system. Since the human ear is not sensitive to these frequencies, it is not damaged by ultrasonics even at reasonably high intensities.

Each of the speech frequencies was used to test a large number of young, presumably normal-hearing people to find the intensity that could be considered as an attribute of normal hearing.

EXAMINATION OF REFERENCE HEARING THRESHOLD LEVELS

The present reference level of zero db (0 db) on American audiometers was derived from studying "normal" individuals in a national hearing survey in 1936. Since this was an average value, some subjects had better than average normal hearing, causing some otologists to complain that it was awkward to express the results of a hearing test on a person with above-normal hearing in minus figures (as —5 or —10 db). It was also cumbersome to have to speak in terms of "hearing loss" rather than "residual hearing." In view of these complaints and because the reference hearing level used in some European countries was lower (or better) than the American standard, the International Standards Organization, of which the American Standards Organization is the United States member body, undertook to study the problem. It proposed recently that the American standard be changed to conform to the European standard.

. In order to change an American standard, various member organizations in this country must approve the proposed modifications. The councils of several major otolaryngologic societies already have moved that the new proposal be accepted and have recommended its adoption in clinical practice. Other member organizations of the ASA, however, recently have rejected the new ISO proposal because of certain specific shortcomings. Until these objections are resolved and the proposed ISO standard is approved by a sufficient number of its members, it cannot become an ASA standard. Deliberations and discussions are still in progress. Table 2 shows the changes in decibel readings that would result according to the standard suggested by the ISO.

TABLE 2. A COMPARISON OF ASA-1951 AND ISO-1963
REFERENCE HEARING THRESHOLD LEVELS

	Reference Threshold Level, db		
FREQUENCY, CPS	ASA-1951*	ISO-1963	DIFFERENCE
125	54.5	45.5	9.0
250	39.5	24.5	15.0
500	25.0	11.0	14.0
1,000	16.5	6.5	10.0
1,500	(16.5)	6.5	10.0
2,000	17.0	8.5	8.5
3,000	(16.0)	7.5	8.5
4,000	15.0	9.0	6.0
6,000	(17.5)	8.0	9.5
8,000	21.0	9.5	11.5

* The figures in parentheses are interpolations.

THE NEED FOR TESTERS WITH SPECIALIZED TRAINING

At the present time the most reliable and accepted method of testing hearing is by using a standard pure tone audiometer. To use this instrument satisfactorily requires specialized training, because the testing necessitates the voluntary cooperation of the subject.

One of the most important aspects of every training program is to instruct the tester in how to make the responses of the subject a reliable indication of whether or not he is hearing the test tone. This can be accomplished best by adhering to these principles: (1) the method of testing should be explained to the listener in a simple and positive manner, and he should be given a practical demonstration if he never has had a hearing test before; (2) the method of response should be as simple as possible; raising a finger or a hand, for example, or pressing a button is simpler than writing down an answer; (3) the subject should be conditioned to give a positive response and encouraged to give reliable answers quickly and concisely; and (4) the subject should be given just enough time to respond after the presentation of each sound signal.

One of the responsibilities of a trained tester is *to be certain* that the responses he is obtaining from the subject are reliable and an accurate indication of the patient's hearing. Frequently, the experienced tester develops an intuitive feeling as to the reliability of the test and can change the technic when there is any question about the cooperation of the subject. For example, if a tester notes that the finger of the subject seems to be indecisive and does not give precise answers, he may ask the subject to raise his entire hand or to say, "Yes," instead of using the finger response.

METHODS OF TESTING HEARING

There are a number of methods of using pure tones to test hearing. The best technic and the one recommended for all physicians is the procedure for performing an individual audiogram based on the technic described in Chapter 22.

SCREENING METHOD

In industry, the armed forces and school systems a large number of people have to have their hearing tested in a short period of time; occasionally it may be necessary to use a technic called a screening method when individual audiometry would be too time-consuming and impractical. In this screening test the intensity of each frequency is set at a specific level, such as 20 db, and the individual is asked if he hears the tone—yes or no. If he hears the tone, he is passed; if he does not, he may be rejected from school or employment or referred to his physician, or perhaps he may be held for individual testing. Such screening audiometry, using above-threshold levels, does not meet the proper requirements of medical practice or industrial medicine.

GROUP PURE TONE TESTING

Another method of testing hearing is group pure tone testing, in which many subjects are given the same tones at the same time through multiple earphones; the subjects then are asked to fill out certain coded forms establishing whether or not they hear the levels tested. This method may have some usefulness in the military and in certain school systems, but here again it is recommended that when opportunity presents itself later, all personnel so tested should be rechecked by individual audiometry.

SELF-RECORDING AUDIOMETRY

Self-recording audiometry with either individual pure tones or continuous tones is a slight modification of the standard individual technic. Self-recording audiometers are being used in increasing numbers, and admittedly they have some advantage in many situations. The advantage of a so-called automatic audiometer is that it does not require a hearing tester in constant attendance. The sounds are presented to the subject in a standardized manner using electronic controls, and the subject can record a written record of his auditory acuity by pressing the button in response to the on-and-off signal of the audiometer.

These questions are asked frequently: Why is special training necessary for performing hearing tests? Why cannot one become proficient by just following the directions supplied with the audiometer or be trained by the salesman who sells the audiometer? The answers already have been suggested in part when it was emphasized that audiometry is a subjective test requiring the response of the subject, and that subjects are not always anxious or able to give reliable responses. It requires a very carefully trained tester to determine when these instances occur.

Experience also has shown that in many instances testers without adequate audiometric training, though they have performed many hundreds or even thousands of audiograms and consider themselves to be authorities on audiometry, are in fact making serious mistakes of which they are unaware, and they are producing hearing tests that are neither reliable nor valid. This experience has been verified in every phase of audiometry in otologic practice, industry and school systems. It was demonstrated very dramatically by a report of a subcommittee of the American Standards Association in which only a few hundred audiograms were found to be reliable out of many, many thousands performed in industry by presumably trained people.

To perform satisfactory audiometry, a tester must be thoroughly trained to understand the importance of his responsibility and to take pride and interest in his work. Without this training unsatisfactory hearing studies may be obtained that may prove to be more of a liability than an asset. Such training in hearing testing is available in numerous institutions throughout the country, or it can be supplied by well-trained audiologists and otologists.

WHO SHOULD DO AUDIOMETRY?

Ideally, the physician should do his own audiometry, for in this way he can make a good appraisal of the hearing level of his patient. Unfortunately, this is not always possible because of the time factor in the busy schedule of the general practitioner, the pediatrician, the industrial physician or the school physician. Nurses, hospital technicians and other personnel available in industry can be trained to perform excellent audiometry. The training may take several days or weeks, depending on the individual aptitude and the manner in which the program is organized. The principal purposes of the training program are to teach the tester to utilize the best available technic, to be completely aware of the potential pitfalls in hearing testing, and to understand the serious consequences of an incorrect report. It is not the responsibility of the tester, unless he is a physician, to interpret results, but rather to do his work so that his hearing tests are valid and reliable. Among the subjects that every teaching program for training hearing testing technicians should include are: acoustical terminology, audiometric technic and its pitfalls and limitations, malingering, psychology of hearing, calibrating equipment, record keeping and some anatomy and physiology of hearing.

HOW TO SELECT THE TEST ROOM

CRITERIA

Since it is well known that in a noisy room it is difficult to hear very soft sounds, and since audiometers are calibrated on subjects tested in a very quiet room, all testing of hearing should be done in a reasonably quiet room with a noise level so low that it will not interfere with an accurate test. Therefore, a most important criterion in selecting a room is its ambient noise level, that is, the level of noise that prevails in the room at various times. If there is excessive noise in the room where hearing tests are done, the subject invariably has difficulty hearing the weaker threshold tones and gives inaccurate responses. Prefabricated soundproof rooms are desirable but expensive and are not purchased generally either by the practitioner or even by all otologic specialists. Some schools and some industries have purchased such rooms, but in many instances efforts are made to find a satisfactory test room without spending a great deal of money.

In selecting the location for testing hearing, the physician should bear in mind that the room should be close to his regular examining office. The test room should be as far away as possible from ringing telephones, elevators, air conditioning systems, air ducts, water pipes, drain pipes, and other sources of disturbing and extraneous noise, particularly the clicking heels of women walking on hard floors. The ceiling should not transmit the noise of people walking on the floor above. The room should have as few windows as possible and only one door. In spite of these apparent limitations, a satisfactory test room can be found in almost every physician's office. Although it is advisable to purchase a prefabricated test room, it generally costs more than a practicing physician wishes to spend; but if he does a great deal of hearing testing and is interested in the work, he should purchase a prefabricated hearing testing booth.

TESTS FOR AMBIENT NOISE

Sound-Level Meter. Several methods can be used to determine whether or not a room is satisfactory for hearing testing. One of the best methods is to use a sound-level meter, an instrument to measure the ambient noise level in a room. The physician can obtain the services of a local engineer, particularly if there are large industries in the area, to do the testing for him. Most major industries have both engineers and sound-level meters to use in their own plants and would be very glad to cooperate with physicians. If the sound-level meter shows that the ambient noise levels fall below the following levels, then the room can be considered to be satisfactory for testing hearing:

TABLE 3. SUGGESTED MAXIMUM AMBIENT NOISE LEVELS FOR AUDIOMETRY ROOMS FOR PHYSICIANS. (In many instances a satisfactory test room environment can be achieved by earphone cushion protectors.)

	OCTAVE BAND				
	300 to 600	600-1200	1200-2400	2400-4800	4800-
Decibels on C scale of sound-level meter	45	45	50	55	60

The readings on the sound-level meter should be taken several times during the day, especially when the outside environment is noisiest. This will give the physician an idea as to when is the best time for him to do hearing tests.

A Comparison of Hearing Tests. If a sound-level meter is not available, another method, which is very satisfactory, can be used. The physician should do hearing tests with his audiometer on 3 or 4 subjects who have normal hearing as determined in a very quiet test room, perhaps available at a local institution or university. These subjects then should be retested by the physician in the room that he desires to use for testing. If it can be determined by the same tester that the hearing of the individual is still normal, then it may be assumed that the room is suitable for obtaining satisfactory audiograms. It is important that the hearing of the subjects be normal for this type of pilot study.

REDUCING AMBIENT NOISE

If there is a significant difference in the thresholds of the tests performed in the room in question as compared with the very quiet room, and if other variations have been ruled out, the ambient noise level of the test room is open to question and probably *too high*. Some measures have to be taken to reduce it. Most of the time the interference occurs in the low frequencies at 250 and 500 cycles. In comparing the thresholds, it should be recalled that a 5-db difference is within expected variation in doing audiograms and not necessarily is due to the masking effect of the ambient noise. If, however, it is more than 5 db, something will have to be done to quiet the room before it can be used. These steps can be taken: make sure there is a tight-fitting and solid door or, better yet, a double door at the entrance to the room, a soft rug on the floor and perhaps acoustic tile on the ceiling. Putty up cracks around the window and put a sign outside the test room: "Quiet, please." In most instances physicians will find a room suitable for hearing testing in their own offices without going to unreasonable expense.

FURNITURE AND REGULATIONS

The test room should be furnished as simply as possible with a table, a chair and lighting fixtures that do not produce a loud hum. If air conditioning units or electric fans are in the room, shutoff switches should be easily accessible, so that they may be silenced during the testing period. Smoking should not be permitted in the test room because of ventilation problems.

THE KIND OF AUDIOMETER TO PURCHASE

An audiometer is a precision instrument that produces pure tones of known intensity. The instrument is very delicate and must be handled with great care and with particular attention to the earphones. Although standard specifications for approved audiometers are established by the American Standards Association, audiometers differ in many features. These differences help to determine which audiometer is best suited for a particular use. For the general practitioner, the pediatrician or the director of a school testing program it is advisable that the audiometer be as simple as possible, since it is likely that only air and bone conduction tests are to be done. If bone conduction audiometry is to be performed, it is essential that a good masking device of known intensity be available. In industry bone conduction rarely, if ever, is done, and only air conduction aspects of the audiometer are of importance. Most commercial audiometers are now of reasonably high quality, but certain features are essential in all audiometers:

1. They should meet the standards of the American Standards Association.

2. They should be simple to operate and should have as few complicating and intricate extras as possible.

3. They should be able to test the following frequencies: 250, 500, 1,000, 2,000, 4,000, 6,000 and 8,000 cycles.

4. Unless the physician intends to use more complicated tests, accessories such as speech testing apparatus, loudness balance testing, etc., should not influence the purchase of the equipment.

5. The interrupter switch should work in such a manner that no click is produced when it is pressed down or released.

6. When the interrupter switch is pressed down, the tone should come on immediately without any lag, and it should stop rapidly when the switch is released.

7. The audiometer should be purchased from a manufacturer who will guarantee prompt attention in case of repairs and supply a substitute audiometer in case the purchased instrument has to be sent to the factory for repairs. This last feature is of utmost importance; otherwise a physician may be without an audiometer for long periods of time.

THE AUDIOMETER

Every audiometer has a series of switches and controls to direct its operation (Fig. 120). The on-and-off switch controls the power on the audiometer. This should be turned on at least 15 minutes before use, and if possible, it should be left on all day rather than turned on and off as the need dictates. A frequency selector dial designates the tone that is produced in the earphones.

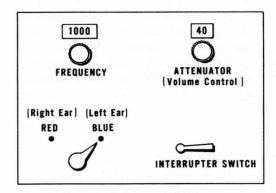

Fig. 120. Main switches and dials of a typical clinical audiometer. Included are the frequency dial, which controls the tonal output, in this case set at 1,000 cps; the attenuator, which controls the volume output in decibels, here set at 40 db; the earphone selector switch; and the interrupter switch, which turns the signal on and off. The interrupter is left in the "off" position and pressed to the "on" position when the tone is to be presented. (E. A. Irvin, M.D., Medical Director, Ford Motor Company)

The volume control dial or the attenuator determines the intensity of the tone produced. Attenuators usually are calibrated in 5-db steps from −10 to 100 db, with the exception of the very low and high frequencies, for which the maximum usually is around 80 db. Readings should not be made between the 5-db steps. Since the maximum output at 250 cycles and 8,000 cycles generally is not more than 80 db, one should bear in mind in testing that exceeding 80 db does not increase the intensity of the tone produced. A small interrupter switch is used to turn the tone on and off. The tone always should be off unless the tester wishes to turn it on for testing purposes. Many instruments will have other switches on the panel. One may be marked "microphone switch." This is used when it is desired to speak through a small microphone on the control panel or a microphone accompanying the audiometer connected so that the patient can hear the examiner through the earphones. This rarely is necessary and is of little value in most testing situations. Another switch is used to connect the bone conduction vibrator. When this is done, a different calibration system may be turned on, and one should be sure to read the bone conduction intensity scale rather than that for air conduction.

Two wires leading from the audiometer are attached to earphones connected by a spring headband. These are very delicate and should be handled with extreme caution, for they easily can be thrown out of adjustment. They are part of a mechanism to convert electric current into sound, which then impinges on the eardrum. A switch enables the operator to shift the sound from one earphone to another. The ear receivers are equipped with a rubber cushion that has considerable importance. It must be of a specified size so that the volume of air that it encloses is precisely that provided when the instrument was calibrated (approximately 6 cc.). The cushion cannot be replaced by a larger or smaller one for reasons of comfort without disturbing the calibration of the instrument. If a type of cushion is purchased to provide better attenuation, the receiver then must be recalibrated with the cushion in place. One can now obtain a type of cushion that fits the head so closely that it protects the ear from higher ambient noise levels than those generally permissible in test rooms. One company calls such cushion "Otocups" and calibrates the earphones for the purchaser.

A push-button cord also accompanies most audiometers so that the patient may signal his response by pressing the button. When the subject hears the tone, he presses the button, causing a light to appear on the instrument panelboard. This is one way of getting a response from the subject. Many experienced testers prefer to rely on the patient's raising a finger or a hand.

CALIBRATION OF AUDIOMETER

Before using an audiometer for testing, one always should determine whether it is accurately calibrated for frequency and intensity. So many factors can affect the calibration of an audiometer that routine checks are essential. Such a check always should be made before using the instrument and again at the end of the day. If the calibration is not checked frequently, the tester may perform many tests without being aware that the audiometer is out of adjustment.

The object of a calibration check is to determine whether the frequencies and the intensities produced by the receivers coincide with the readings indicated on the frequency and the attenuator dials of the audiometer.

FREQUENCY

Rarely is any difficulty in calibration encountered with the frequency component. However, in some instruments the frequency control may become loose with continued use and produce a significantly different tone from that indicated. Some audiometers are so constructed that this difference may result also in a false intensity measurement.

To determine whether the frequency has been calibrated properly, an oscilloscope is most desirable and readily available in most radio repair shops and electronic laboratories. If the tester has a good ear for pitch, he sometimes can compare roughly the tones on the audiometer with corresponding tones on a tuning fork or a piano. If the instrument is found to be inaccurately calibrated in its frequency output, it should be returned to the factory for adjustment.

INTENSITY

The audiometer is much more likely to go out of calibration in intensity than in frequency, and therefore it is more often necessary to verify the intensity calibration. Unfortunately, a simple and practical device for measuring the intensity of a tone has not yet been developed. The best device is an artificial ear, which is expensive and not readily available. A few companies produce a special calibrator for audiometers that could be purchased by hospitals and lent to physicians.

CHECKING

A simple and practically useful technic is to test the audiometer on a number of known normal and abnormal ears before and after using it daily. The experienced tester certainly will know his own hearing threshold and can get a rough idea from a knowledge of his own audiogram whether or not the instrument is in reasonable calibration. For example, if the tester has normal hearing and suddenly finds one morning that he has a 15-db loss at 2,000 cycles in either one or both ears, he should first switch the earphones around and retest himself. Then he should test at least 3 or 4 other subjects with stabilized and known hearing thresholds: If all of them show similar defects at 2,000 cycles, it is apparent that the instrument is out of adjustment and cannot be relied upon. Switching the earphones may localize the trouble and show the defect to lie in only one earphone. In any event, the instrument requires recalibration and should not be used until the inaccuracies have been corrected.

Sometimes in testing normal ears it is found that all of them show "too good" hearing; that is, all will have thresholds of −10 or better. Or all of the presumably normal ears may show a consistent 5- to 10-db "loss," and hardly any will have a zero threshold. Such findings indicate that the zero threshold on the audiometer is established inaccurately, and the instrument should be returned to the manufacturer for correction. If the deviation from zero threshold occurs only in the lower and the middle frequencies, it may be due to the masking effect of ambient noise in the room. This can be determined by rechecking the same subjects in a very quiet room.

When a tester observes that he is obtaining audiograms indicating a persistent unexplainable hearing impairment either at all or specific frequencies, he should stop testing patients and test several ears known to be normal in order to assure himself that the instrument is calibrated properly.

After testing a group of subjects each day, the tester should recheck his instrument on himself and on several normal ears. This final check is necessary, because the tester may have been testing many abnormal ears and may not have been aware that at some time during the day the audiometer has gone out of adjustment. By establishing the calibration of the audiometer at the end of the day the tester will know whether he needs to retest any subjects, and he will have also an important confirmation for medicolegal purposes in case it should be required.

When a tester uses his own or other normal ears to verify the calibration of an audiometer, he is testing only the calibration at threshold and assuming that the attenuators are working properly and producing accurate readings at above-threshold levels. However, a special calibrator can test above-threshold levels.

Adjustments

When the tester suspects that an audiometer is out of adjustment, he has several alternatives. If an artificial ear and qualified electronic engineers should happen to be available to handle the problem, as in certain universities, research centers or industries with electronic laboratories, then the tester should turn over the instrument to them for prompt attention. Generally, these facilities are not available. The next alternative is to return the instrument to the company from which it was purchased. For this reason it is advisable to keep the original shipping crate in which the audiometer was received. When sending the instrument, it is well to include a note to the manufacturer as to the exact difficulty encountered.

Sometimes the tester may not be using the instrument properly and erroneously may assume that it is out of adjustment. It may be wise to discuss the problem with the salesman through whom he obtained the instrument to determine whether a simple solution is available. Generally it is not wise to permit the salesman to attempt major adjustments himself, or to allow such adjustments to be made by a local electronic or radio repairman who does not have access to the calibrated artificial ear necessary to insure the accurate calibration of the audiometer. Furthermore, it should not be taken for granted that because an instrument has just been received following a factory adjustment, it is perfectly calibrated. The instrument must be tested clinically before use, as was recommended previously. It is quite possible that in shipping, packing or in some other manner the calibration has become faulty.

A Second Audiometer or Prompt Repair. The need to ship the audiometer back to the manufacturer and to be without an instrument for weeks can create a very trying and unsatisfactory situation. In industrial programs and certain school programs it may be necessary to have two audiometers or some readily accessible facility for prompt repair of an audiometer. The manufacturer from whom the instrument was purchased should lend another instrument during repair periods. If a loan audiometer is being used, its calibration must be established carefully and a note made on each audiogram as to the change in instruments. This record should be considered when results are compared if there is a consistent variation between the two audiometers.

RECORD OF CALIBRATION TESTING

It is important that testers keep a separate daily record of their calibration testing, indicating the exact time and manner in which the audiometer in use was checked for calibration. This is an important precaution, particularly in cases with medicolegal aspects.

Chapter 22

How To Do an Audiogram and Avoid Pitfalls

AIR CONDUCTION

It has been demonstrated repeatedly that though hearing testers without adequate training may have performed many hundreds of audiograms and may consider themselves to be experts, many of them are making mistakes of which they are unaware, and they are producing test results that often are inaccurate.

Although audiometric testing may appear to be disarmingly simple, it is by no means easy to obtain accurate thresholds consistently. Reliable and valid audiograms are of such great diagnostic importance, such a valuable guide to therapy and so decisive in medicolegal cases that it has seemed worth while to present in this chapter an outline of basic technic, with emphasis on the essential features of good audiometry. This presentation is followed by a discussion of the more common pitfalls that beset routine audiometry.

HOW TO PERFORM A ROUTINE AUDIOGRAM

Before starting the audiogram the tester should consider the following preliminary steps:
1. Seating the subject
2. Testing the earphones
3. Checking the audiometer
4. Instructing the subject
5. Placing the earphones on the subject

Seating the Subject

If the tester and the subject are in the same room, the subject should be seated in a comfortable (nonsqueaky) chair so that his hands can rest on the arms of the chair or on the far end of the tester's table. The examiner must be able to observe the subject's response with care. He should be able to watch the subject's hands and also his face and head.

The subject should face the tester obliquely, but he should not be able to observe the hands or the arms of the tester or the control panel of the audiometer.

Having the subject close his eyes during listening helps him to concentrate more on threshold sounds and prevents him from receiving possible signal cues from the examiner's hands or face.

Although some technicians advocate having the subject sit with his back to the tester, the author feels this is unsatisfactory even if the push button is used to register the response. It divorces the tester from numerous indications that help him to establish an opinion as to the validity of the threshold and the cooperation of the subject, and it prevents him from forming a judgment as to the possibility of malingering.

Testing the Earphones

To be certain that the earphones are in proper working order, the tester should place both earphones over his own ears before beginning a series of tests and at routine intervals. He should determine quickly whether the thresholds are within reasonable calibration and the earphones in their proper jacks. One earphone usually is marked "Right" and the other "Left" to correspond with the control switch on the panel of the audiometer. The tester should try a tone in each ear to ascertain that the earphones correspond with the switch.

In addition to checking the tones at normal threshold levels, the tester should try the loud tones as well, carefully noting whether the interrupter switch makes a clicking noise when it is depressed, since on occasion subjects will respond to such a click instead of to the pure tone. There should be no clicking noise in a properly functioning instrument.

The earphones should be treated with care at all times, and precautions should be taken against dropping them. One should clean the earphones after testing industrial personnel whose heads or ears are likely to be dirty from their occupations. Should an ear of a subject be discharging, it is important to clean the cushion carefully. Intrusion of water or dirt into the diaphragm of the earphones must be avoided meticulously.

CHECKING THE AUDIOMETER

A routine check of the audiometer controls before placing the earphones on the subject will improve considerably the efficiency of the tester in performing repeated audiograms. One of the more frequent errors that thus can be avoided is a loud blast in the subject's ear because the attenuator inadvertently was left at 100 db—a mishap that not only may cause ear discomfort for the subject but also may destroy his confidence in the tester.

A routine check of all the panel controls can be made in a very short time. The tester should be certain that:

1. The frequency selector is placed at 1,000 cycles, if this is the first tone to be tested.

2. The attenuator is turned down to about 10 decibels.

3. The audiometer is given time to warm up.

4. The earphone plugs are tightly inserted into their jacks.

5. The microphone switch, if there is one, is turned off.

6. The interrupter switch is adjusted so that a tone is produced only when the interrupter switch is pressed down.

If the audiometer has a switch for converting to bone conduction, this switch also should be turned off. If a masking device is present, this, too, should be turned off.

INSTRUCTING THE SUBJECT

After the subject is seated, the tester should make certain that the subject has a clear and complete understanding of what is expected of him. The tester may say: "You will hear certain tones in each ear. When you hear the tone, no matter how weak it is, raise your finger and hold it up as long as you hear the tone. When it stops, put your finger down. We shall test your right ear first."

PLACING THE EARPHONES

It is most important that the earphones be placed snugly on the subject's ears so that there is no leakage between the phones and the side of the head, and that the headband be adjusted to the size of the head so that the phones are comfortable. Women subjects must remove earrings and push back their hair from over the ears. All eyeglasses, particularly horned-rimmed glasses, also should be removed in all instances. If the subject puts on the earphones himself, the tester personally should check them to be certain they are applied properly. The auricle of the ear should not be bent over by the phone, and the center of the phone should be aligned directly with the opening of the ear canal.

The cord leading from the earphones must not be draped over the front of the subject, where it might be rubbed by his movements.

Be certain that the phone marked "Right" is placed on the right and not on the left ear.

The earphones should not be applied until directions have been given to the subject, and the tester is ready to proceed with the actual performance of the audiogram.

THE AUDIOGRAM

Sample Tone. After the earphones are applied, if the subject has not previously been tested, allow him to listen to a sample tone, such as the 1,000-cycle tone set at about 40 db, or louder, if necessary. Avoid too loud a sample tone, which could startle the subject or produce a temporary auditory fatigue following exposure to the loud tone. The tone is produced by setting the frequency selector at 1,000 cycles, the attenuator at 40 db, and pressing down on the interrupter switch for an interval of about a second or less. If necessary, the subject again should be reminded to raise his finger when he hears the tone and to hold up his finger as long as the tone persists. When the tone stops, he should lower his finger immediately.

Occasionally, the subject may be asked in which ear he hears the sample tone, so that the tester may verify that the tone is being applied to the ear indicated by the selector switch on the audiometer.

Procedure. The author usually tests the right ear first, because it is generally more natural for the subject to respond with the right hand. Not infrequently, subjects indicate their responses with the right hand to tones in the right ear and with their left hand to tones in the left ear. It often is helpful in testing difficult cases for the tester deliberately to use such a method.

The tester is to determine the subject's hearing for the frequencies of 1,000, 2,000, 3,000, 4,000, 6,000, 8,000, 500 and 250 cycles per second (if desired), preferably in the order listed. The 1,000-cycle tone is tested first, because this is usually the easiest one for which to establish a definitive threshold.

With the frequency dial at 1,000 cps, set the intensity at about 20 db above the estimated threshold and press down the interrupter switch gently for less than a second. If the subject responds, reduce the intensity to 0 or —5 db and present the tone again. If the subject responds at —5 db twice, the examiner may go to —10 if he desires, but in most practices two out of three responses at —5 db are considered to be far enough down the scale to record the patient's threshold at this level.

If the subject did not hear the 1,000-cycle tone at 20 db, the tester should increase the intensity to 40 db. If this is heard, then the tester may presume that the threshold lies somewhere between 40 and 20 db, and so the next tone is presented at 30 db. In this manner the threshold can be narrowed down by the use of irregular intervals of intensity and time, and in most cases this procedure definitely establishes the existing hearing level.

All tones presented should be brief bursts of sound and held for no longer than 1 second. It is also wise to check that the recording of the threshold is being done properly for the tested ear and not for the opposite ear.

Caution should be exercised to avoid a rhythmic presentation of the tones either in intervals of frequency or of intensity. Some testers have developed the habit of beginning at 50 db and of reducing the tone regularly at intervals of 5 db until the subject indicates he can no longer hear the tone. This regular reduction in intensity should be avoided, as it is an excellent means of producing an inaccurate threshold in routine testing. An inaccurate threshold also may be obtained if the tester presents the tones in rhythmic, equally spaced time intervals, since the subject may continue to respond rhythmically to the tone long after it has ceased to be presented to the ear. This is particularly common in situations in which many subjects are to be tested daily by a tester who is unfamiliar with the importance of his responsibility. It is essential to vary constantly the time and the intensity intervals between the tones.

When the threshold for the 1,000-cycle tone has been determined and recorded for one ear, the frequency selector is moved to 2,000 cycles, and the threshold for the same ear at this frequency then is determined in the manner outlined above. This procedure is repeated for the frequencies of 3,000, 4,000, 6,000, 8,000, 500 and 250 cycles, and the thresholds in turn are recorded. Then the threshold again is checked for the original 1,000-cycle tone.

When the tester has completed the recording of thresholds for one ear, the test tone is switched to the opposite ear, and the identical procedure is repeated, starting with 1,000 cycles and returning finally to check again on the 1,000-cycle threshold as was done on the other ear.

It also is advisable to recheck the thresholds for those frequencies that indicate a loss greater than 20 db. This recheck is particularly essential in industrial pre-employment or preplacement tests. The examiner always should record on the audiogram all thresholds independently obtained.

When the thresholds for all frequencies have been determined properly and recorded for both ears, the routine audiogram is complete.

Modifications Based on Experience. As the hearing tester becomes more experienced, he will be better able to judge the initial intensity at which each tone should be presented in order to obtain the threshold as rapidly and reliably as possible. For example, he will observe that if a subject has a threshold of about 30 db at 2,000 cycles, then in all likelihood the threshold at 4,000 and 8,000 cycles will be greater than 30 db. If a hearing loss is present at 500 cycles, the threshold at 250 cycles is likely to be on about the same general level.

The experienced tester tends to start each tone about 10 or 15 db above the estimated threshold and rapidly narrows down the difference. Except in rare instances (to check reliability) it is time-consuming and of no value to recheck intensities at higher or lower levels than those to which the subject already has given reliable responses. For example, if a subject definitely hears at 30 db, there is no reason to test 50 and 60 db. Of if he does not respond at 25 or 20 db, it is not necessary to test 10 and 5 db.

However, validity and reliability are of prime importance in all audiometry and should not be sacrificed for the sake of saving time or effort.

Because many of the audiograms obtained will demonstrate normal hearing, a trained and experienced tester can expedite the manner in which an audiogram is obtained. By slightly modifying his technic, he can save considerable time and do many more tests without sacrificing accuracy.

A modification of the previously described method becomes logical when the tester obtains a threshold of 5 db or less on the 1,000-cycle tone. This result justifies the assumption that the subject may have normal hearing in all frequencies. Consequently, the tester now can move the frequency to 2,000 cycles and the attenuator to 0 or even −5 and test for threshold. If the subject responds to either of these at least twice, then this response is recorded as threshold. The same is done for all other frequencies in both ears, starting at 0 db instead of working down from a louder tone. In this manner it is possible to obtain an accurate threshold in a very short time on a subject with normal hearing.

The procedure should be done with as much careful attention as any other test, even though less time is consumed. The tendency to rush all subjects through the test by using this modified method should be avoided, since in the end more time will be consumed if there is a large number of abnormal ears among the patients to be tested.

INDUSTRIAL TESTING. Part of this technic has a special application in industrial testing. Since most of the hearing losses in industrial personnel will be found in the frequencies above 1,000-cycles, the thresholds at 1,000 and below will in most instances be normal. Therefore, it is wiser when numerous audiograms are to be performed, to spend more time establishing the thresholds in the higher frequencies than in the lower ones. By setting the attenuator at 0 or 5 db (depending on the ambient noise in the room during the testing at 1,000, 500 and 250 cycles), it generally will be found that the vast majority of the subjects will respond to threshold at this low intensity. This will save much time in each test. Sometimes the ambient noise level is disturbing, particularly if it is of the low frequency type. In such instances the subject seldom will respond to very low intensities at 250 cycles, and he will require a louder tone for recognition before he can work his way down to a reliable threshold.

The importance of accurately testing the low tones should not be overlooked, since they often are the sole indication that the subject has some damage in the middle or the inner ears and should receive further study.

Another word of caution is in order about modifying standard audiometry. A modified technic is most conducive to the neglect of vital precautions in audiometry. For example, the tester may have a tendency to look up after each frequency or to ask the subject methodically if he heard the tone. Such errors must be avoided carefully, particularly in industrial hearing programs in which the test is one of a pre-employment or preplacement nature.

IN GENERAL, if the threshold at 2,000 cycles is not close to 0, there is a strong possibility that at higher frequencies the threshold also will be higher, and the modified method should not be utilized.

RECORDING AUDIOGRAMS

Graph. A number of methods for recording the results of audiometry are in use at the present time. The predominant method is to record the threshold at each frequency on a graph, such as that supplied by manufacturers of audiometers (Fig. 3). Such a graph shows a curve of the individual's threshold. For air conduction tests it is customary to record threshold for the right ear with an O, and to use a red pencil to connect the circles with a continuous line. The results for the left ear are recorded with an X, and a blue pencil is used to connect the X's with a broken line. For bone conduction the use of a different color for each ear is not essential, but it helps to distinguish more readily the thresholds of one ear from those of the other. If no threshold is obtainable at a certain frequency because the audiometer cannot be made loud enough for the subject to respond, this lack of response should be recorded by an arrow pointing downward to signify "out"; red is used to indicate the right ear, and blue, for the left ear. At the bottom of each graph should be a statement that O is for the right and X for the left.

One of the chief disadvantages of this type of graph in industry and otology is that if 8 or 10 audiograms are done in a year on a certain subject, the record becomes bulky, and it becomes difficult to compare one curve with another performed on a different date.

Serial Audiogram. Another manner of recording audiograms, one that obviates the use of an individual graph, is a serial audiogram sheet for each individual. A sample is shown in Figure 121. Here, instead of using a sym-

DATE	TESTER	RIGHT EAR AIR CONDUCTION								LEFT EAR AIR CONDUCTION							
		250	500	1000	2000	3000	4000	6000	8000	250	500	1000	2000	3000	4000	6000	8000
6-1-55	J	5	10	0	25	25	60	40	10	5	0	0	0	15	40	20	0
		10	10	0	35	30	60	35	10	5	0	0	0	20	50	20	0
															45		

FIG. 121. Serial record of hearing thresholds. Independently determined thresholds at each frequency are recorded separately.

bol for the right and the left ears, the numerical number of decibels desig-
nating the threshold is recorded at each frequency. If there is no response
to the test tone at maximum intensity, an arrow pointing downward or the
notation NR is used to indicate no response. Each new audiogram is
recorded below the previous one, so that a serial record over a period of
months or even years can be compared carefully by a glance at the serial
audiogram. Furthermore, a place for comments and a brief history is available on this type of serial audiogram.

Serial audiograms make it easier to record all thresholds obtained independently. For example, if the hearing test is started at 1,000 cycles and a
threshold obtained, and at the conclusion of the test another threshold is
obtained at 1,000 cycles, both these thresholds, even if alike, should be
recorded one on top of the other in the space provided for the threshold
at 1,000 cycles. In legal situations these multiple numbers will confirm that
the threshold was rechecked several times. It is important to record *every*
threshold that is derived independently, even if there is considerable variation, for this may have considerable significance. It is important that every
serial audiogram include the date and the initials of the tester, as well as
other information that can be placed under Comments.

Securing Objectivity. Since there is always a possibility that the tester
in an attempt to complete the test quickly may be influenced by a previously obtained threshold, it is advisable for the tester not to have before
him the previous audiogram on the serial chart. For this reason it is helpful
to have an assistant record while the tester calls off the threshold obtained
at each frequency. If a tester cannot obtain a satisfactory assistant for this
purpose, he should place a card over every previously obtained audiogram
so that it does not influence him in any way. A specially prepared mask
which allows only the blank spaces on the audiogram to be seen also can
be prepared. This type of self-restriction will insure to the tester's satisfaction that he is performing as objective a test as possible.

Preserving Records. Original audiograms should not be destroyed, even
if they are transcribed from one form to another. They are important written records of a subject's hearing. Recording of thresholds never should be
erased when on a repeat check the original threshold is found to differ from
the new. Instead, all thresholds should be recorded. The difference may be
significant, and this may have important bearing on the interpretation of
any hearing loss.

REVIEW OF COMMON ERRORS IN AUDIOMETRY

Despite careful training in audiometry, hearing testers routinely should
evaluate their technic with critical detachment. To aid the tester in this

self-criticism a checklist is presented of the most common errors and pitfalls that the author has encountered among testers:

1. Taking too much time to do an audiogram will fatigue the subject
and result in an inaccurate response. Adjustments from one frequency to
another and from one intensity to another should be made quickly, and the
entire audiogram should be completed as rapidly as possible without sacrificing the validity of the threshold.

2. Rushing through the test so rapidly that accurate thresholds are not
obtained equally must be avoided. The tester should understand that some
subjects take longer than others to respond. Sufficient time must be given
to each to respond to the stimulus. Faster and more definitive responses
can be obtained if the directions are concise and explicit prior to testing.

3. Allowing the subject to sit so that he can watch the control panel
of the audiometer or motions of the operator may result in inaccurate
responses and enhances the possibilities of malingering.

4. Placing the wrong receiver on the ear and recording the threshold
for the wrong ear is another common error that should be avoided.
Repeated checks should be made to see that the earphones are placed
correctly, and that they correspond with the switch on the control panel.

5. Presenting the signal and then looking up at the subject as if to ask
if he has heard the tone or giving other visual clues that the tone is on
should be avoided. This is poor audiometric technic, and frequently the
subject will respond even though he does not hear the tone.

6. Making intensity readings in less than the 5-decibel steps in which
most audiometer attenuators are calibrated is incorrect, and most likely it
will result in inaccurate thresholds. Readings always should be made on
the intensity dial in multiples of 5 decibels.

7. Presenting the sound signal for a long period of time, particularly
if it is loud, may produce temporary fatigue and result in an inaccurate
threshold. The tone should be produced in short bursts, and each tone
should be presented for about the same length of time (½ to ¾ second).

8. Taking too long to determine whether the threshold is at 0, −5, and
−10 decibels is unjustified in a conservation of hearing program. The
insignificance of such a determination as compared with other factors does
not warrant the time it consumes for medical or industrial purposes. A
5-decibel threshold on either side is often an expected variation and does
not indicate an uncooperative patient or a defective instrument. Occasionally, accurate threshold readings at the 8,000-cycle tone may be very
difficult to obtain. Often such difficulty is caused by the short wavelength
at this high frequency and the possible presence of so-called standing
waves. As a result, the threshold may fluctuate widely, particularly if the
subject presses the earphone closer to his ears in an attempt to hear better.

9. If during the testing of many subjects significant hearing losses are found repeatedly in the same frequencies on consecutive subjects, it is wise for the tester to recheck the earphones on himself to ascertain whether anything has gone wrong during the testing procedures.

10. Avoiding a rhythmic presentation of the signals either in intensity or in time intervals is necessary.

11. If during the testing of a subject or a number of subjects, the ambient noise level in a room increased so that it interfered with the threshold obtained, the tester should make a note to that effect on the audiogram to show that the test was done under adverse conditions.

12. Occasionally, a subject's responses are so varied that an accurate threshold is not obtainable at that particular time. Rather than delay the entire testing procedure of many other persons who may be waiting to be tested, it is wiser to recall this subject at a time when he can receive more individual attention. It is unsatisfactory for a tester to report a vague general threshold on such a subject when accurate responses are not attainable. Such responses may be an indication of functional hearing loss, malingering, or some organic condition that requires further study.

13. In recording hearing losses at the frequencies of 250 cycles and 8,000 cycles, it should be remembered not to record higher or lower levels than the maximum output of the audiometer. The tester should be familiar with the limitations of his instrument.

14. When the tester is depressing the interrupter switch, he must be particularly careful not to press down this switch so hard or let it spring back so quickly that it makes a clicking sound, which may result in a subject's responding to the click rather than to the pure tone presented.

15. Neither the examiner nor the subject should do any unnecessary talking during the test procedure, as this disturbs the subject's concentration. If instructions are given properly before the test, only rarely should a discussion be necessary during the test procedure.

Chapter 23

Masking and Bone Conduction Tests

SHADOW CURVE

When an individual wishes to test vision in only one eye, he merely closes the other eye or covers it with a patch to exclude it from the test. To test hearing in only one ear is not quite so simple, because sound waves, unlike light waves, travel in all directions and are not stopped easily by merely plugging the opposite ear. When a person hears normally in both ears, it is easy to test each ear separately, because he hears the very weak threshold tones in one ear long before they become loud enough to be heard in the opposite ear. However, when the ear to be tested has no hearing, and the opposite ear has normal hearing, there is a problem. Though the normal ear is covered with an earphone, after the tone applied to the deaf ear reaches 50 db or more, it becomes loud enough to be carried through and across the head to be heard in the normal ear. In such a case the subject would raise his finger to indicate that he heard the sound, and so he would mislead the tester, who would record hearing as present in the ear being tested when in fact that ear is totally deaf. This type of false audiogram is called a shadow curve.

MASKING

WHEN TO USE

Whenever an audiogram shows a difference in threshold between the two ears of roughly 35 db or more in most frequencies, it is essential to mask out the better-hearing ear during the testing of air conduction in the worse ear. Masking is achieved by introducing a sound or noise into the good ear and thereby occupying its nerve pathway so that it is prevented from responding to the test tones applied to the opposite ear.

Before proceeding with the discussion of a satisfactory technic for masking in testing air conduction, we wish to re-emphasize certain points mentioned in Chapter 3; there an explanation was given of how bone conduction could be tested with tuning forks. Although it takes about 50 db of sound intensity for a tone heard by air to cross from one ear to another via the bones of the head, a tone applied directly to one mastoid bone can be heard equally well in the opposite ear. The skull attenuates bone-conducted sounds very little, if at all; it makes practically no difference to what point on the skull a bone vibrator or tuning fork is applied. In any case the sound will be heard at threshold levels only in the ear with the better bone conduction, i.e., with better sensorineural function. For this reason the opposite ear always must be masked out in testing for bone conduction; otherwise, the examiner could not be sure which ear he really was testing.

A good rule to follow is that in air conduction testing no masking is is required unless there is a difference between the hearing thresholds of the two ears of 35 db or more at most frequencies. For bone conduction tests masking should be used routinely.

Bone Conduction Testing. PURPOSES. If a patient has normal air conduction thresholds or a hearing loss of 10 db or less, there is no need to perform bone conduction tests; the results would not be of diagnostic value, since the patient has normal hearing. The two chief purposes of bone conduction testing are: (1) to obtain a rough assessment of sensorineural function, and (2) to compare bone conduction threshold levels with air conduction threshold levels. The information so obtained is helpful in determining whether a hearing loss is conductive, sensorineural or mixed. The procedure is similar to that used in tuning fork tests, but it is more accurate and quantitative.

PROCEDURE. Testing for bone conduction is done very much like testing for air conduction. The bone vibrator is placed snugly on the mastoid process, care being taken not to let the vibrator touch the auricle of the ear being tested. The spring wire headband is fitted comfortably on the opposite side of the head, and the patient is told that he is to raise his finger and hold it up as long as he hears the tone in the ear tested. If he hears the tone in the opposite ear, he should tell the examiner. The patient also will be told that he will hear a loud masking noise in the opposite ear, but he should disregard this and listen for the tone.

Then the earphone that supplies the masking noise is placed over the ear opposite to that being tested with the bone vibrator (without an earphone). At this point the person operating the audiometer should ascertain that the switch marked "bone conduction" on the instrument panel is in the proper position for bone conduction testing. He gradually turns up the masking volume control until the "white noise" reaches 100 db (i.e., .0002 dyne/cm²). This is done by easy stages so that patients with sensitive ears and others with recruitment may not be made acutely uncomfortable by sudden exposure to such loud noise.

With the pure tone frequency for bone conduction set at 1,000 cycles, the hearing threshold is determined in the same way as in air conduction testing, and then the identical procedure is repeated for 2,000, 4,000, 500 and 250 cycles. After that the masker is shut off, and the positions of the bone vibrator and the masking earphone are switched. The vibrator is applied to the mastoid of the opposite ear, now to be tested, and the ear previously tested now is masked with the white noise. With the instruments in these positions, the bone conduction threshold values for the second ear are recorded for the same range of frequencies.

INTENSITIES AND FREQUENCIES. It is to be noted that whereas in air conduction testing the tone intensities may be increased to as high as 100 db for most frequencies, the vibrator used in bone conduction attains a maximum of only 50 or 60 db, as specified on the audiometer panel. Furthermore, in bone conduction testing, the highest frequency usually included in the test is 4,000 cycles. At 250 cycles there is some question of validity, because the tactile sense plays a role, especially at higher intensities.

Resolution of Divergent Opinions and Reference Levels. There is some difference of opinion as to when masking should be used, and there is considerable disagreement on how much and what type of masking is necessary. Some advocate that the extent of masking should be determined for each individual patient by means of a formula based on his air conduction audiogram, whereas others propose fixed masking levels for all.

To add to the confusion, the dial settings on many commercial audiometers have no absolute reference levels, so that it is difficult to know the real intensity of the masking noise. The calibration often is arbitrary, representing what the manufacturer considers to be "effective masking," and this may vary from producer to producer. The same decibel setting for a masking noise on four commercial audiometers may differ by as much as 20 decibels, and the reference levels generally are not designated. Even the spectrum of the noise is not described clearly on some instruments. Obviously, much clarification is needed in the problem of masking. One cannot rely on lateralization as observed in the Weber test for determining whether an ear should be masked.

IN CLINICAL PRACTICE all these differences can be effectively narrowed down by arbitrarily using white noise as a masker at a fixed level of 100 decibels (based not on the audiometer scale but on "acoustical zero," which is a sound pressure level of 0.0002 dyne per square centimeter; incidentally, this is equivalent to 85 db on the audiometer scale).

AIR CONDUCTION													
		RIGHT						LEFT					
DATE	LEFT MASK	250	500	1000	2000	4000	8000	RIGHT MASK	250	500	1000	2000	4000	8000
		-5	-5	-10	-10	-10	-10	-	55	60	60	50	65	60
								60	75	NR	NR	NR	NR	NR
								80	NR	NR	NR	NR	NR	NR
								100	NR	NR	NR	NR	NR	NR

BONE CONDUCTION												
		RIGHT						LEFT				
DATE	LEFT MASK	250	500	1000	2000	4000	TYPE	RIGHT MASK	250	500	1000	2000	4000
								-	5	5	10	15	15
								60	25	35	50	60	NR
								100	NR	NR	NR	NR	NR

Fig. 122. Patient with left total deafness due to mumps. Right ear is normal. Without masking the right ear in testing the left, a threshold of about 60 db seems to be present by air conduction, and bone conduction appears to be almost normal. These are shadow curves. With 60-db white noise masking (WN) in the right ear, the shadow curve for air almost disappears but not for bone conduction. With 80-db WN in the right ear, the shadow curve for air is gone. With 100-db WN in the right ear, there is no hearing for air or bone in the left ear. If, however, the 100-db white noise is put into the left ear during testing of the right normal ear, there is overmasking, and the right ear will show a reduced threshold. White noise in this case was measured above the zero average on the audiometer.

Although this is not the very best type of masking noise available, it is used most commonly in commercial audiometers and fulfills the two most important requirements: (1) it must be loud enough to mask out the ear not being tested, and (2) it must not be loud enough to interfere with the ear being tested. The testing results shown in Figure 122 exemplify some of the problems associated with masking and bone conduction testing.

THREE TYPES OF MASKING NOISE

Two types of masking noise are generally available on commercial instruments: (1) *sawtooth noise* and (2) *white noise*. A third type, *narrow band noise*, is beginning to appear on the market.

Narrow band noise is considerably more efficient than the other two, but most commercial audiometers in use today do not provide it. White noise or thermal noise contains all the frequencies in the audible spectrum at approximately equal intensities. In narrow band noise the frequencies lie within a narrow band around the frequency of the tone used for testing the opposite ear. Narrow band noise usually is produced by selectively filtering white noise until the frequency band is at least twice as wide as the critical band width. Because of its proved effectiveness in masking, it is likely to supersede the old types of masking noise now found in commercial audiometer design.

CLINICAL TESTING OF RESIDUAL HEARING

Too frequently a patient with unilateral deafness is tested with inadequate masking or no masking at all and is told he has residual hearing in an ear that is essentially deaf. In some instances he even may be misdiagnosed as having otosclerosis and be operated on without having a chance of success.

Simple Methods of Masking. In clinical practice several simple methods of masking are available to determine grossly whether an ear has some useful hearing or is practically totally deaf, as is commonly the case in unilateral deafness due to mumps and in some ears postoperatively. These methods employ three different sources of noise: (1) the air hose available in most nose spray apparatus, (2) douching the ear with water at body temperature, and (3) a Barany noise apparatus. Patients frequently are seen in practice who have conductive hearing loss in both ears, usually due to otosclerosis but occasionally to bilateral chronic otitis media. In some instances these patients have had mastoid, fenestration or stapes surgery in one ear only, and they seek the physician's help to determine whether it is possible to restore hearing in either ear. If the hearing level in both ears is around 50 or 60 decibels, it is very difficult to mask out either ear with commercially available masking devices. The important question to be determined is whether the ear that had the surgery now is totally deaf or actually does have a good amount of residual hearing. The most effective way of determining this in everyday practice is to strike a 500-cycle tuning fork, apply it to the operated ear by both air and bone conduction, and ask the patient whether he still hears it while the open end of the air hose is slanted into the opposite ear, and the air is turned on to make a loud masking nose. If, while the fork is still vibrating, the patient's hand comes down when the air hose is turned on and then reappears when the air hose is turned off again, in all likelihood the operated ear has little or no residual hearing, and further surgery is not warranted. Incidentally, under such circumstances it would be very injudicious to operate on the opposite ear, for in the event of a surgical complication the patient might lose his hearing in his one remaining useful ear and become totally deaf. The same masking effect can be obtained by douching the unoperated ear with tap water warmed to body temperature to avoid inducing vertigo. A Barany noise apparatus is an inexpensive and simply operated piece of equipment. It merely is wound up, inserted into the ear with a small tip and a button pressed. The noise produced is of a high level and can mask out most conductively deafened ears.

Sensorineural Acuity Level, a Supplementary Procedure. In order to overcome some of the difficulties in testing by bone conduction in conductively deafened ears, Rainville, Jerger and others developed a test called SAL (sensorineural acuity level). In this technic the bone conduction vibrator must be connected to a noise generator and applied to the patient's forehead. First the earphones of the audiometer are applied to both ears, and the air conduction threshold is obtained for each ear with no noise produced by the bone vibrator. Then the air conduction thresholds are obtained with the noise vibrator turned on to a specific level. The noise is supposed to be in signal strength of two volts across the vibrator. From these two air conduction thresholds, by comparing the results with a level that presumably is considered to be normal, it is possible to determine the level of sensorineural hearing loss. This technic avoids masking in a bone conduction test, but it is really not a substitute for standard bone conduction testing. It does not actually assess the bone conduction level in some patients any better than the standard technic, but it is a useful supplementary procedure.

PROBLEMS OF BONE CONDUCTION TESTING

Intensity of Masking in Conductive Hearing Loss

Masking for neutralizing a normal-hearing ear or an ear with sensorineural deafness is relatively easy (the latter can be masked out almost as easily as an ear with normal hearing), but a much higher intensity of masking noise is required to mask out an ear with conductive hearing loss. In such a case a number of problems emerge, since commercial audiometers generally do not provide higher masking noise levels. Even if such higher noise levels were available and used, they then would be transmitted through the skull by bone conduction and also affect the ear being tested, consequently producing a spurious threshold. There is no direct relationship between the amount of conductive deafness and the amount of masking necessary. Unfortunately, the relationship is not one to one.

Effectiveness of Media. The masking presently available in commercial audiometers is not effective in masking out the ear with a handicapping

AIR CONDUCTION

			RIGHT							LEFT					
DATE	Exam.	LEFT MASK	250	500	1000	2000	4000	8000	RIGHT MASK	250	500	1000	2000	4000	8000
Air hose Noise		100	70	80	70	80	80	NR		45	55	50	35	50	50
			NR	NR	NR	NR	NR	NR							

BONE CONDUCTION

			RIGHT						LEFT				
DATE	Exam.	LEFT MASK	250	500	1000	2000	4000	RIGHT MASK	250	500	1000	2000	4000
		–	5	10	10	30	30	–	–5	–5	5	30	30
		80	5	10	10	35	30						
		100	20	30	20	40	35						
Air Hose		35	NR	NR	NR	NR							

FIG. 123. The right ear in this patient actually has no hearing and gives no caloric response; yet it gives a measurable threshold by air and bone conduction despite large amounts of masking. The reason is that the masking noise is not enough to overcome the conductive hearing loss in the left ear. Discrimination tests with masking are more helpful. The use of compressed air noise, a Barany noisemaker, or narrow band noise through an insert receiver effectively masks out the left ear. With the present findings a misdiagnosis of right conductive deafness with an air-bone gap could be made, and the patient could be operated on without there being any chance of success.

level of conductive deafness, that is, over 25 or 30 db in the speech frequencies. Narrow band noise is considerably more effective and may help to solve some serious problems now confronting audiometry. This is particularly true if the narrow band masking can be delivered through an *insert type of receiver*, such as that used in hearing aids, instead of through a conventional earphone. The small insert receiver produces far less cross mask. The results shown in Figure 123 illustrate the difficulty in masking out an ear with conductive hearing loss.

At the time of purchasing an audiometer it is advisable to have a clear understanding of the spectrum of the noise and its absolute intensity at every level indicated on the volume control. If the physician now has an audiometer that does not provide these data, they can be obtained with the help of a nearby sound laboratory, or the intensity can be measured by a loudness balancing of the noise against a pure tone of 1,000 cycles on several normal-hearing subjects.

CALIBRATION OF THE BONE CONDUCTION VIBRATOR

Several major problems still exist in bone conduction testing. The first involves calibration of the bone conduction vibrator and the second concerns the relation of bone conduction threshold levels to the actual function of the sensorineural mechanism.

As yet there is no basic standard manner of calibrating tone vibrators. A satisfactory artificial ear has not yet been developed to accomplish this, and consequently there is no acceptable reference level for bone conduction testing. The result is that bone conduction testing is not nearly as reliable as air conduction testing. Each manufacturer of audiometers calibrates his instruments in his own way, and the results in different instruments are not always comparable. Two biologic technics for calibration are in common practice. In one the manufacturer sets the bone conduction reference threshold level at 0 decibels, using normal ears in a very quiet room, so that the subjects with a 0 air threshold level get a 0 bone threshold level. In the other technic the same reasoning is applied to patients who have true sensorineural hearing losses, so that the air and the bone conduction thresholds match. None of these technics is really quite satisfactory, but for the time being they must be used until a more sophisticated and reliable method is developed.

The problems of bone conduction audiometry are numerous and complex. They include such factors as placement and pressure of the oscillator, thickness of the skin and underlying tissue, density of the petrous bone, frequency being tested, noise conditions of the test room, condition of the ear not under test, masking occlusion effect and the vibrations of the skull and the bony capsule. Another important factor that has been overlooked is that of the air factor arising from the bone vibrator, especially when testing in the higher frequencies and higher intensities is done. A strong air signal emanating from the bone vibrator may be detected by air conduction before actual bone vibration takes place to elicit responses.

If a bone vibrator is calibrated on normal ears or ears with pure sensorineural impairment, and there is a strong air signal emanating from the bone vibrator, then when the bone vibrator is used on ears with conductive hearing impairment, it may not be of proper calibration at the higher frequencies and intensities. In these ears the air signal may be suppressed, with the result that the higher readings then obtained on the hearing loss dial would produce poorer bone thresholds than the actual conductive impairments of these patients would warrant.

Caution Needed in Interpretation of Bone Conduction Audiograms. The difficulties in standardizing calibration of audiometers and the numerous problems associated with bone conduction testing require great caution in the interpretation of bone conduction audiograms. Let us consider some examples showing how bone audiograms should be interpreted.

If an air conduction audiogram shows a loss of about 40 db in the speech frequencies, and the bone conduction audiogram shows a practically normal level, it is obvious that the patient has a conductive hearing loss. The patient is said to have an air-bone gap of about 40 db (i.e., the spread between the air and the bone conduction thresholds). Further-more, it is a safe conclusion that the patient's sensorineural mechanism is not impaired. In such a patient, if the conductive lesion is corrected, it should be possible to restore his hearing to normal.

In another patient with a similar air conduction threshold the examiner may find that the bone conduction threshold is not normal but still is better than the air threshold. Here there is an air-bone gap of roughly 20 db. This implies that the sensorineural mechanism is not normal, and that there is in addition a conductive deafness because of the air-bone gap, so that the maximal effect of surgery would be to bring the hearing level back to the bone conduction threshold. This is an example of mixed deafness.

In still another patient with a similar air conduction curve the bone conduction might be at about the same level as the air conduction; the condition then would be diagnosed as sensorineural deafness. There is no significant air-bone gap. In general, there should be at least a 10-db spread between air and bone thresholds in the speech frequencies to warrant considering the air-bone gap to be significant. In an air-bone gap of 10 db or less, the air factor of the bone vibrator may produce a false and misleading bone conduction threshold, and such an air-bone gap should not be considered to be significant.

Relation of the Bone Conduction Threshold Levels to the Function of the Sensorineural Mechanism

In patients whose audiograms have isolated dips, as at 3,000 or 4,000 cycles, there is no need to test bone conduction, for in these cases the classification is almost invariably sensorineural deafness. It is not likely that a conductive or a mixed hearing loss can produce such an isolated dip. However, this statement does not hold for all high tone hearing losses. One may find that in a patient with a high tone hearing loss whose bone conduction may be even somewhat reduced, the cause is not in the sensorineural pathway but in the middle ear. Fluid in the middle ear is the most common cause.

In interpreting bone conduction audiograms it is essential to bear in mind that the threshold obtained by bone conduction testing provides only a rough approximation of the function of the sensorineural mecha-nism. In certain cases of conductive deafness, especially in adhesive otitis and in the presence of fluid in the middle ears, the lower bone conduction values that frequently are obtained do not indicate necessarily true sen-sorineural deafness but rather impaired mobility of the oval and the round windows.

Bone conduction audiometry on the mastoid bone often shows a marked reduction that is not borne out by testing on the upper incisor tooth with a 500-cycle tuning fork. In such instances the sensorineural function is more likely to reflect the better bone conduction by teeth than the poorer bone conduction via the mastoid bone. Of course, it is important to rule out tactile sensation in evaluating these conflicting findings. Another important factor in assessing bone conduction thresholds is to bear in mind that the maximum intensity obtainable on commercial audiometers for bone vibrators is about 55 or 60 db. The failure to obtain any bone conduction in routine testing does not indicate necessarily that the sensorineural mechanism is dead. It indicates only that the mechanism does not respond at the maximum intensity of the tone.

Since bone conduction testing really consists of a vibratory stimulus, it has created a problem in interpretation. Many patients with very severe air conduction hearing losses give responses to bone conduction at 250 and 500 cycles as low as 20 or 25 db. This creates the impression that an air-bone gap exists in these low frequencies. Such an impression is not justified. Actually, in most patients with severe nerve deafness, the thresholds at these low frequencies are probably a response to tactile sensation and not to auditory stimuli. On the basis of these findings alone, middle ear surgery is not warranted.

Chapter 24

Special Hearing Tests

For the majority of patients who complain of hearing loss, the history, the ear examination, the tuning fork tests, and air and bone conduction audiometry provide sufficient information to make a diagnosis. This information tells the physician how much hearing is lost, what frequencies are affected, and even helps him to determine whether the loss is conductive or sensorineural in nature.

These tests are particularly adequate in most cases of conductive hearing loss. However, there are some cases of conductive hearing loss and many cases of sensorineural loss in which these tests do not disclose enough information to make an accurate diagnosis possible, and additional hearing studies may become necessary.

Since air and bone conduction audiometry measures only thresholds of pure tones, it provides limited information. For instance, it does not help the physician to detect certain phenomena that aid in localizing the site of a lesion in sensorineural involvements or to assess a patient's capacity to use his residual hearing. Phenomena such as recruitment, tone decay, tonal distortion, and the patient's ability to discriminate speech, to localize sound or to understand speech in a noisy environment give clues to the site of a lesion. To obtain this information special hearing tests have been devised. These rarely are done by general practitioners or pediatricians, but many are carried out in an otologist's office, and most are performed in hospital or university hearing centers.

Though family doctors and otologists may not perform all these tests, they should know when they are indicated, and they should be able to interpret the results as an aid in evaluating a patient's complete hearing status.

THE DIFFERENCE BETWEEN AUDIOMETRIC THRESHOLD LEVELS AND DISCRIMINATION ABILITY TO HEAR SPEECH

It is common practice to interpret a patient's ability to hear speech by averaging his pure tone thresholds in the three speech frequencies in the audiogram. For example, if his hearing loss was 30 db at 500, 40 db at 1,000, and 50 db at 2,000 cps, his average hearing loss would come to 40 db for the speech frequencies, and this would be called his hearing loss for pure tones and for speech. It is also common practice to express this as an average and to tell the patient that he has a 40 per cent hearing loss. This latter procedure has serious shortcomings and should be avoided in clinical practice. The only place it has some application is in determining hearing impairment in compensation problems, but this is not the same as using it to describe a patient's hearing capacity.

Let us consider several problems associated with this procedure. If a patient is told that he has a 40 per cent hearing loss, he naturally infers that he has only 60 per cent of his hearing left, which, of course, is not true, for maximum hearing does not stop at 100 db (maximum output of most audiometers), but the ear continues to respond to much higher intensities. Percentages as a means of expressing hearing loss are most seriously at variance with the facts in cases of sensory hearing loss due to Ménière's disease and other sensorineural handicaps. When the physician tells a patient with Ménière's disease that he has only a 40 per cent hearing loss, the patient has a right to reply that the calculation may be perfectly correct, but as far as he is concerned, his hearing loss is nearly 100 per cent, because he cannot use his ear on the telephone at all, and he gets little or no use of it in daily communication. The problem exists because the threshold determination shows a 40-db hearing level for pure tones, whereas what the patient is referring to is his ability to distinguish or to discriminate what he hears. In some patients with Ménière's disease the ability to discriminate may be impaired so completely as to make the ear useless even with only a 40-db threshold level in the speech frequencies.

Still another shortcoming of expressing hearing loss on the basis of speech frequency is demonstrated in Figure 124. Both patients, whose audiograms are shown as A and B, have an average hearing loss of 40 db;

AIR CONDUCTION						
	250	500	1000	2000	4000	8000
(A)	15	20	40	60	65	NR
(B)	50	50	40	30	30	35

Fig. 124. Patients A and B have an average pure tone loss of 40 db, but patient A can get along well without the use of a hearing aid, whereas patient B will need amplification.

but patient A can get along quite well without the use of a hearing aid, whereas patient B badly needs a hearing aid to get along reasonably well.

The physician should explain to his patient the difference between audiometric threshold levels and discriminating ability. The patient also should be told the facts about his other difficulties, such as sound localization in unilateral hearing losses, recruitment, hearing in the presence of noise, etc.

FIG. 125. LISTS OF SPONDEES*

LIST A	LIST B	LIST C	LIST D	LIST E	LIST F
greyhound	playground	birthday	hothouse	northwest	padlock
schoolboy	grandson	hothouse	padlock	doormat	daybreak
inkwell	doormat	toothbrush	eardrum	railroad	sunset
whitewash	woodwork	horseshoe	sidewalk	woodwork	farewell
pancake	armchair	airplane	cowboy	hardware	northwest
mousetrap	stairway	northwest	mushroom	stairway	airplane
eardrum	cowboy	whitewash	farewell	sidewalk	playground
headlight	oatmeal	hotdog	horseshoe	birthday	iceberg
birthday	railroad	hardware	workshop	farewell	drawbridge
duckpond	baseball	woodwork	duckpond	greyhound	baseball
sidewalk	padlock	stairway	baseball	cowboy	woodwork
hotdog	hardware	daybreak	railroad	daybreak	inkwell
padlock	whitewash	sidewalk	hardware	drawbridge	pancake
mushroom	hotdog	railroad	toothbrush	duckpond	toothbrush
hardware	sunset	oatmeal	airplane	horseshoe	hardware
workshop	headlight	headlight	iceberg	armchair	railroad
horseshoe	drawbridge	pancake	armchair	padlock	oatmeal
armchair	toothbrush	doormat	grandson	mousetrap	grandson
baseball	mushroom	farewell	playground	headlight	mousetrap
stairway	farewell	mousetrap	oatmeal	airplane	workshop
cowboy	horseshoe	armchair	northwest	inkwell	eardrum
iceberg	pancake	drawbridge	woodwork	grandson	greyhound
northwest	inkwell	mushroom	stairway	workshop	doormat
railroad	mousetrap	baseball	hotdog	hotdog	horseshoe
playground	airplane	grandson	headlight	oatmeal	stairway
airplane	sidewalk	padlock	pancake	sunset	cowboy
woodwork	eardrum	greyhound	birthday	pancake	sidewalk
oatmeal	birthday	sunset	greyhound	eardrum	mushroom
toothbrush	hothouse	cowboy	mousetrap	mushroom	armchair
farewell	iceberg	duckpond	schoolboy	whitewash	whitewash
grandson	schoolboy	playground	whitewash	hothouse	hotdog
drawbridge	duckpond	inkwell	inkwell	toothbrush	schoolboy
doormat	workshop	eardrum	doormat	playground	headlight
hothouse	northwest	workshop	daybreak	baseball	duckpond
daybreak	greyhound	schoolboy	drawbridge	iceberg	birthday
sunset	daybreak	iceberg	sunset	schoolboy	hothouse

* Auditory Test W-1, Spondee Word Lists, Central Institute for the Deaf.

TESTING HEARING WITH SPEECH

SPEECH RECEPTION TESTS

In addition to pure tones for testing threshold and for calculating hearing acuity the physician can use speech of electronically controlled intensity. What is measured by this test is called a speech reception threshold (SRT). This represents the faintest level at which speech is heard and repeated. The patient's hearing loss for speech is the difference in decibels between his threshold and that for normal ears tested with the same speech material (the reference level on the speech audiometer). The results obtained with this test are equivalent to averaging the hearing levels obtained at 500, 1,000, and 2,000 cycles, the range that comprises the so-called speech frequencies.

Several types of speech material can be used to determine SRT. These include isolated words, individual sentences and connected discourse. The most commonly used material is the standardized word list composed of spondaic words (spondees). These are 2-syllable words equally stressed on both syllables, prepared in several lists (Fig. 125).

Administration. The test can be administered by phonograph records or by monitored live voice through a microphone attached to the speech audiometer. Earphones are placed on the patient's ears to test the hearing in each ear separately, or the patient may be tested through a loud speaker, in which case binaural hearing is tested. The patient is instructed to repeat the spondee words or sentences as they are presented. He should be told also that the words or the sentences will become fainter as the test proceeds, but that he should repeat them until they are no longer audible.

The Significance of Various Speech Reception Thresholds. The point at which 50 per cent of the items are heard correctly as the intensity is reduced is considered to be the speech reception threshold. In clinical practice 5-db steps of attenuation for every 3 words is a satisfactory rate.

A normal-hearing person has an SRT of between 0 and 10 db. An SRT up to about 25 db usually presents no important handicapping hearing impairment in cases of conductive hearing loss. However, when the loss exceeds this level, the patient experiences difficulties in everyday communication, and a hearing aid usually is necessary.

In general, thresholds for speech tests and thresholds obtained by averaging the pure tones in the speech frequency should differ by no more than 6 db. Discrepancies may be found between the two in cases in which there is a sharp drop-off in pure tone thresholds across the 500 to 2,000 frequency range, with resulting discrimination problems. Discrimination difficulty may exist in cases of Ménière's disease or acoustic nerve tumor.

in which there is a wide disparity between SRT and pure tone average losses. There may be also a wide disparity in cases in which the loss is produced by emotional rather than organic causes.

DISCRIMINATION TESTING

Determining the speech reception threshold is a rather imperfect measure of a person's ability to hear speech. Generally, it does not tell whether the patient is able to distinguish sounds that he hears, particularly difficult sounds. A special test to measure speech discrimination, devised to satisfy this need, differs from tests previously described in that it does not measure a minimal sound level but the *ability to understand speech* when it is amplified to a comfortable level.

Discrimination testing usually is done at 30 or 40 db above the speech reception threshold. This level has been found to yield maximum discrimination scores. In some patients with a severe hearing loss a level of 40 db above the speech reception threshold is very difficult to obtain, since most instruments cannot go above 100 db. In other subjects such a level might be painful or uncomfortable, or it might cause distortion in the instrument or the ear itself, resulting in invalid scores. In such cases the level of presentation of the test material should be adjusted to a comfortable listening level for the particular subject.

Materials used to test discrimination ability are known as phonetically balanced word lists (PB lists). These are lists of monosyllabic words balanced for their phonetic content so that they have about the same distribution of vowels and consonants as that found in everyday speech. The lists are made up of 50 words each, and because each list is balanced in a particular way, it is necessary to administer the full list of 50 words when the test is performed (Fig. 126). Occasionally, the list is cut in half, but this leaves the resulting scores open to some question.

Administration. The test usually is administered through each earphone in order to test the discrimination ability of each ear individually. Testing can be done by means of a phonograph record on which the PB word lists have been recorded or by monitored live voice testing through a microphone. Each word is preceded by an introductory phrase, such as, "Say the word —— —," and the subject is asked to repeat the word that he thinks he hears.

Rating. Only those words understood perfectly are counted as correct. Each word has a value of two points, so that a perfect score would be 100 points. If 10 of the 50 words are repeated incorrectly, the patient has an 80 per cent discrimination score. It is obvious, then, that an individual can suffer not only from a quantitative reduction in his ability to hear sounds but also from a reduction in discrimination, so that even when the

Fig. 126. Phonetically Balanced Word Lists (PB Lists)*

	List 4E	List 4F	List 3E	List 3F
1.	ought (aught)	our (hour)	add (ad)	west
2.	wood (would)	art	we	start
3.	through (thru)	darn	ears	farm
4.	ear	ought (aught)	start	out
5.	men	stiff	is	book
6.	darn	am	on	when
7.	can	go	jar	this
8.	shoe	few	oil	oil
9.	tin	arm	smooth	lie (lye)
10.	so (sew)	yet	end	owes
11.	my	jump	use (yews)	glove
12.	am	pale (pail)	book	cute
13.	few	yes	aim	three
14.	all (awl)	bee (be)	wool	chair
15.	clothes	eyes (ayes)	do	hand
16.	save	than	this	knit
17.	near	save	have	pie
18.	yet	toy	pie	ten
19.	toy	my	may	wool
20.	eyes (ayes)	chin	lie (lye)	camp
21.	bread (bred)	shoe	raw	end
22.	pale (pail)	his	hand	king
23.	leaves	ear	through	on
24.	yes	tea (tee)	cute	tan
25.	they	at	year	we
26.	be (bee)	wood (would)	three	ears
27.	dolls	in (inn)	bill	ate (eight)
28.	jump	men	chair	jar
29.	of	cook	say	if
30.	than	tin	glove	use (yews)
31.	why	where	nest	shove
32.	arm	all (awl)	farm	do
33.	hang	hang	he	are
34.	nuts	near	owes	may
35.	aid	why	done (dun)	he
36.	net	bread (bred)	ten	through
37.	who	dolls	are	say
38.	chin	they	when	bill
39.	where	leave	tie	year
40.	still	of	camp	nest
41.	go	aid	shove	raw
42.	his	nuts	knit	done (dun)
43.	cook	clothes	no (know)	have
44.	art	who	king	tie
45.	will	so (sew)	if	aim
46.	tea (tee)	net	out	no (know)
47.	in (inn)	can	dull	smooth
48.	our (hour)	will	tan	dull
49.	dust	through (thru)	ate (eight)	is
50.	at	dust	west	add (ad)

* Central Institute for the Deaf.

speech is made sufficiently intense to be well above his threshold, he still cannot distinguish what is being said.

ARRANGEMENT OF EQUIPMENT

Ideally, pure tone and speech tests should be conducted via a 2-room arrangement, which provides a soundproof room with the necessary earphones, microphone and loudspeakers, in which the patient is seated, and an adjacent control room housing the pure tone audiometer, the speech audiometer and the examiner's microphone. The examiner conducts the tests from this room. All electrical connections are accomplished through wall plugs, and the addition of an observation window between the 2 rooms permits the examiner to watch the patient's reaction during the testing period. The 2-room arrangement is essential when monitored live voice testing is done through a microphone; otherwise the subject might very well hear the speech directly from the tester's voice rather than through the equipment that electronically controls the intensity of the speech. One other precaution is to have the subject seated so that he cannot observe the tester's lips during the procedure. Even a fair lipreader can render the speech tests inaccurate if he is allowed to complement the auditory signals with lipreading.

Evaluation of Discrimination Score. It is essential to remember that the

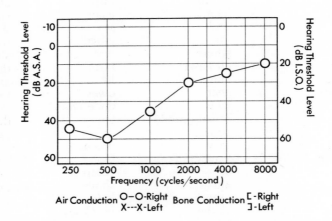

Fig. 127. One patient had this audiogram due to otosclerosis. The discrimination score was 98%.

Another patient had this same audiogram due to acoustic neuroma. The discrimination score was 42%.

Still another patient had this same audiogram due to Ménière's disease. The discrimination score was 62%.

discrimination score cannot be translated directly into the percentage of difficulty that the patient will have in everyday life. A discrimination score provides only a rough idea of the patient's ability to distinguish certain sounds in a quiet environment. With experience a broader interpretation can be made, but when this is done, other factors such as the effects of environmental noise must be taken into consideration.

Figure 127 compares the discrimination scores in a series of patients with about the same speech reception threshold but with different diagnoses.

Clues to Discrimination. These tests require electronic equipment that may not be available in the offices of many practitioners. Nevertheless, even a careful history and examination will give a rough estimate of a patient's ability to hear and to distinguish speech. For example the patient should be asked how he gets along with each ear when using the telephone. He may volunteer that though voices come over loud enough, he cannot understand conversation on the telephone. This usually indicates a reduction in discrimination ability.

Another important clue to discrimination ability is whether the patient experiences more difficulty in noisy environments. If he does, it is probably because he has reduced discrimination, which is further aggravated by environmental noise that masks out the normally weak consonants. The physician who has no hearing testing equipment in his office may obtain a fair idea of a patient's discrimination score by asking him to repeat words in the phonetically balanced lists when the physician presents them without letting the patient see the examiner's face. The words should be spoken at a normal level of intensity and enunciated normally. If the loss is unilateral, the better ear must be masked with noise intense enough to prevent its participation in the test. The same precaution is necessary during testing with audiometric equipment. Scores obtained without masking the opposite ear can result in a diagnosis of doubtful validity.

RECRUITMENT

The phenomenon of recruitment has been defined elsewhere in this book as a disproportionate increase in the sensation of loudness of a sound when its intensity is raised. The principal value of detecting recruitment is that it helps to trace the site of the lesion in the auditory pathway to the hair cells of the cochlea. The patient often provides clues to the presence of cochlear damage when he is questioned about his hearing difficulty. He may say that loud noises are very bothersome in his bad ear, or that the sound seems to be tinny and harsh and very unclear. Or he may volunteer that music sounds distorted or flat. These complaints should not be confused with the annoyance voiced by a neurotic patient who hears well but is bothered by such noises as the shouting of children. A well-defined sensorineural hearing loss always should be present before recruitment can be accepted as a basis for localizing an auditory deficit to the cochlea.

DEMONSTRATION

Tuning Fork. Recruitment can be detected in some cases with the aid of a 500-cycle tuning fork if a hearing loss affects the speech frequencies, as often occurs in Ménière's disease. The test is done by comparing the growth of loudness in the good ear with that in the bad ear. The fork is struck once gently and held up to each of the patient's ears, and he is asked in which ear the tone sounds louder. Naturally, he will say the tone is louder in the normal-hearing ear. Then the intensity of the tone is increased by striking the fork once again quite hard (but not too hard, or the tone will be distorted). The patient then is asked again to indicate in which ear the tone now sounds louder, with the fork held first near the good ear and then quickly moved about the same distance from the bad ear. If complete or hyperrecruitment is present, the patient will now exclaim in surprise that the tone is as loud or louder in his bad ear. This means there has been in his bad ear, in spite of a hearing loss, a larger growth in the sensation of loudness, since the same tone now sounds as loud or louder in the bad ear as in the good ear.

Alternate Binaural Loudness Balance Test. Testing for recruitment with a tuning fork is a rather rough technic, but it may help in diagnosing recruitment. More precise tests have been devised to test for recruitment, but most of these are suitable for use only when one ear is impaired, and the other is normal. The technic in common use is called the alternate binaural loudness balance test, which matches the loudness of a given tone in each ear.

This test is done with an audiometer and involves presenting a tone of a certain intensity to the good ear and then alternately applying it to the bad ear at various intensities; the patient is asked to report when the tone is equally loud in both ears. Initially, a brief tone 15 db above threshold is applied to the good ear. Then the tone is presented briefly to the bad ear 15 db above its threshold, and the patient is asked if the tone was louder or softer than that heard in the good ear. According to his response, necessary adjustments are made to the intensity going to the bad ear until a loudness balance is obtained with the good ear. Then the intensity to the good ear is increased by another 15 db, and another balance is obtained with the bad ear. Loudness balancing is continued in 15-db steps until sufficient information is obtained about the growth of loudness in the bad ear. This technic requires that the same frequency be balanced in the two ears, and that the tone be presented alternately to the good ear, which serves as the reference. Also, the difference in threshold between the two ears should be at least 20 db for this test to be valid.

If the difference in loudness level between the two ears is maintained unchanged at higher intensities, recruitment is absent. On the other hand,

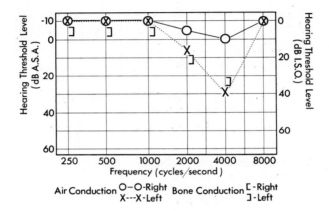

Air Conduction O–O-Right Bone Conduction ⌐-Right
X---X-Left   ⌐-Left

Fig. 128. Male, 21, with acoustic trauma of the left ear caused by explosion of a firecracker. Two methods of recording results of loudness balance tests are shown:

4,000 cps

R	L
0	30
5	30
10	35
30	40
45	50
70	70
85	85
100	100

4,000 cps

o Right ear threshold
x Left ear threshold

if the loudness difference gradually decreases at higher intensities, recruitment is present. If the loudness difference completely disappears between the two ears at higher intensities, the condition is called complete recruitment and is indicative of damage to the inner ear. There may be complete

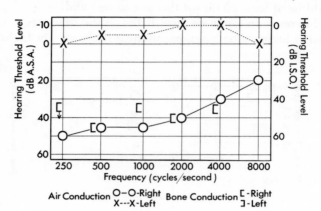

Fig. 129. Patient with Ménière's disease in right ear.
Discrimination score: 62% at 70 db
42% at 80 db
30% at 90 db

Note that not only does the 1,000-cps tone sound equally loud in both ears at 80 db, but that an 85-db tone in the bad right ear sounds as loud as a 95-db tone in the normal left ear. This is called hyperrecruitment. Diplacusis is marked, with the higher sounding and distorted tone in the right ear.

1,000 cps	
L	R
0	45
15	50
25	55
35	60
50	65
60	70
70	75
80	80
85	80
95	85

o Right ear threshold
x Left ear threshold

or even hyperrecruitment, in which case the tone in the bad ear sounds even louder than the tone in the good ear at some point above threshold. Recruitment may occur at varying speeds. If it continues regularly with each increase of intensity, it is called continuous recruitment, and this is indicative of inner ear damage. Recruitment that is found only at or near threshold levels is not characteristic of inner ear damage but occurs often in sensorineural hearing impairment. Figures 128 and 129 show two cases that exhibit recruitment, with methods of recording the result.

Detection of Small Changes in Intensity. Another method of demonstrating recruitment involves the patient's ability to detect small changes in intensity. A recruiting ear detects smaller changes in loudness than normal ears or those with conductive hearing loss. At levels near threshold a normal ear is likely to require a change of about 2 db to recognize a difference in loudness, but in an ear that recruits, only a ½-db increase may be necessary to detect the loudness change. As the intensity of the tone then increases in normal ears, the change necessary for detecting the difference in loudness becomes smaller, whereas the recruiting ear requires about the same change as it did near threshold level.

SISI Test. Another test for localizing the site of damage to the cochlea is the short-increment sensitivity index (or SISI) test. It measures the patient's ability to hear small, short changes of sound intensity. The test is done monaurally by fixing the level of a steady tone at 20 db above the patient's threshold at each frequency to be tested, and superimposing on this steady tone 1-db increments of about 200 milliseconds' duration, interspersing the increments at 5-second intervals. The patient is to respond each time he hears any "jumps in loudness." If he hears 5 of the 1-db increments, his sensitivity index is 25 per cent. A score of between 60 and 100 per cent at frequencies above 1,000 cps is positive for cochlear disorders, whereas a score below 20 per cent is considered to be negative. Scores between 20 and 60 per cent are infrequent but are observed most commonly in presbycusis.

Other tests using speech discrimination and Bekesy audiometry testing also help to determine the presence of cochlear damage; these are supplementary to the basic tests described here. They are especially helpful when both ears have a hearing loss, because a "control" ear is not essential to the test procedure.

DIPLACUSIS—DISTORTION OF PITCH

Another simple and fairly reliable office test can be done with a tuning fork to help to localize the site of auditory damage in the cochlea. This test explores not distortion of loudness (recruitment) but distortion in pitch, which is called diplacusis. It seems that distortion is the keynote of hair cell damage.

A 500-cycle tuning fork is struck and held near the normal ear and then to the opposite ear. If the damage is localized in the cochlea, the patient may report that the same tuning fork has a different sound when it is heard in the bad ear. Usually, he will say that the pitch is higher and not as clear, but rather fuzzy.

HEARING TESTS USING SPEECH TO DETECT, CENTRAL DEAFNESS

Special tests using modified speech are becoming very useful in deciding whether a hearing loss is due to damage in the central nervous system. Lesions in the cortex do not result in any reduction in pure tone thresholds, but brain stem lesions may cause some high tone hearing loss. Routine speech audiometry is practically always normal in cortical lesions, and sometimes it is impaired in brain stem lesions, but without a characteristic pattern. Since neither pure tone nor routine speech tests help to localize damage in the central nervous system, more complex tests have been developed to help to provide this information.

A chief function of the cortex is to convert neural impulses into meaningful information. Words and sentences acquire their significance at the cortical level. Because quality, space and time are factors governing the cortical identification of a verbal pattern, the tests are so designed that they explore the synthesizing ability of the cortex when one or more of these factors is purposely changed.

Binaural Test of Auditory Fusion

One such test of central auditory dysfunction is the binaural test of auditory fusion. Speech signals are transmitted through two different narrow band filters. Each band by itself is too narrow to allow recognition of the test words. Normal-hearing subjects show excellent integration of test words when they receive the signals from one filter in one ear and the other filter in the other ear. Poorer scores are made by patients with brain lesions and are indications of a functional failure of the synaptic connections within the cortex.

Sound Localization Tests

Sound localization tests also are being used in the diagnosis of central lesions. Deviation of the localization band to one side points to a cerebral lesion on the contralateral side or to a brain stem lesion on the homolateral side.

OTHER TESTS

Distorted voice, interrupted voice and accelerated voice tests likewise are used in detecting central lesions. In the distorted voice test phonetically balanced words are administered about 50 db above the threshold through a low pass filter that is able to reduce the discrimination to about 70 or 80 per cent in normal subjects. Patients with temporal lobe tumors present an average discrimination score that is poorer in the ear contralateral to the tumor.

The interrupted voice test presents at about 50 db above threshold phonetically balanced words that are interrupted periodically 10 times per second. Normal-hearing subjects obtain about 80 per cent discrimination; those with temporal lobe tumors have reduced discrimination in the ear contralateral to the tumor.

In the accelerated voice test, when the number of words per minute is increased from about 150 words to about 350 words, the discrimination approaches 100 per cent in normal-hearing subjects, but threshold is raised by 10 to 15 db. In patients with tumors of the temporal lobe there is a normal threshold shift, but the discrimination never attains 100 per cent in the contralateral ear. In cortical lesions the impairment seems always to be in the ear contralateral to the neoplasm and moderate in extent. Brain stem lesions exhibit severe bilateral impairments.

INTERPRETATION OF DISCRIMINATION SCORES

Discrimination scores between 90 and 100 per cent are considered to be normal. Scores between 90 and 100 per cent are obtained usually by patients who have conductive hearing losses or those who have dips at high frequencies, such as a 40-db dip at 3,000 cps; these scores are common also in cases in which the losses encompass only the higher frequencies of 4,000, 6,000 and 8,000 cps. Discrimination usually is not affected adversely when the loss is in this higher frequency range, because most speech sounds are in the area below 4,000 cps. A slight reduction in the discrimination score occurs in patients with sensorineural deafness involving 2,000 cps and above. Generally, patients with these high tone losses experience more difficulty in daily conversation than their discrimination score would suggest.

In the interpretation of a discrimination score it should be recalled that the test was done in a quiet room and therefore does not measure the patient's ability to discriminate against a noisy background. In such an environment the discrimination score probably would be worse, because consonants are masked out by the noise. At present there is no completely reliable method of measuring an individual's ability to get along in every-day conversation under varied circumstances.

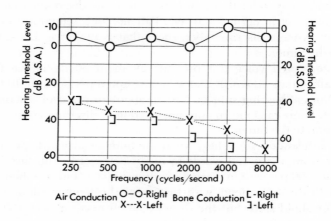

Fig. 130. Patient has an acoustic neuroma. There was abnormal tone decay in the left ear during the 60-second test (right ear masked).

500 cps	1,000 cps	2,000 cps
*35 to **70	*35 to **75	*40 to **80

* Threshold at start of the 1-minute tone presentation.
** Threshold after 1 minute of continual stimulation.

The Bekesy tracing revealed a large gap between the pulsed and the continuous tracings.

	1,000 cps	
	R	L
	0	35
No recruitment	15	50
	30	60
	45	75
	50	80

The discrimination score in the left ear was 92% when the right ear was not masked. With masking in the right ear, discrimination dropped to 22%, an indication that the first result was incorrect, because the test material was being heard in the good ear.

LOWER SCORES

Discrimination scores are moderately lower in patients with deafness due to **presbycusis** or **congenital causes.** Severe reductions in discrimination are associated with two principal causes, Ménière's disease and acoustic neuroma.

In Ménière's disease the discrimination difficulty generally is attributed to the distortion produced in the cochlea, i.e., distortion in loudness, pitch and clarity of speech. The characteristic finding in marked Ménière's disease is that the discrimination score becomes even worse as speech is made louder (Fig. 129).

In acoustic neuroma the damage to the auditory nerve fibers may produce very little reduction in the hearing threshold level for pure tones but a disproportionately large reduction in the discrimination score. This disproportion is an important clue to the presence of acoustic neuroma, one that should be watched for in every case of unilateral sensorineural deafness.

IMPORTANT POINTS IN DISCRIMINATION TESTING

Masking. Because masking often is overlooked in discrimination testing and speech reception testing, its importance must be reiterated. Without proper masking of the nontest ear serious errors in diagnosis can be made (Fig. 130).

Etiology. From the examples in Figures 127, 129 and 130 it is obvious that it is not possible always to predict the discrimination score from the pure tone audiogram. The etiology is of the utmost importance in assessing the discrimination.

TESTS FOR FUNCTIONAL DEAFNESS

Whenever a patient claims to have a hearing loss that does not seem to be based on organic damage to the auditory pathway, or whenever the test responses and the general behavior of the patient appear to be questionable, a variety of tests can be performed to help to determine whether the loss is functional rather than organic.

SUGGESTIVE CLUES

The most suggestive findings are inconsistencies in the hearing tests. For instance, a patient has a hearing threshold level of 70 db in one test and then gives a 40-db threshold when the test is repeated several minutes later; or the audiogram of a patient shows a 60-db average hearing loss bilaterally, but the patient inadvertently replies to soft speech spoken behind his back; or he has a speech reception threshold of 20 db in contrast with a 60-db pure tone average; or the patient gives poor or no responses in bone conduction tests, indicating severe sensorineural involvement, but has suspiciously good discrimination ability for the apparent degree and type of loss.

Also, the patient's behavior may not be consistent with the degree of loss claimed, especially in cases of bilateral functional deafness. Usually, a patient with severe bilateral deafness is very attentive to the speaker's face and mouth in order to benefit from lipreading. A functionally deaf person may not show this attentiveness. He also may have unusually good voice control, which is not consistent with the degree of loss. Occasionally, a functionally deaf person will assume a moronic attitude or repeat part of a test word correctly and labor excessively over the last half of the word. These and other subtle clues should alert the examiner to the possibility of the presence of a purely functional deafness or a functional overlay on an organic deafness.

LOMBARD OR VOICE-REFLEX TEST

When a patient claims deafness in one ear, but it is suspected of being functional, several simple tests are available to determine the validity of the loss. The patient is given a newspaper or a magazine article to read out loud without stopping. While he is reading, the tester takes a stiff piece of typing paper, such as onion skin paper, holds it flat over the patient's good ear, and briskly rubs it against the ear in a circular motion. If the patient's voice does not get significantly louder, it is highly suggestive that he can hear in his supposedly "bad" ear. Since hearing is partly a feedback mechanism that informs the speaker how loud he is speaking, a person with normal hearing will speak more loudly in a very noisy area so that he can hear himself and be heard above the noise. If the patient does not raise his voice when noise is applied to one ear, it means that he is hearing himself speak in the other ear, and consequently that ear does not have the marked hearing loss indicated on the pure tone or speech audiogram. Instead of rubbing paper against the patient's ears as the source of noise, a Barany noise apparatus or the noise from an audiometer noise generator is extremely effective in this test, because the level of the noise can be controlled. This type of test is called the Lombard or voice-reflex test, and although it does not help to establish thresholds, it does give the examiner some idea of whether or not the loss is exaggerated.

STENGER TEST

The Stenger test also is used for detecting unilateral functional deafness and evaluating the approximate amount of residual hearing. This test can be done with tuning forks or with an audiometer, the latter being the more reliable. The test depends on the fact that if two equally sensitive ears receive an identical stimulus at the same time, the sound will be localized somewhere near the center of the head. If the sound in one ear is made louder, then the listener will hear it only in that ear. He will not even realize that the weaker sound exists in the other ear. A tone is presented to the good ear about 10 db above its threshold, and the patient will localize it naturally in that ear. Then the tone is presented also to the bad ear at the same number of decibels above its threshold. If the hearing loss is authentic in his bad ear, the patient should localize the sound somewhere in the center of his head. If the threshold is better than has been admitted in the bad ear, the tone will sound louder in that ear and should be localized there. If he admits that he does hear the sound in his bad ear, then obviously the hearing level in that ear is better than at first indicated. Or the patient may claim that he hears no sound at all, even though the tone is still on in his good ear, in which case the intensity in the bad ear gradually is lowered until the patient says he again hears the sound in his good ear. The fact that the tone in the "bad" ear had to be reduced to allow the sound to localize to the good ear indicates that the bad ear has better hearing than previously was admitted.

Also, the fact that the patient reports hearing no sound, even though the tone is still on in his good ear, indicates his confusion and his method of trying to solve it by ceasing to respond.

REPETITION OF AUDIOGRAM WITHOUT MASKING

Still another test to indicate whether a patient really has a total unilateral deafness or may be malingering is to repeat the audiogram but this time without masking the good ear. Since a pure tone presented to the test ear can be heard also in the nontest ear when the loudness of the tone is 50 to 55 db above the threshold of the nontest ear, at least some shadow curve should be present in the absence of masking. If the patient does not respond when the intensity levels reach this point, then the chances are that he has a functional deafness in the test ear, because there should be shadow hearing from the good ear. If the patient does report hearing the tone, he should be questioned carefully about its location. Again, total lack of response is an indication of the dilemma that the functional patient faces when he feels that his claim is threatened with exposure.

Delayed Talk-Back Test

The monitoring effect of an ear can also be disrupted if a person listens to himself speak through earphones while the return voice is delayed in time. A delay of 0.1 to 0.2 second causes symptoms similar to stuttering. If this occurs when the feedback level is lower than the admitted threshold, functional loss is present. In the delayed talk-back test, which is done through a modified tape recorder, it is possible to detect hearing losses of sizable degree but not the minor exaggerations that occur occasionally in medicolegal situations. This is so because delayed feed-back affects the rhythm and the rate of the patient's speech at levels averaging 20 to 40 db above threshold.

PGSR Test

A great deal of testing has been done with the psychogalvanic skin response (PGSR) test, which is as close to being an objective test of hearing as presently is available, though it still has many shortcomings. This test is done with special equipment and is based on the conditioned response mechanism. The patient is conditioned so that each time that he hears a tone, it is followed about a second later by a definite electric shock in his leg, to which is strapped an electrode. Through electrodes placed on the patient's fingers or palms it is possible to measure the change in skin resistance or the so-called electrodermal response excited by the electric shock in the patient's leg. Each time that the patient receives a shock, the skin resistance is altered and can be read on a meter or recorded on a moving graph. After the patient is well conditioned, the electric shock is stopped, and only the sound is given. In a well-conditioned patient, about a second after the sound is applied, he will "expect" the shock again and show a typical change in his electrodermal response through the movement of the meter dial or the pen tracing the responses. It can be concluded, then, that each time the patient gives a positive reading on the recording equipment after a sound is given, he hears the sound. By lowering the intensity of the stimulus, a threshold level can be obtained. At certain intervals it is necessary to reinforce the conditioned response mechanism by reapplying the electric shock.

This is an excellent technic based to some extent on the traditional lie detector method, but many complicating factors make it far from a completely reliable method of measuring a hearing threshold level objectively and reliably. It is excellent, however, if it is used in conjunction with a battery of other tests, in helping to establish the organic or the nonorganic basis of any hearing threshold.

USE OF EXCELLENT AUDIOMETRIC TECHNIC

One of the most effective methods of obviating functional deafness, particularly in industry and in school hearing testing programs, is to use excellent audiometric technic. Malingering and inaccurate responses are discouraged by a tester who uses excellent technic. Malingering normal hearing also is possible. If a patient is given a sound and is asked repeatedly, "Do you hear it?" he will be tempted to say, "Yes," even if he does not hear it, whenever some advantage or remuneration is at stake, such as obtaining employment.

Responsibility of the Tester. The question as to what a tester in industry or in a school system should do when he suspects or detects a malingerer or someone with functional deafness is of importance. It is not the tester's responsibility to accuse or even to imply to the subject that he is suspected of giving inaccurate responses. Quite often inaccurate responses are the result of disturbances in the auditory tract or nervous pathway, or the loss may be a true hysterical deafness. The tester may not be qualified to express so sophisticated a judgment. The tester's only responsibility is to suspect that the audiogram does not represent the accurate threshold of hearing of the individual tested. The subject should be handled in a routine manner, and subsequently the findings should be brought to the attention of the physician in charge of the hearing testing program. If the physician is suitably trained to study the patient on a more comprehensive basis, he should proceed to do so. If not, the patient should be referred to an otologist or a hearing center that is equipped to study the problem more intensively.

AUDITORY TONE DECAY

Just as marked recruitment usually is indicative of damage in the inner ear, abnormal tone decay (abnormal auditory fatigue) usually is a sign of pressure on or damage to the auditory nerve fibers. This phenomenon may be of particular importance in that it can be an early sign of an acoustic neuroma or some other neoplasm invading the posterior fossa.

ADMINISTRATION OF TEST

The test for abnormal tone decay is very simple to perform and should be done routinely in every case of unilateral sensorineural deafness, especially when no recruitment is found.

The test is based on the fact that whereas a person with normal hearing can continue to hear a steady threshold tone for at least 1 minute, the patient who has a tumor pressing on his auditory nerve is unable to keep hearing a threshold tone for this length of time. The test is performed monaurally with an audiometer. A frequency that shows reduced threshold is selected, and the patient is instructed to raise his finger as soon as the tone comes on and to keep his finger raised as long as he can hear the tone. The tone then is persented at threshold or 5 db above threshold, and a stop watch is started with the presentation of the tone. Each time that the patient lowers his finger, the intensity is increased 5 db, and the time is noted for that period of hearing. The tone interrupter switch never is released from the "on" position during any of the intensity changes. The test is 1 minute in duration.

FINDINGS

A person without abnormal tone decay usually will continue to hold up his finger during the entire 60 seconds. Occasionally, he may require a 5- or 10-db increase during the first part of the test, but he then maintains the tone for the remainder of the time. A patient who has abnormal tone decay may lower his finger after only about 10 seconds, and when the tone is raised 5 db, he may lower his finger again after another 10 seconds and continue to indicate that the tone fades out repeatedly, until after 60 seconds there may be an increase of 25 db or more above the original threshold. Some patients may even fail to hear the tone at the maximum intensity of the audiometer after 1 minute, whereas originally they may have heard the threshold tone at 25 db. This finding of abnormal tone decay is highly suggestive of pressure on the auditory nerve fibers. Figure 130 describes a typical case. Unfortunately, a tuning fork cannot be used to perform this test, because its sound decays rapidly, and the test requires a continuous tone at a constant intensity.

BEKESY AUDIOMETER

Another method of measuring abnormal tone decay is with a Bekesy audiometer. This is a type of self-recording audiometer that does not require the tester to be in constant attendance during the test. It is being used with increased frequency for threshold and special testing, and physicians should be acquainted with its operating principles and the information that it can supply.

SELF-RECORDING OR AUTOMATIC AUDIOMETRY

PROCEDURE AND MECHANISM

This method of establishing pure tone thresholds permits the patient to trace his own audiogram as the tone or tones are presented to him automatically. Each ear is tested separately. The patient holds a hand switch and has on a set of earphones through which he hears the tone. As soon as he hears the tone he presses the switch, which causes the sound to decrease in loudness, and holds it down until the tone is no longer audible. When he can no longer hear the tone, he releases the switch, which will allow the tone to increase in intensity until it can be detected again, at which time he again presses the switch and holds it until the tone is gone. This procedure continues until the full range of frequencies has been tested.

The switch controls the attenuator of the audiometer that decreases or increases the intensity of the tone. A pen geared to the attenuator makes a continuous record on an audiogram blank of the patient's intensity adjustments. The audiogram blank is placed on a table which moves in relation to the frequency being presented. Several methods of frequency selection are available. The audiometer can be set up to produce the frequency range continuously from 100 to 10,000 cycles, or it can be arranged to test hearing in a 2-octave range or, if desired, to test threshold for a single frequency for several minutes.

The test signal can be continuous, that is, without interruption, or pulsed at a rate of about 2½ times per second. Operation of the patient's hand switch attenuates the signal at a rate of about 2½ to 5 db per second according to the speed selection made by the examiner. Thus a test routinely performed with Bekesy self-recording audiometry can determine thresholds with both pulsed and continuous tone presentations. If the pulsed tone is used first, a pen with a specific colored ink is placed in the penholder, and the thresholds are recorded. When the pulsed tone testing is completed, a pen with a different color is placed in the penholder, the frequency is reset to the original point, and the switching is changed to provide a continuous tone. The patient traces another audiogram, as he did for the pulsed tones. It is important that the patient not see the equipment in operation, because awareness of the movements of the pen and the action of the hand switch may affect his responses and result in an invalid audiogram.

VALUE

With proper instruction to the patient, automatic audiometry not only

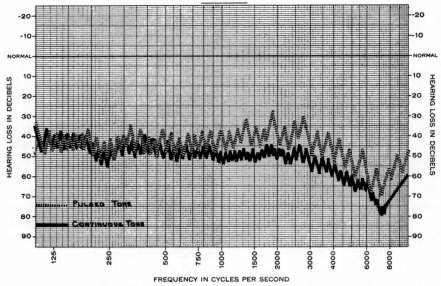

FIG. 131. Bekesy tracings of a patient with Ménière's disease. A slight separation of the pulsed and the continuous tone tracings appears only in the higher frequencies.

provides an accurate picture of thresholds but also supplies other valuable information and helps to determine the site of lesions within the auditory system. By comparing the thresholds for the pulsed and the continuous tone, the physician can get a reasonably good indication of the site of the lesion or at least additional information that will contribute to this determination.

TYPES OF AUDIOGRAMS

In normal or conductively impaired ears the pulsed and the continuous tracings overlap for the entire frequency range tested. This a Type I audiogram. In the Type II audiogram the pulsed and the continuous tones overlap in the low frequencies, but between 500 and 1,000 cycles the continuous frequency tracing drops about 15 db below the pulsed tracing and then remains parallel with the high frequencies. Type II audiograms occur in cases of cochlear involvement. Sometimes the pen excursions narrow down to about 5 db in the higher frequencies. Cases of cochlear involvement sometimes also show Type I tracings.

In the Type III audiogram the continuous tracing drops suddenly away from the pulsed tracing, and usually continues down to the intensity limits

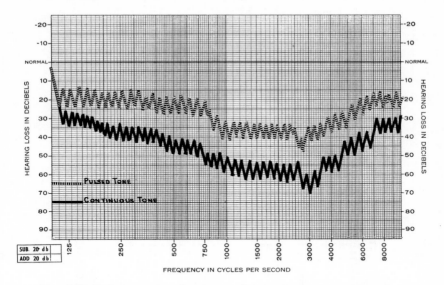

FIG. 132. Bekesy tracings in a case of acoustic neuroma. Tone decay is demonstrated by a large gap between the pulsed and the continuous tone tracings. In some cases the continuous tone tracing may break completely away at around 500 cps, and the tone may not be heard even at the maximum output of the audiometer.

of the audiometer. Eighth nerve disorders usually show Type III audiograms. Another type of audiogram found in 8th nerve disorders is the Type IV tracing, in which the continuous tone tracing stays well below the pulsed tracing at all frequencies.

INTERPRETATION OF THE BEKESY AUDIOGRAM

There is some feeling that the amplitude of the Bekesy audiogram provides considerable information about the presence or the absence of recruitment. For example, tracings of very small amplitude might lead one to believe that the patient can detect changes in intensity much smaller than the average subject, and that he therefore has recruitment. Unfortunately, this is not the case. It is more likely that tracings of small amplitude are suggestive of abnormal tone decay rather than of recruitment. A great deal of the interpretation depends on the on-and-off period of the tone presented. Figures 131 and 132 show examples of Bekesy audiograms.

RUDMOSE SELF-RECORDING AUDIOMETER

Whereas the Bekesy audiometer presents a continuously varying fre-

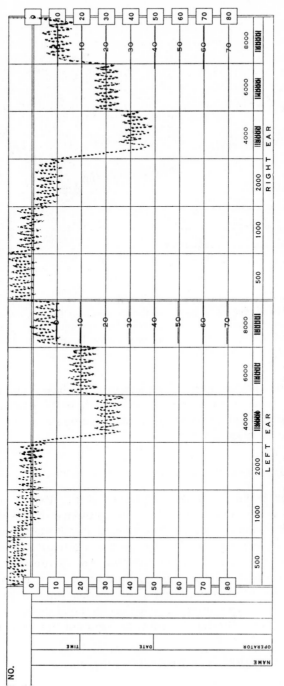

Fig. 133. Rudmose discrete frequency audiogram showing normal hearing in low frequencies and at 8,000 cps, and a loss at 4,000 and 6,000 cps.

quency (unless it is purposely set up to deliver a discrete frequency), the Rudmose self-recording audiometer presents discrete individual frequencies that are changed automatically at about 60-second intervals. The newer types of Rudmose Bekesy type audiometers present both pulsed or continuous tones at the option of the operator. Figure 133 shows an example of an audiogram obtained with a Rudmose self-recording audiometer.

Chapter 25

Handicapping Effects of Hearing Losses

Although the most obvious of the effects of hearing loss is that on communication through sound media, far more serious is the damaging effect of hearing loss on the individual's confidence in his ability to function effectively in his social and business life. His natural optimism and belief in his personal competence to deal with his fellowman in a successful manner are undermined, and he finds himself unsure, apprehensive and resentful.

EFFECT ON THE PERSONALITY

No other physical handicap has so many and such serious repercussions on the personalities of people as hearing loss, and, interestingly enough, some of the worst effects are associated with hearing losses that are comparatively mild in degree, almost negligible on the basis of physical measurements alone. Conversely, many profound hearing losses may produce severe disruption of communication without seriously affecting the personality. The reasons for such differences are found in the strength of character of the individual and in his mental, spiritual and economic resources to triumph over adversity and to make the most of his ability to find self-fulfilment, economic security and the joy of living.

Hearing loss cannot be restricted to the ear itself. It is not possible to divorce the ears from what lies between them. Hearing is a phenomenon that utilizes the pathways between the ears and the brain and is an essential part of human response pathways. In any discussion of hearing, communication, deafness and handicap it is necessary to think of the person as a whole and not merely as a pair of ears. For this reason hearing loss concerns not only the otologist but also the general practitioner, the pediatrician, the psychologist, the psychiatrist and many others, including, more recently, members of the legal profession.

THE RELATIONSHIP BETWEEN HEARING AND SPEECH

To understand the basis for the personality changes and communication handicaps that hearing loss may produce, it is necessary to recall the relationship between hearing and speech. The reader now is well aware that the ear is sensitive to a certain frequency range, and obviously speech falls within that range. Speech can be divided into two types of sounds: vowels and consonants. Roughly speaking, one could say that vowels fall into the frequencies below 1,500 cps, and consonants above 1,500 cps. Also the vowels are relatively powerful sounds, whereas consonants are weak, and quite often these are not pronounced clearly or even are dropped completely in everyday speech. Vowels give power to speech; that is, they signify that someone is speaking, but by themselves they give very little information about what the speaker is saying. To give specific meaning to words, consonants are interspersed among the vowels. Thus, it can be roughly stated that vowels tell that someone is saying something whereas consonants help the listener to understand or to discriminate what the speaker is saying.

For example, the hard-of-hearing individual whose audiogram is shown in Figure 124B would have difficulty hearing speech unless it was quite loud. His difficulty lies in the low tones, and so he cannot hear vowels. For example, he would not be able to hear soft voices. However, if the voice was raised, he would hear it and understand it clearly. His principal problem is one of loudness or amplification.

The person whose hearing impairment is portrayed in Figure 124 A has a high tone loss with almost normal hearing in the low tones. This means that he hears vowels practically normally but would have difficulty in hearing and discriminating consonants. If the speaker raised his voice, the patient might find it disturbing, since it would emphasize the missing consonants only slightly, though it would increase the loudness of the vowels to a disturbing degree. This individual's chief problem is not *hearing* but *distinguishing* what he hears. He hears the vowels, and so he knows someone is speaking; but he cannot distinguish some of the consonants, and thus he is unable to tell what is being said. This type of person would want the speaker to enunciate more clearly and to pronounce the consonants more distinctively rather than to speak in a loud voice.

Hearing loss of this type with its accompanying handicaps is found commonly in presbycusis, occupational deafness and in certain types of congenital deafness.

REACTIONS TO HEARING LOSS

The manner in which people react to hearing loss varies considerably. Some may try to minimize or to hide their defect. Such a person, to keep up with a conversation, makes strenuous listening efforts and fills in hearing gaps by guessing, while he carefully conceals his frustration by acting particularly pleasant and affable. His effort to "save face" leads to numerous embarrassing situations, becomes fatiguing and leads to nervousness, irritability and instability. He sits on the edge of his chair and leans forward to hear better. From the strain of listening his brow becomes wrinkled, and his face serious and strained. Toward evening he is worn out from his efforts to hide and to deny his handicap. The sense of humor in which he once took great pride falters in a losing effort to maintain a pretense of normalcy and makes way for a desperate show of sham amiability and a grim smile.

Some people react to hearing loss, particularly that of slow and insidious onset, by becoming withdrawn and losing interest in their environment. This, the most common type of reaction, is reflected in an avoidance of social contacts and in a preoccupation with the subject's own misfortunes. He shuns his friends and makes excuses to avoid social contacts that might cause his handicap to become more apparent to his friends and to himself.

Economic and Family Aspects. This reaction may be seen in a businessman who has to sit at board meetings and planning or training meetings for salesmen and executives. The handicapped person soon realizes that he cannot keep up with what is going on, and rather than tolerate the criticism and suspicious remarks reflecting on his alertness and proper interest in the business, he may resign his responsibilities and step down to a position less worthy of his potential.

When a salesman becomes hard of hearing, his business usually suffers, and his ambitions frequently are suppressed or completely surrendered. A hearing impairment may cause no handicap to a chipper or a riveter while he is at work. His deafness may even seem to be to his advantage, since the noise of his work is not as loud to him as it is to his fellow workers with normal hearing. Because there is little or no verbal communication in most jobs that produce intense noise, a hearing loss will not be made apparent by inability to understand complicated verbal directions. However, when such a workman returns to his family at night or goes on his vacation, the situation assumes a completely different perspective. He has trouble understanding what his wife is saying, especially if he is reading the paper, and his wife is talking while she is making noise in the kitchen. This kind of situation frequently leads at first to a mild dispute and later to serious family tension.

The wife accuses the husband of inattention, which he denies, while he complains in rebuttal that she mumbles. Actually, he eventually does become inattentive when he realizes how frustrating and fatiguing it is to strain to hear. When the same individual tries to attend meetings, to visit with friends, or to go to church services and finds he cannot hear what is going on or is laughed at for giving an answer unrelated to the subject under discussion, he soon, but very reluctantly, realizes that something really is wrong with him. He stops going to places where he feels pilloried by his handicap. He stops going to the movies, the theater or concerts, for the voices and the music are not only far away but frequently distorted. Little by little his whole family life may be undermined, and a cloud overhangs his future and that of his dependents.

High tone hearing loss and distortion, common features of sensorineural deafness, often cause serious deterioration in a person's ability to understand speech. Music, certain voices and especially amplified sound often will sound hollow, tinny and muffled. The hard-of-hearing person so affected may first ask his companion to speak louder, but in spite of the louder speech he seems to understand even less. Loudness actually may reduce discrimination in such individuals. Distortion is the factor that causes the greatest difficulty. It is natural that people who do not hear clearly should become confused and annoyed.

The Plight of the Aged Deaf. Hearing losses in older persons, whether from causes associated with aging or owing to other sensorineural etiologies, are often quite profound. All too often the unfortunate oldster begins to believe that his inability to hear and to understand a conversation, particularly when several people are talking, is due to deterioration of his brain. This belief generally is forced on him by his family and friends, who disregard him in group conversations and assume the attitude that he does not know what is going on anyhow. So why include him in the conversation? Occasionally, he will overhear a remark or notice a gesture signifying that he is getting old and slowing down. Such talk and such attitudes further undermine the old person's already weakened self-confidence and hasten the personality changes so common in deafness and more particularly in the aged deaf. What a great injustice thus is done to all concerned!

Effect of Mild Hearing Losses. Strangely enough, some of the most profound personality changes and communication handicaps occur in people who have comparatively mild hearing losses. This effect is particularly evident in otosclerosis. It is seen also in occupational deafness of moderate degree and in that accompanied by distortion and tinnitus. Often, such an individual is constantly disturbed not only by the noises in his ears, the artificial tinny sound of music, amplified sound and certain voices, but even more by the haunting fear that he will not be able to understand what someone is going to say to him. Sometimes he may hear very well and at other times he cannot make out what is being said. The feelings of uncertainty and insecurity that result from so-called borderline hearing loss may lay the foundation for profound changes in a subject's personality structure. They lead to irritability and suspicion. Frequently, catching only stray words of a nearby conversation, he comes to feel that others are talking about him in a critical and derogatory manner. This makes him feel resentful and tends to bring out in him latent neurotic tendencies for which he otherwise might have compensated successfully.

Effect of Profound Hearing Losses. In general, people with profound hearing losses are somewhat easier to help than the borderline cases, since the former are under greater compulsion to admit that they have a handicap. People with borderline losses tend to hide their handicap and to deny it even to themselves. They conceal their deafness just as they try to conceal their hearing aids if they can be induced, or are able, to use them. Of course, the major handicaps in the severe losses are with communication as well as some personality problems. Often these individuals cannot hear warning signals, such as a fire bell or a telephone bell. They cannot maintain their job on engines if they are required to use their hearing to detect flaws in the motor. This is particularly true in persons working with airplanes and diesel engines or other noisy motors. Another important handicap in the more severe losses is the inability to tell the direction from which a sound is coming. This difficulty is particularly prominent when the deafness exists in only one ear, or when the hearing loss in one ear is much worse than in the other, because two ears with reasonable normal hearings are needed to localize the source and the direction of sound.

Another interesting aspect of profound hearing loss is that after a while the person so handicapped tends to speak less clearly. His speech deteriorates; he begins to slur his s's, and his voice becomes rigid and somewhat monotonous. This frequently happens when a person can no longer hear his own voice. He cannot hear himself speak, so at first he raises his voice, often to the point of shouting. After a while he may find this still unsatisfactory, and then he loses interest in his ability to speak clearly, and he will not even realize that his speech is deteriorating. The reason is that one of the important functions of the ear is to serve as a monitor for speech. Hearing his own voice tells a person not only how loud he is talking but also whether he is modulating and pronouncing his words correctly. With the loss of this important monitoring system in nerve deafness, various speech and voice changes often occur.

EFFECT ON SOCIAL CONTACTS

Unlike the blind and the crippled, the deaf have no outward signs of disability, and strangers are apt to confuse imperfect hearing with imperfect intelligence. This hurts the hard-of-hearing person's feelings; this and similar attitudes make for a strained relationship between a speaker and a listener. As a result, the hard-of-hearing person frequently limits his social contacts, and this often leads to moods of frustration, insecurity, and even aggression.

The hard-of-hearing person misses the small talk about him. He does not get the flavor of a conversation so much enriched by side-remarks and innuendoes. This eventually makes him feel shut off from the normal-hearing world around him and makes him a prey to discouragement and hopelessness. Until a person loses some hearing, he hardly can realize how important it is to hear the small background sounds around him, and how much these sounds help him to feel alive, and how their absence makes life seem to be rather dull. Imagine missing the sounds of rustling leaves, footsteps, keys in doors, motors running and the thousands of other little sounds that make human beings feel that they "belong."

A Personal Tragedy With Dynamic Aspects

When people become aware, if only to a small degree, of the possible effects of hearing loss, they wonder how a money value can be placed on such a handicap. Although the compensation aspects of occupational deafness demand standardized values on hearing losses, from a medical and a social aspect a hearing loss is a personal tragedy to each individual. Furthermore, the handicapping effects of hearing loss are dynamic. They are changing even as this book is being written. With the development of new media for sound communication, an individual's hearing comes to assume ever greater importance. For example, a hearing loss today is far more handicapping than it was before TV, radio and the telephone began to play such major roles in education, leisure and the business world. Today the inability to understand on a telephone is indeed a major handicap for the vast majority of people. The loss of even high tones alone to a professional or an amateur musician or even to a high-fidelity fan also is handicapping. The hearing loss of tomorrow will have a different handicapping effect from the hearing loss of today.

AUDITORY REHABILITATION

Although it is true that there is no medical or surgical cure for sensori-neural deafness, a great deal can be done to help the individual to compensate for his hearing handicap and to lead as normal a life as possible with minimal undue effects on his personality or his social and economic status. This is all done through a method emphasized during World War

II and described as "auditory rehabilitation." Thousands of servicemen with hearing impairments were successfully rehabilitated through the large hearing centers established by the Army, the Navy and the Veterans Administration. Although few such centers are now available to civilians, many private otologists, university centers and hearing aid centers can provide rehabilitation measures for persons with handicapping hearing losses that cannot be corrected medically or surgically.

Despite the serious limitations of modern knowledge and therapy of so-called nerve deafness, it can be stated truthfully that practically everyone with a handicapping hearing loss can be helped greatly by effective auditory rehabilitation. The principal objective of such a program is to help the individual to overcome his hearing handicap in every way possible. The program includes (see numbered paragraphs following):

1. Giving the individual a clear understanding of his hearing problem and explaining to him why he has trouble hearing or understanding speech. This requires the otologist or audiologist to demonstrate to the patient on a large diagram of the ear just how the hearing mechanism works, and where the patient's pathology lies. The patient also should be given a clear understanding of the difference between hearing trouble and trouble in understanding what he hears. He should be told that the difficulty lies in his ears and not in his brain. It also should be explained to him why he has more difficulty in understanding speech when there is much noise around, or when several people are speaking simultaneously. The problems that might easily lead the patient to develop frustrations and personality disorders should be explained clearly so that he can meet these problems forthrightly and intelligently. Personality changes that otherwise might develop from hearing loss thus can be prevented or mitigated.

2. Psychological adjustment for each patient. This involves giving the patient a more penetrating insight into the personality problems that are already in evidence or likely to develop as a result of his hearing loss. The individual must be treated in relation to his job, family, friends and way of life. This is not a generalized technic but one that must be specifically designed to meet the needs of the individual whose hearing is impaired. Frequently, it is advisable to carry out this part of the program not only with the patient himself but also with his wife or family, for it is impossible to separate a man's personality problems from the problems of his family. At this point in the program the patient must accept his hearing disability as a permanent situation and not sit idly by, waiting for a medical or surgical cure. Above all, confidence and self-assurance must be instilled in the patient. He must be encouraged to associate with his friends and not to isolate himself because of difficulties in communication. It must be impressed on him that by using the hearing he has left

effectively, he can achieve his ambitions and carry on as usual with only minor modifications.

3. The fitting of a hearing aid when it is indicated. This is a vital part of the program, but before a patient can be expected to accept a hearing aid, he must be psychologically prepared for it. Many people are reluctant to use hearing aids, and many who have purchased hearing aids never use them or use them ineffectively. Before recommending a hearing aid, it is necessary to determine whether the patient will be helped by it enough to justify his purchasing one. This is particularly important in sensorineural deafness in which the problem is more one of discrimination than of amplification. Usually a hearing aid does very little to improve a person's ability to understand, but it does improve his ability to hear by making sounds louder.

It generally is felt that when an individual has a speech reception loss greater than 30 decibels, he requires help with a hearing aid. At this level he starts to have trouble in comfortably hearing speech unless the speaker keeps his voice raised under circumstances that ordinarily would call for whispers or soft tones.

A hearing aid is essentially a miniature amplification system which serves to make the speaker's voice louder when it reaches the ear of the hard-of-hearing user. The hearing aid actually has no effect on the user's hearing. It makes it neither worse nor better, as some people are wont to believe. It just helps the individual to hear better by amplifying the sounds that enter the microphone of the hearing aid. In many instances when distortion is present in the listener's ear, amplification will aggravate the distortion, and under these circumstances a hearing aid will be of limited usefulness.

One of the most important things that a hearing aid does in types of hearing losses commonly found as a result of noise exposure is to permit the individual to hear what he already hears but with greater ease. It removes the severe strain of listening. Although the individual may not be able to understand more with an aid than without one, he nevertheless receives great benefit from the device, because it relieves him of the tension, the fatigue and some of the complications of hearing impairment.

Some hearing aids sound better than others to certain ears because of their amplifying pattern and frequency range; in addition, hearing aids vary in their amplifying power and in important special features, such as tone control and telephone circuits. Since a hearing aid represents a substantial investment and in many cases can make a tremendous contribution to a patient's welfare, it is in the interest of the purchaser to go to a hearing center where he is encouraged to compare many different types of aids without being rushed into an unsuitable selection, and where he will find the personnel to be experienced, patient and considerate.

The patient who seeks early medical attention for his hearing loss is wise in many respects. If his condition can be benefited by medical or surgical means, he has a better chance of being helped. If a hearing aid is necessary, the sooner the patient acquires it, the less severe will be the shock to his "nerves" when the aid obliges him to listen to environmental noises that the patient may have been shielded from too long, such as the barking of dogs and the crying of a baby.

Thousands of hearing aids, bought and paid for and given too brief and halfhearted a trial, are relegated to a bureau drawer. Overlong postponement in acquiring the aid is sometimes a factor. Often, too, the patient expects to hear normally with a hearing aid, when the condition of his hearing makes such a result impossible. Both the physician and the hearing aid dealer should make it clear to the patient that a hearing aid never can be a perfect substitute for a normal ear, especially in a patient with sensorineural deafness. Other common causes of disappointment with a hearing aid are incompetent hearing aid salesmen, and the patient's preoccupation with an "invisible" or inconspicuous aid, when what he should look for is an aid that will enable him to understand conversation with maximal effectiveness.

4. Auditory training to teach the patient how most effectively to use his residual hearing with and without a hearing aid. If the patient can be aided with a hearing aid, he also should be made to realize that merely putting on the aid will not solve all of his hearing and psychological problems. He has to learn to use the hearing aid with maximum efficiency in such situations as person-to-person conversation, listening to people in groups and at meetings, and on the telephone. Above all, he must recognize the limitations of an aid, so that he will use it when it can be helpful and not use it or turn down the volume when it is more of a detriment than a help, as in certain noisy situations.

If the individual cannot use a hearing aid, he can be taught to use his hearing more effectively by looking more purposefully at the speaker's face and to develop an intuitive grasp of conversational trends so that he can fill in the gaps better than the average person.

5. Speech reading—a broader concept of lipreading. This is particularly important in patients who have profound hearing losses. It teaches the patient to obtain the information from the speaker's face that cannot be obtained by sound communication. All people do a large amount of speech reading naturally, and by excellent training a person can develop this faculty extremely well, though some individuals have a greater aptitude for speech reading than others.

By cooperating with a carefully planned and competently presented rehabilitation program, practically all people with handicapping deafness can be aided not only to hear better, but, more important, they can be helped to overcome the many personality problems and psychological difficulties that result from deafness.

One factor that often complicates the problem of helping the hard of hearing is that they delay so long in obtaining medical attention. It is difficult to get some obviously deafened people to admit that they have a hearing problem at all, and even more difficult to convince them that they should see a physician about it. This is one of the reasons that physicians often do not see patients until their deafness has for years created marked social and communicative problems both to the patient and to his family and friends.

Although in older people this delay is usually due to pride (they think, "This couldn't happen to me!"), it is more often due to lack of observance on the part of parents when hearing handicaps are neglected in children. In children the delay is the more regrettable, since many of the conditions that cause hearing losses in the young can be cured if they are detected early enough, whereas in other cases they can be prevented from becoming worse. Too often the failure of children to answer when they are spoken to is attributed to childish inattention, and the possibility that hearing impairment may be playing a part is overlooked.

The emphasis in this chapter on rehabilitative measures short of medical or surgical cure reflects the fact that a total cure—especially in adults—is not possible in the great majority of cases of hearing loss. The often dramatically successful middle ear surgery is limited mainly to the treatment of otosclerosis having a reasonably good spread between air and bone conduction (air-bone gap); for such surgery to have a chance of success the patient must have a cochlea in at least fair working order and a functioning auditory nerve. Unfortunately, these requirements are not met by a majority of hard-of-hearing patients. Yet for them rehabilitation often can do a great deal.

The physician can play an important part in helping patients over their psychological hurdles after a hearing aid, speech reading and similar measures have done all that can be expected of them. The patient still may need help in adjusting socially, economically and emotionally to his continuing handicap. The hard-of-hearing patient must learn "how to live with a hearing handicap." A patient of ours chose these very words as a title for his book for the hard-of-hearing public. In a nutshell his thesis is that "above the ears there is a brain," an organ of often inadequately explored possibilities but one that can solve many problems if properly used. He points out that people who do not use their brain for all it is worth really suffer from a handicap far more severe than a mere hearing impairment, and this leads him to a series of case histories of men, women and children who have lived successfully with their hearing losses, sometimes with the help of understanding parents and marriage partners, but in other cases in the face of misunderstanding and discouragement. Sometimes I prescribe this book for my patients.

The informed physician is the ideal person to share with his patients his knowledge of the causes of their hearing handicap, and to help them to overcome the psychological hurdles that loom so much larger in the average patient's mind than the hearing loss itself.

Chapter 26

Prevention of
Occupational Deafness

Numerous factors have combined in recent years to make occupational deafness of importance to physicians. The industrial revolution during and after World War II vastly increased the number of employees exposed to intense noise in defense industries. As a result the incidence of occupational hearing loss rose markedly, probably affecting millions of persons.

GROWTH OF AN INCREASED SENSE OF RESPONSIBILITY

Before 1948 hearing loss caused by industrial noise was not considered important enough to be included in workmen's compensation in the majority of states. In those in which compensation for deafness was provided for, it was included incidentally in paragraphs pertaining to explosions and injuries; the text usually specified as a condition for recovery that deafness must be total in one ear or both ears. Little or no mention was made of partial hearing losses due to prolonged exposure to excessive occupational noise. The chief reason for this omission was that lawmakers were not aware of the far-reaching consequences of hearing loss. Since it did not seem directly to cause loss of wages or loss of earning power, legislators felt it did not warrant being considered an occupational disease.

Beginning in New York in 1948 and extending into Wisconsin and Missouri, a series of legal precedents was established that made partial loss of hearing resulting from exposure to industrial noise compensable though no wages might have been lost. Since then many other states, as well as the Federal Government, have made partial hearing loss due to noise exposure compensable. Some states even have passed specific laws defining partial hearing loss as a disease: occupational deafness. In states

351

in which this entity is not specifically included under workmen's compensation or in special laws, redress for industrial hearing loss still can be obtained by recourse to the common law. Large sums of money have at times been awarded by jury verdicts to workers suing employers in this manner.

The possibility of claims for compensation and the high incidence of deafness are not the sole factors motivating the present interest in the problem of industrial deafness. Management and labor as well as physicians are genuinely concerned about employee health. The threat of hearing loss to the well-being of people generally and to skilled industrial workers in particular is receiving increasing recognition.

The very serious repercussions that deafness may have on the individual and the damage it may inflict on his personality also are becoming more widely understood. Physicians throughout the country are being called upon in sizable numbers to assume vital roles in advising local industries on medical problems and in determining the cause and the degree of hearing impairment in personnel—especially in industrial compensation cases.

BASIS OF JUDGMENT BY A PHYSICIAN

In order that a physician may be able to provide a considered judgment in such cases, he must have the best available scientific information at his fingertips in this highly specialized field.

The characteristic audiometric findings in noise-induced hearing loss are discussed and illustrated by audiograms in Chapter 14. In this field it is essential that a physician be able to make a specific diagnosis. He must be competent to differentiate a hearing loss produced by exposure to noise from hearing losses of other sensory and sensorineural etiologies, including most cases of presbycusis.

EFFECT OF PROLONGED EXPOSURE TO INTENSE NOISE

In its early stage prolonged exposure to intense noise affects the outer hair cells of the organ of Corti and produces a slight dip at about 4,000 cps. Actually, the hearing loss affects a range from 3,000 to 4,000 cps, but measurements do not always cover this frequency spectrum. At this early stage the hearing loss rarely exceeds 40 db. As the exposure to noise continues, inner hair cells also become affected, and the hearing impairment becomes greater than 40 db. As long as only the hair cells are damaged, the impairment is classified as sensory. As exposure to intense noise continues, and the impairment gets worse, the supporting cells in the cochlea also may become damaged, and subsequently the nerve fibers themselves become affected. The case then falls into the sensorineural classification. As a matter of fact, most cases of occupational deafness that physicians see in their offices are of the sensorineural type, since patients generally seek medical attention only after their losses have become handicapping. By this time the nerve fibers usually have become involved.

Factors in Making a Diagnosis

Distinguishing Noise-induced Sensorineural Deafness. How does one go about making a diagnosis of sensorineural deafness due to prolonged exposure to intense noise and distinguishing it from other possible causes? Reference already has been made to the points of distinction between early occupational deafness and presbycusis. In the former the audiometric pattern is a dip at 4,000 cps, with better hearing in the higher frequencies. Testing at 8,000 cps and above shows fairly good residual hearing in occupational deafness. In presbycusis the higher frequencies almost invariably are more depressed than the lower ones. Furthermore, complete and continuous recruitment is present in early cases of occupational deafness but not in presbycusis. In addition, a diagnosis of occupational hearing loss requires a proven history of many months' exposure to a damaging noise level. Age, too, must be given consideration in making this distinction. A diagnosis of premature presbycusis in patients below 45 should be made with great caution. There are so many more likely causes than the questionable diagnosis of "premature presbycusis."

It is not always possible to distinguish more advanced cases of occupational deafness, i.e., cases of the sensorineural type, from cases of presbycusis. Evidence of damaging noise exposure must exist. If, in addition, the patient hears much better at 8,000 cps and above than at lower frequency levels, the principal cause of hearing loss is probably exposure to intense noise rather than aging. The presence of continuous recruitment also favors a diagnosis of noise-induced deafness, provided that the patient worked in a very noisy area. The subject's age is a vital diagnostic criterion, since a marked hearing loss in a young man would not be expected without other corroborating items such as heredity, ototoxic drugs, Ménière's disease, etc. Another point of distinction is that occupational deafness does not seem to progress when noise exposure stops, whereas presbycusis generally progresses, though very slowly. Of course, it may take many months or years to make this comparison.

Figure 134 illustrates a typical case of sensorineural deafness due to noise exposure. Figure 135 typifies an even more advanced case in a boilermaker. Because of his age, we assumed that some portion of the latter case was due to presbycusis, but the patient claimed his hearing had been bad for many years and had become slightly worse during the past year.

Unilateral Deafness Not Occupational Deafness. The likelihood that prolonged exposure to intense noise may be the cause of severe deafness in only one ear, while the other ear remains practically normal, is in conflict with available facts. Patients with unilateral total or subtotal deafness who work in noisy industries may claim that their deafness was produced by many years' exposure to intense noise. Since many physicians have heard of a link between noise and hearing loss, some are likely to assume such a connection. However, all evidence reported by competent investigators and extensive clinical practice agrees that a severe sudden or even insidious hearing loss in only one ear cannot result from prolonged exposure (for months or years) to intense industrial noise that is heard in both ears. *Sudden acoustic trauma is a different story entirely.*

Even if severe unilateral deafness develops over a period of several weeks, the probability of its being caused by prolonged exposure to

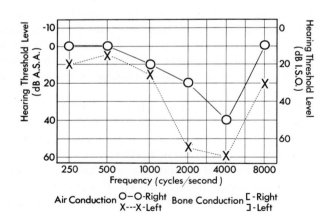

Fig. 134. *History:* 39-year-old male with 7 years' exposure to small-arms gunfire as instructor on police rifle range. Does not wear ear protectors. Bilateral ringing tinnitus. Complains of discrimination difficulty.

Otologic: ears normal

Audiologic: Both ears exhibit the characteristic C-5 dip as the result of exposure to intense noise. The fact that frequencies below 4,000 cps are starting to be affected explains the complaint of discrimination difficulty.

Classification: sensorineural hearing loss

Diagnosis: repeated exposure to small-arms gunfire

intense industrial noise is almost negligible. Since both ears are almost equally sensitive in an individual, and industrial noise usually reaches both ears with almost equal intensity, it is unlikely that one ear could be seriously affected and the other not at all.

HIGH AND LOW TONE HEARING LOSS IN INDUSTRIAL DEAFNESS

The employee who develops industrial deafness has in the early stages a high tone hearing loss without involvement of the frequencies below 2,000 cycles. Consequently, he has little difficulty in hearing ordinary conversation, but he may on occasion have some difficulty in understanding poorly enunciated speech or whispers. He also may have hearing trouble in the presence of much noise, because the noise would mask out some of the discriminating characteristics of the consonants and make

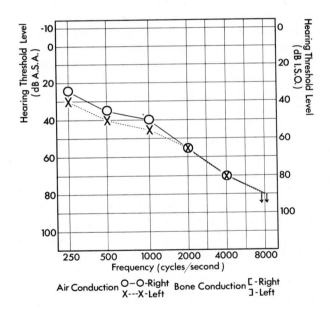

FIG. 135. *History:* 62-year-old male who worked as boilermaker for 31 years. Patient has no tinnitus, and he claims he gets along well without a hearing aid.

Otologic: normal

Audiologic: Note that both ears have about the same degree of hearing loss. Presbycusis probably plays only a minor role in this hearing loss, since the intense noise over so many years is capable of producing this degree of damage. Not many industrial noises cause such a degree of hearing loss.

Classification: sensorineural hearing loss

Diagnosis: noise-induced

them even more difficult for him to distinguish. And he may find it difficult to understand some voices on the telephone, television, records, movies or even radio, because the reproduction of voices through amplification systems often reduces their clarity.

The word "deafness" commonly used to refer to industrial or occupational hearing loss may be somewhat misleading when the term is applied to its early phases, since "deafness" implies obvious difficulty in hearing speech. Actually, the difficulty lies not so much in hearing speech as in understanding it. Hence, unless one specifically looks for this lack of consonant discrimination, he is likely to miss the diagnosis of industrial deafness in its early stages, the more so since the employee usually tries hard to compensate for his handicap.

Because of these factors many representatives of management deny the presence of occupational deafness in their plants, since they can walk repeatedly through their noisy shops and converse satisfactorily with all the employees. Too frequently, management fails to recognize that conversing in a noisy environment requires one to speak above the level of the noise, and that the vocabulary used in these brief conversations is such that an employee might be able to carry on that kind of limited and stereotyped conversation even though he had very serious deafness.

When Extended, a Serious Handicap. It is not until the hearing loss extends to the lower frequencies and becomes more profound in the higher ones that poor hearing and poor understanding of speech become a prominent symptom. By then the damage to hearing is severe, irreversible and often seriously handicapping. Furthermore, it assumes medicolegal importance as grounds for compensation.

The major handicaps in the severe cases are in communication, and because this enters into every phase of personal and business life, the psychic fallout very easily can cause personality problems. Often these individuals cannot hear warning signals, such as a fire alarm or a telephone bell. If they should happen to be employed in automobile repair work and are expected to detect the need for adjustment by listening to a motor, they cannot do this work any more, and they may lose their jobs. The situation is even more acute for men who work with airplane and diesel engines and still other noisy motors.

Another handicap for those with more severe hearing losses is the inability to tell the direction from which a voice or other sound is coming. People who are deaf in but one ear have the same problem, because it takes two ears with normal function to localize the direction of sound.

RECRUITMENT

A factor often present in industrial deafness is a reduction of a person's ability to understand speech because of distortion due to recruitment. Reverberations of the voice of a train announcer at a railroad station that make the message hard for everybody to understand become completely unintelligible blurs to the person with sensorineural deafness, and the louder they are, the less he understands. Like letters written with ink on blotting paper, the sounds of "Coach S 231 on Track 9 on the Panama Limited" dissolve and diffuse to a throbbing roll of thunderous sound signifying nothing.

Persons with recruitment often will ask a person to speak a little louder, but when he raises his voice a trifle more than necessary, they understand even less. Instead of helping them to understand better, loudness—for such individuals—actually may reduce discrimination. This symptom of distortion is in itself one of the major causes for annoyance. It is natural that people who do not hear clearly should become frustrated and irritable.

THE PHYSICIAN'S ROLE IN INDUSTRIAL DEAFNESS

EXAMINATION OF CANDIDATES FOR EMPLOYMENT

Physicians living in industrialized areas may be called on to examine candidates for employment by local plants and to advise whether the applicant's hearing is such that he should be considered for a noisy job. Medical men also may be called on to recommend measures for the mitigation of noise problems and for protecting the hearing of factory workers.

CONSERVATION OF HEARING PROGRAM

The most effective means by which noisy industries can meet the immediate and future problems of occupational deafness is to establish a conservation of hearing program. Initiating and maintaining such programs requires the cooperation of the physician, the safety engineer, the hygienist, the nurse, the industrial relations manager, a consulting otologist and still others.

To be really successful, the purposes and the operating details of a conservation of hearing program must be understood fully by both management and labor. The orientation of management and the provision of a broad perspective of all aspects of occupational deafness generally require an educational program. Since there is at present no satisfactory treatment for industrial deafness, it is the responsibility of both management and labor to do everything possible to prevent hearing loss among industrial employees.

It seems almost inevitable that every noisy industry sooner or later will need to develop some sort of conservation of hearing program to protect both itself and its employees. Reports in the literature reveal that the following occupations produce noise sufficient to affect the hearing of high frequencies and to produce occupational deafness: boilermaking, weaving, aircraft manufacture and maintenance, chipping, riveting, blasting, machine manufacturing, gunfiring, metal working, drop forging, and many other industries utilizing large presses, high pressure steam, large wood and metal saws, and heavy hammering operations as in steel and iron works.

PHYSICAL MEASUREMENT OF NOISE

Taking physical noise measurements in an industry is primarily the responsibility of the safety engineer or the industrial hygienist. Small plants that have very noisy machinery may find it more advantageous and less expensive to hire a consulting engineer or another qualified person to make the noise measurements. Large plants having their own engineering departments generally have an individual who can take noise measurements with equipment already available or easily obtainable. Simply measuring the intensity of the noise is not enough to determine its effect on the hearing of exposed personnel. The spectrum of the noise also must be determined—i.e., the relative intensities of the various frequencies of which the noise is composed. It is important also to consider the type of noise being measured. Is it continuous or intermittent? Is it a shock pulse? Does it repeat itself once a day or once every second? All these aspects of a noise are important in helping to evaluate its potential effect on hearing.

The effect of any noise on hearing cannot be judged by a single number of decibels. For example, to state that 100 decibels of noise is harmful to hearing is an incomplete concept that requires other information to make it meaningful. If the noise has most of its energy in the frequency range below 300 cycles, then a noise of that intensity is *not* harmful; but if it owes its energy mainly to frequencies above 2,000 cycles, then a noise of 100 decibels certainly is harmful. Furthermore, the duration of exposure and other factors must be considered in determining the effect of noise on hearing.

Another complicating factor is individual susceptibility. It is common experience that two individuals working on the same job and exposed to the same noise will not show the same type or degree of hearing damage. Often one individual shows little hearing loss, whereas another working at the same job suffers some impairment at the higher frequencies that reasonably can be attributed to his exposure to noise. This subject of individual susceptibility requires much clarification, but it does not mean that in a comparatively mild noise, such as 90 db, a person will show a marked hearing loss.

The primary purpose in making accurate sound measurements of the various noises in an industrial plant is to classify broadly which noisy jobs are innocuous, potentially hazardous or definitely hazardous to the hearing of the exposed personnel.

HEARING TESTING

MOST ESSENTIAL PHASE

The most essential phase of any conservation of hearing program is *to measure the hearing of employees, both before employment and routinely thereafter.* This is particularly true from the medicolegal aspect, since physical noise measurements alone are of little value if an employee enters a claim for occupational deafness. The testing program generally is the responsibility of the physician, though he himself may not do the testing. That duty may be assigned to the plant nurse or to any well-trained person who has taken a comprehensive course in industrial audiometry.

It is often better to do no hearing testing than to perform audiometry in an inaccurate manner. Hearing tests to be useful medically and a protection in medicolegal situations must be carried out by expertly trained technicians interested in their work, using calibrated equipment in a suitable test room, and observing the best technic of audiometry.

The over-all hearing testing program should be supervised by an otologist thoroughly familiar with the problems encountered in performing hearing tests and in the characteristics of occupational deafness. Small industrial plants in which only a small number of persons need to be tested may find it advantageous to make an agreement with a local otologist to take charge of the hearing tests, to assume general supervision of the program and to work with management in interpreting audiograms and making individual recommendations. The management of a large industrial corporation will find it worth while to train a responsible person to undertake the hearing tests and to provide reliable equipment and satisfactory test room facilities.

PRE-EMPLOYMENT OR PREPLACEMENT AUDIOGRAM

An employee's pre-employment audiogram establishes his hearing status before he is exposed to noise in his new job. It has been estimated that about 20 per cent of applicants for noisy industrial jobs already have some hearing loss at the time they present themselves for employment.

The importance of securing an accurate initial hearing threshold record is obvious, but the author's experience as a consultant in examining the adequacy of hearing testing programs in several industrial plants shows that accuracy and reliability in such testing cannot be taken for granted.

When the author checked what was being done in one of these plants, he found that the hearing of employees had been tested by an inadequately trained technician, unfamiliar with the pitfalls of industrial audiometry. At the time the records were studied in association with another audiologist, it was discovered that a significant number of employees whose initial audiograms showed them to have normal hearing in reality had been afflicted then by hearing losses of long duration, quite unrelated to their present employment.

The inaccuracy of the initial pre-employment audiogram was in most instances confirmed by the employees themselves, who admitted having had long-standing hearing losses prior to employment and acknowledged giving false responses to the previous tester. Some of the employees felt they would lose their jobs if their hearing were found to be defective, and by carefully watching the tester's technic they had devised methods for giving a false impression of normal hearing.

The production and the recording of audiograms with a false appearance of validity by testers inadequately trained in the art of industrial audiometry is by no means of uncommon occurrence, particularly in instances in which the subjects had accumulated previous experience with audiometric testing in the Armed Services and the Veterans Administration.

Instances are certain to arise in which so many new employees are hired in one day that it is impossible to test them all before they report for work. For this and other reasons it may be advisable to do preplacement audiometry in addition to pre-employment testing. This means that initial tests are performed on employees when they are assigned to a job that has been classified as potentially hazardous to hearing.

The importance of the initial pre-employment or preplacement audiogram as a document of legal importance should be considered carefully. Several thresholds at different frequencies should be established to provide a base line with which future comparisons can be reliably made.

EAR PROTECTORS

When an industrial machine is found to produce sound of an intensity that may be harmful to hearing, the best procedure is to try to reduce

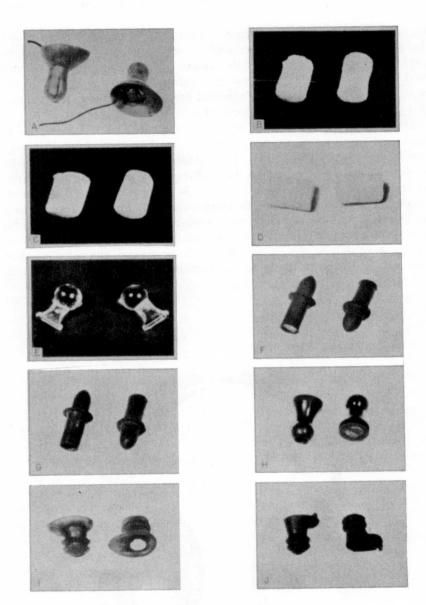

Fig. 136. Insert type of ear protectors.

(A) Baums mega eardrum protectors. (B) Nods noise mufflers.
(C) Fleats antinoise ear stoppers.   (D) Olygo noise absorbers.
(E) Nelson ear stoppers.   (F) Sepco safety ear protectors.
(G) SMR ear stoppers.   (H) Mallock-Armstrong ear defenders.
(I) MSA ear defenders.   (J) NDRC wardens (type V-29 r).

the noise at its source by quieting or isolating the machine. This is not always possible or practical. In such instances adequate protection to employees may be provided by the proper use of ear protectors. Under ideal conditions an ear protector can attenuate air-borne sound by as much as 40 decibels. However, in actual practice the attenuation realized by a protector is generally not more than 30 db.

Sound may reach the inner ear by air conduction via the external ear canal, and when sound intensity exceeds a certain critical level, it may pass directly through the bones of the skull—i.e., by bone conduction. In normal ears the sound energy in the midfrequency range that reaches the ear by bone conduction alone is about 50 db weaker than that which reaches it by air conduction. In employees with sensorineural hearing loss (those who have reduced bone conduction), the difference may be even greater than 50 db. On the other hand, employees with conductive hearing losses have some degree of built-in protection against damaging noise reaching the inner ear by air conduction.

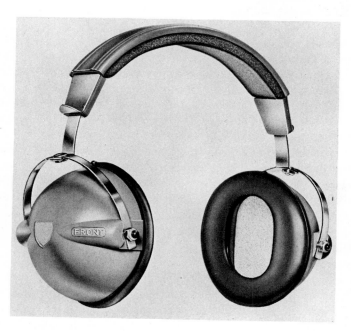

Fig. 137. Muff type of ear protectors. (American Optical Company, Safety Products Division, Southbridge, Mass.)

Best Known Types

Ear protectors generally are classified according to the manner in which they are worn. The three best known types are inserts, muffs and helmets (the latter are seldom used).

Insert Type. Figure 136 illustrates some of the many varieties of ear insert protectors, which differ widely in construction and in their mode of action. One of the least effective protectors is the cotton ball, generally fashioned by the employee himself from absorbent cotton or cotton waste; this provides very little if any protection and should not be recommended or permitted. On the other hand, good protection is afforded by some insert protectors or earplugs. The earplugs are designed to occlude the external ear canal completely and may be made of soft rubber, hard rubber, wax, plastic, or a combination of these materials.

The muff type of protector, shown in Figure 137, is designed to cover both ears and to be held snugly to the sides of the head by a headband. The cups may be made of rubber and plastic and are so constructed that they encompass the ear without compressing it. It is important that the headband be springy enough to hold the earmuffs snugly without causing discomfort. If safety glasses and hard hats are worn at the same time, an adaptation is required to permit the earmuffs to fit snugly.

The helmet type of ear protector, which is used to cover most of the bony portion of the head to prevent bone conduction, is necessary only in extremely intense noise levels. These are seldom found in industry. Occasionally, an industrial noise may be so intense that it cannot be reduced satisfactorily by any single type of ear protector. It is possible in such rare instances to use both an insert and an earmuff in combination.

Under experimental conditions the insert and the muff protectors provide about the same degree of attenuation, but in practice the muff type is generally much more effective. The maximum protection is afforded in the higher frequencies above 1,000 cycles per second. The attenuation below 1,000 cycles is considerably lower, generally being of the order of 15 or 20 db. If the insert and the muff types are combined, a possible maximum of about 50 db can be realized under ideal conditions. It is fortunate that ear protectors give most efficient attenuation in the higher frequencies, since noise in these frequencies is most harmful to hearing.

Values and Relative Merits. When employees are told that an ear protection program is about to be instituted, one of their chief complaints is that they cannot wear ear protectors, because then they could not hear sounds and voices essential to the operation of their equipment. Though such an objection may seem to be reasonable, it is actually contrary to the facts, because ear protectors in very noisy areas often make it *easier*—not harder—for employees to understand conversation and instructions necessary in the operation of their machines. This has been demonstrated conclusively in the experimental laboratory and in many tests under actual working conditions.

To carry on conversation, employees wearing proper ear protectors do not need to raise their voices as much as those with no ear protection in the same noisy environment. This advantage is of considerable value if extensive daily communication is necessary.

Before instituting an ear protection program it is first necessary to "sell" its desirability to both management and workers. In the past there has been a difference of opinion about the relative values of ear plugs and earmuffs. More recently, this controversy gradually has died down, as the disadvantages of earmuffs have been overcome. Ear inserts are good only if they are worn all the time, and if they are inserted properly in the ear. They do not always provide the necessary protection, because some workers often are tempted to insert the plug loosely; even if they have been properly inserted, normal jaw movements tend to loosen the plug and to make it ineffective. Their use is difficult to police in practice.

The chief disadvantage of earmuffs has been their very high price. Increased production resulting from greater demand for earmuffs has made it possible to obtain effective earmuffs at greatly reduced cost. The consensus today seems to be that earmuffs are usually the ear protector of choice.

It must be admitted that the wearing of earmuffs is uncomfortable in industries in which workers are exposed to very high temperatures and humidity, as in foundries. It is possible, even then, to use earmuffs if their use is confined to several hours a day at intermittent periods. There are times when a person cannot wear muffs because they become filled with perspiration; special consideration should be given to circumstances of this type.

In summary, an ear protection program monitored by audiometric tests offers the best and the most economical hearing protection.

SOME BASIC QUESTIONS AND CRITERIA

APPLICANTS WITH A HEARING HANDICAP

One of the most important decisions that a physician may be called on to make in examining a worker on behalf of a prospective industrial employer is whether or not to recommend his employment if he has a hearing handicap. In general, it is inadvisable to adopt a blanket policy not to hire individuals with mild high tone hearing losses. To do so would deprive industry of many skilled workers and create an unwarranted labor scarcity. The decision not to hire should be made on an individual basis and after careful consideration has been given to these questions:

1. Will the applicant's hearing be further damaged to a handicapping degree by exposure to the noise? If it will be, then he should not be hired for that job unless adequate ear protection can be provided.

2. Is his hearing loss now at the point at which a small degree of further loss will place him in the handicapped classification and make him a compensation problem? If the answer is "yes," the individual should be so advised and not hired for his own good and that of the industrial employer.

3. Is the employee so highly skilled that he is essential in the job under consideration, and is the risk of further hearing damage unavoidable because of his vocation—such as that of a drop forge operator or a chipper? In such a case one must take a calculated risk, since any employee who has experience in this line of work almost certainly has some hearing loss. It would be only good sense to hire him, but he should be provided with the very best possible protection for his work.

NOISE: DAMAGE RISK CRITERIA

It has not been possible to establish a sharp, clear-cut level between a hazardous and a nonhazardous noise because of the many complex variables that enter into the equation. Nevertheless, certain "damage risk criteria" have been suggested to help to determine whether a noise should be considered to be harmful to hearing. These proposed criteria are only guides and not inflexible or firmly established rules. They are based on projections of the results of very short exposures to noise, and considerable field work and further research are necessary to verify their validity. For the present, however, these criteria prepared by the American Academy of Ophthalmology and Otolaryngology are the best available and should be used as guides in industry. The criteria apply only to steady-state noise exposures of more or less constant intensity and are based on full daily exposure. They are expressed in this fashion:

The effects of continuous exposure to steady noise may depend on the way the sound energy is distributed in the noise. Early noise-induced hearing losses are usually confined to the frequencies around 4,000 cycles per second. As the exposure lengthens the losses spread to lower frequencies, whose audibility is more directly involved in the understanding of speech. Data on noise-induced hearing loss, both temporary and permanent, indicate that the losses occur at frequencies above those that characterize the exposure sounds. Since the most important frequencies to be protected are in the range of 500 to 2,000 cycles per second inclusive, it follows that the 300-600, 600-1,200, and 1,200-2,400 cycles per second bands deserve our major attention if we are trying to protect man's hearing for speech.

Our knowledge of the relations of hearing loss to noise exposure permits us to propose guidelines for establishing standards for preventing significant noise-induced hearing loss in the majority of exposed persons. These recommended standards have been proposed by the International Organization for Standardization. They are presented below in brief modified form. They do not apply to exposure to impulsive noise but *only* to *steady* noise.

(1) When the exposure to broad-band noise is habitual and the noise is continuous during the working day (5 or more hours) the average of the levels at 300-600, 600-1,200, and 1,200-2,400 c/s should not exceed 85 db. If this average exceeds 85 db, hearing conservation measures should be initiated.

Example:

Octave Band	300 to 600	600 to 1,200	1,200 to 2,400
Level	95	95	$92 = \dfrac{282}{3} = 94$ db average level

(2) When the exposure to broad-band noise is habitual and the noise is continuous for less than 5 hours per day, Table II should be consulted for recommended allowable exposures.

TABLE II

Average Level of 300- 600 600-1,200 and 1,200-2,400 c/s Bands	On-time per Day (minutes)
85 db	Less than 300
90 db	Less than 120
95 db	Less than 50
100 db	Less than 25
105 db	Less than 16
110 db	Less than 12
115 db	Less than 8
120 db	Less than 5

So far there is no good guide for noise that is intermittent, such as a drop hammer or forging or metal working. In general, however, it would be safe to consider that any intermittent noise that produces an over-all sound pressure level of 125 db or greater should be considered to be hazardous, and ear protective measures should be instituted.

SUMMARY

Industry must be encouraged to prevent occupational deafness from compromising the speech frequency range, so that plant employees can be protected from a handicapping hearing loss in everyday communication, but it must be borne in mind that some high tone hearing losses occur in population that is not exposed to noise, and that some high tone hearing loss must be considered to be part of the unavoidable risk of living in an industrialized society.

Chapter 27

Hearing Loss in Children

Hearing loss in children is of special importance because it often goes unrecognized for a long time and creates serious problems. Many children are compelled to repeat grades in school because of unsuspected and remediable hearing handicaps. Equally important is the social cost of truancy and other forms of antisocial behavior so prevalent among children who are made to feel that they "do not fit in" with their classmates. The severe repercussions that hearing loss has on an individual's personality, both in childhood and in later life, places this problem in the forefront of medical importance. Since the solution or amelioration of the problem depends primarily on the early detection of hearing loss in children, the major responsibility rests on the general practitioner and the pediatrician.

The extent of the problem nationally can be recognized from the reports of many school studies. Most of these show that between 2.8 and 4 per cent of school children have "significant hearing losses." In Chicago 2.8 per cent of pupils tested in 98 public schools had a hearing loss of at least 30 db in two or more frequencies in the speech range. In Philadelphia 4 per cent of school children had hearing losses. These and other reports emphasize further that well over 80 per cent of the hearing losses in these children are curable with adequate medical attention.

In children below the age of 6 the high incidence of mild or even moderate hearing loss is not fully realized, because such losses in preschool children often go unrecognized. In 54 per cent of the cases found by the Chicago audiological screening clinics to have a moderate loss or a severe loss of 35 db or more for the speech frequencies, even the children's own parents had no suspicion of any hearing difficulty. Although the great benefit to be derived from routine testing in a school hearing conservation program is apparent, facilities for testing preschool children with symptoms suggesting deafness also would be extremely valuable.

A distinction should be made between the child with a hearing impairment and the "deaf child." The "deaf child" is one whose hearing is non-functional for ordinary purposes. Even with a hearing aid, he has no real serviceable hearing. His problem is far different from that of the child whose hearing is impaired but useful. The "deaf" present predominantly institutional problems, but this is usually not the case with hard-of-hearing children. Since there are comparatively few deaf children, and facilities for these are well-established, we shall concern ourselves principally with the hard-of-hearing child, except to stress the need for correct diagnosis of deafness as early in infancy as possible and the importance of early efforts to help the child to develop proper speech and to grow up as normally as possible.

CONGENITAL AND INFANT HEARING IMPAIRMENT

A child may be born with a hearing deficit or acquire it in infancy before he develops any speech patterns. In either case the symptomatology is similar, because the deafness occurred before the development of speech. The defect may be conductive, as in congenital fixation of the stapes footplate, ossicular defects, or aplasia of the outer or the middle ear. It may be sensorineural, as in hereditary nerve deafness or in deafness resulting from Rh incompatibility with kernicterus, maternal rubella in the first trimester of pregnancy, anoxia or viral infections. Congenital hearing losses more commonly are bilateral than unilateral. The impairment may run the gamut from very slight impairment to total deafness in both ears.

Conductive hearing loss, especially if bilateral, may retard speech development somewhat and cause inattention, but the child understands and responds to loud speech, and he develops essentially normal speech patterns. However, the child with moderate or severe sensorineural deafness usually shows not only a poor hearing response, but, even more prominently, he may develop no speech, or his speech may be defective. Sensorineural losses involving only the higher frequencies generally cause few symptoms and may therefore go unnoticed until they are detected in a school hearing testing program.

When a mother brings a child to the physician and complains that Johnny is 3 years old and still cannot speak, or that Susan seems to be backward in school, disinterested and inattentive, the first question that should arise in the mind of the physician is: "Can this child hear?" One of the earliest clues to the presence of a hearing loss is retarded or defective speech. Temper tantrums in a speechless child, retarded school work, inattention and many emotional disturbances may be caused by varying degrees of hearing impairment.

HEARING AND SPEECH

To understand the problems associated with hearing impairment in children, one should be aware of the intimate relationship between hearing and speech development. Throughout infancy the child listens to speech, learns to associate sounds with meaningful information, and subsequently mimics what he hears. By the age of 3 a normal child has developed most of his speech patterns. But the child with no useful hearing will form little or no intelligible speech spontaneously, because what he has never heard he cannot imitate. If he passes silently through the early years ideally suited for language development, he is thereby handicapped in developing normal speech, education, and important social and emotional qualities. If he has a partial hearing loss accompanied by distortion, he is likely to develop a defective speech pattern.

When a child is acquiring speech, he learns to pronounce vowels and consonants and to combine them into meaningful sounds. In our audible frequency range the vowels (*a, e, i, o, u*) are low tones, whereas the consonants are high tones. If the child has a high tone hearing loss, he will hear the vowels or low notes, but the consonants will be inaudible or seem to be indistinct or distorted. The way he learns to pronounce these sounds then will be correspondingly distorted.

The child who has difficulty in correctly pronouncing certain sibilant sounds, particularly *s*, was in the past likely to be described as "tongue-tied." Most of these children are in reality not tongue-tied, but due to a high tone deafness they do not hear the sibilant sounds in the high frequency range. To a child with such a high tone loss an *s* may sound like a *t*, and in learning to pronounce words he naturally will repeat only what he is able to hear. If he does not hear accurately, he cannot repeat accurately what is said to him.

DIAGNOSING EARLY DEAFNESS

When a child's mother reports her youngster to be unresponsive and possibly hard of hearing, it is vital that the presence or the absence of hearing impairment be determined accurately, and, in the event of a hearing loss, that its cause be pinpointed. The question often is asked: "How old must a child be before his hearing can be tested?" Today an approximate hearing threshold can be obtained in some children as young as 3 months. Parents never should be told that a child is too young to have his hearing tested if there is sufficient need and justification for such a study. The earlier a hearing defect is detected and treatment begun, the better.

History of Auditory Behavior. Obtaining an accurate quantitative assessment of an infant's or a young child's hearing is frequently a very difficult task. In the case of younger children it is often not possible to do reliable air conduction, let alone bone conduction tests. The principal responsibilities of the physician are: (1) to be on the alert for the possible presence of a hearing loss, and (2) when findings are suspicious, to determine whether more definitive studies are warranted. Many methods are available to the physician to determine whether deafness is a reasonable etiologic possibility. One important measure is to secure from the parents an adequate history of the child's auditory behavior. For example, a child who never answers or never comes when he is called from another room but does react when he can see the face of the caller, may well be deaf. It is important in such cases to ask the parents whether they call the child by voice alone, or whether in addition they stamp their foot or bang the table. The child who cannot be awakened at night by being spoken to in a loud voice should be considered to be in need of hearing tests, especially if his speech development also is retarded or defective. Since similar negative responses often are obtained in the case of emotionally disturbed children or in children with retrocochlear lesions, careful differentiation is essential both through hearing tests and by other consultations.

Certain auditory behavior patterns are prominent during a baby's development, and these should be explored to determine whether deafness is a likely etiology.

During the first 6 months a baby should respond to his mother's voice before seeing her; he should be affected by sounds such as being startled, awakened or amused. He even should be able to localize his mother's voice, and he should start to imitate certain simple sounds. Before the age of 1 year the average child can be expected to obey simple commands and to understand several words, especially familiar names. By the age of 2 the child should start to speak simple words like *all gone, bye-bye*, etc. From then on the child's vocabulary and understanding should continue to increase and become more comprehensive.

A careful history of auditory response can lead the physician to a judgment of whether a mother's concern about her baby's hearing is justified. Simple tests can be made on infants and young children to show whether they hear.

Response to Noisemakers. The reaction of a child under 5 years of age to handclapping behind his back, stamping the feet, or striking pans together does not always prove whether or not he can hear. If he responds, it may be because he feels the vibration. If he does not, it may be for a variety of psychological or physiological reasons though his hearing is normal. If a child has some useful hearing and a vibrating tuning fork of 500 cycles is placed surreptitiously near one of his ears, he may either turn in the direction of the sound or otherwise show that he hears. Handbells also may be used behind the child's back to see whether he consistently turns around when they are sounded. A positive response by the child in carefully conducted noisemaking tests generally is reliable, but in such tests a negative response does not always indicate deafness. Noisemakers of different frequencies should be used to determine whether the response is better in the higher or the lower frequency range. True response to the sound made by the physician must be carefully distinguished from random movement. Children up to 3 months of age respond more consistently to percussion than to voice sounds. Older children respond more readily to voice sounds, and better to moderately loud than very loud voices and sounds. The examiner should remain carefully out of the child's line of sight, to avoid visual reactions being mistaken for auditory responses. Reactions to look for are an eye blink reflex, a pinna reflex, turning of the head or other obvious signs. Responses to noisemakers usually cease after just a few observations. Not only do these gross hearing tests help to determine whether there is a hearing loss; they also warn of neurologic defects.

Abnormal Auditory Behavior in the Nondeaf Child. Whenever a physician suspects a hearing loss, he should seek more definitive and quantitative evaluations. When a child's speech defect involves the enunciation of sibilants, particularly the letter *s*, further hearing tests are in order. This often takes not only considerable time and patience but also special training and equipment. It should be done by an otologist or audiologic center equipped and trained to perform such studies.

The deaf child, the mentally retarded child, and the emotionally disturbed child often develop symptoms so similar that they obscure the diagnosis. Yet it is obviously essential to distinguish among these very different conditions in order to institute proper therapy and to offer a prognosis. Aphasia very frequently is confused with deafness. Damage to the brain may cause an inability to comprehend speech, resulting in a receptive or sensory aphasia. Or the damage could result in inability to give expression to thought (verbal aphasia), even though the receptive areas are intact. Generally, the damage is in both areas but more predominant in one or the other. In contrast with the aphasic child, the deaf child should be able to learn and to repeat speech.

Studies have shown that there is not, as is accepted generally, a high incidence of hearing loss in the mentally retarded population. Initial tests

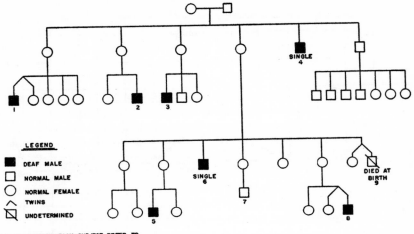

FIG. 138. This family tree seems to indicate some interesting genetic aspects of sex-linked hereditary deafness. Audiograms were available for this family on all of the living persons with profound congenital nerve deafness. Not all the members of this family have been given hearing tests, but those reported as not deaf have normal speech and clinically normal hearing as established from information supplied by close relatives. (Sataloff, J., Pastore, P. N., and Bloom, E.: Sex-linked hereditary deafness, Am. J. Human Genet. 7:201-203, Fig. I, June 1955)

may indicate a hearing loss, but when tests are repeated by a trained listener, they may reveal more hearing than the first tests suggested.

The autistic child also is often confused with the deaf child, because he may not use speech and pay no attention to sounds around him. Such a child and children with other types of disorders that may be confused with deafness must have an accurate differential diagnosis if each is to receive therapy appropriate to his condition. Autistic children often come from homes of professional parents who show little affection for the child. For this reason an evaluation of the home environment may aid in the differential diagnosis.

CONGENITAL DEAFNESS

The term "congenital deafness" merely indicates that deafness was present at birth. It neither specifies the cause of deafness nor suggests its likely cure. In the past most cases of congenital deafness were attributed to heredity or birth injury or to some cause that could not be established.

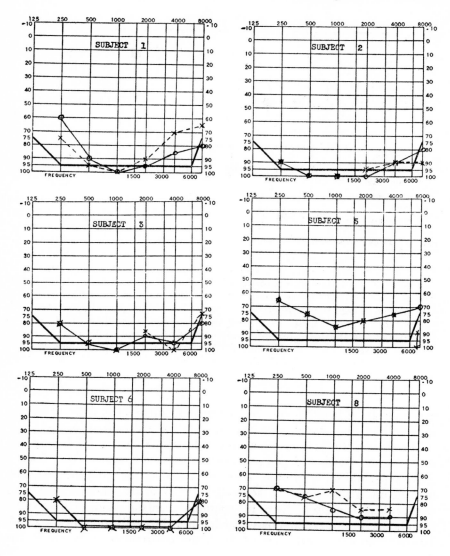

Fig. 139. The audiograms obtained on 6 of the 7 deaf individuals in the family referred to in Figure 138.

Subject 1 (In Figs. 138 and 139) Is now 53 years of age and has little intelligible speech. He was the first born and only male child in his family and has a twin sister.

Subject 2 Is a 44-year-old deaf mute. He is the first born and only male.

Subject 3 Is a 37-year-old first born male who received his education at a school for the deaf.

(*Continued on facing page*)

As otologic research advanced, physicians were enabled to remove from this classification certain cases of hearing loss for which now the cause is known. Deafness caused by Rh incompatibility and that following maternal rubella are examples of congenital hearing loss for which the cause now can be specified rather than merely described as congenital. Although a few cases of congenital deafness now can be further classified into sensory or neural, the majority still fall into the more general sensorineural group. Even in cases definitely felt to be of the neural type, tone decay

---

Fig. 139 (*Cont.*)

Subject 4 Disappeared over 40 years ago at the age of 7. At that time he was known to be deaf and unable to speak.

Subject 5 Is a 16-year-old now attending a school for the deaf. He is the first born son and has a sister, whose hearing is normal. He uses a hearing aid with fair results and has fairly intelligible speech. The usefulness of early amplification and adequate training is evident in this subject.

Subject 6 Is a 37-year-old bachelor classified as a deaf mute with little intelligible speech.

Subject 7 Is a 5-year-old first born male child with normal hearing and speech. He was conceived after a 5-year period of apparent sterility requiring a D & C. The mother denies any miscarriages or abortions prior to subject's birth.

Subject 8 Is a 3-year-old first born male and has a twin sister. He has no speech and has profound nerve deafness. Both his twin sister and older sister have normal hearing and speech development. The hearing threshold on this youngster was obtained with repeatedly consistent psychogalvanic skin resistance tests.

Subject 9 Was a male twin who died at birth.

There are 3 sets of twins in the pedigree. In each set there is a male and female, and the male was the first born son and demonstrated deaf mutism in 2 of the 3 sets.

It is apparent from this pedigree that deafness is manifest only in the male child and is transmitted through the maternal side. There are 7 first born males with profound congenital nerve deafness, a condition not present in subsequently born males or found in any females. There are insufficient subsequent males to establish statistically that deafness is restricted to the first born males. Deafness does not exist in the children of the normal male member of the pedigree.

This family seems to demonstrate sex-linked nerve deafness of the recessive heredity type, similar to that seen in hemophilia. There is no history of any consanguineous marriages in the family. There is an excellent probability in this family that approximately one-half of the males born after an affected male may be expected to be deaf. Although it is possible that there may be other effects of the gene in the heterozygous condition, none was apparent in this family. Allied conditions, such as Rh incompatibility and syphilis, were ruled out as etiologic possibilities.

The family pedigree exhibited demonstrates clearly that profound congenital nerve deafness can be hereditary and sex-linked. Early recognition and adequate educational measures are essential in such instances. (Sataloff, J., Pastore, P. N., and Bloom, E.: Sex-linked hereditary deafness, Am. J. Human Genet. 7:201-203, Fig. II, June 1955)

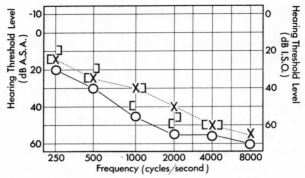

Air Conduction O—O-Right Bone Conduction ⊏-Right
X---X-Left   ⊐-Left

FIG. 140. *History:* 7-year-old male whose mother noted poor hearing when the child was 2. Speech development was slow. Has difficulty pronouncing sibilants, and *s* is slurred. An older brother has a similar hearing loss. The hearing problem is nonprogressive in both children.

Otologic: ears normal

Audiologic: Pure tone air and bone conduction thresholds indicate a bilateral gradually sloping loss with no air-bone gap.

Speech reception threshold: Right, 38 db.   Left, 38 db
Discrimination score: Right, 78%   Left, 80%
There was no abnormal tone decay.

Classification: sensorineural hearing loss

Diagnosis: Menasse type congenital hereditary deafness

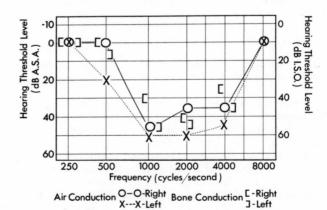

Air Conduction O—O-Right Bone Conduction ⊏-Right
X---X-Left   ⊐-Left

FIG. 141. *History:* This child's father has a similarly shaped audiogram and a deep monotonous voice, which is apparent also in the child. Enunciation is good.

Otologic: ears normal

Audiologic: Air and bone conduction thresholds reveal a bilateral basin-shaped curve with no air-bone gap. Right ear discrimination was 80% at 70 db.

Classification: sensorineural

Diagnosis: congenital and inherited

is about normal, and in most the discrimination score is in keeping with the audiometric findings rather than markedly reduced.

Heredity. The most common cause for congenital sensorineural deafness is heredity. This accounts for most of the children that attend schools for the deaf. The need for early detection of deafness in these children and their educational needs is well-known. A child has a greater risk of being born deaf if both his parents or their families have the same type of hereditary nerve deafness. For this reason intermarriages are discouraged between people in whose families this type of deafness exists. If only one of the parents is deaf or has deafness in his family, the threat that the children will be born deaf is less acute; but the possibility still exists. In considering this point it is important to be sure that the type of deafness that has occurred in the family is of the inherited type and

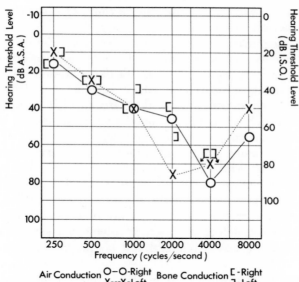

Air Conduction O—O-Right   Bone Conduction ⌈-Right
              X---X-Left   ⌉-Left

Fig. 142. *History:* Marked jaundice noted several days after birth. Cerebral palsy since birth. Marked speech defect, especially with sibilants. Younger brother has similar condition and similar hearing loss.

Otologic: ears normal

Audiologic: Air and bone conduction thresholds reveal bilateral sharply sloping curves with some recovery at 8,000 cps and no air-bone gap.

Speech reception threshold: Right, 40 db   Left, 40 db
Discrimination score: Right, 44%   Left, 48%

There was no recruitment or abnormal tone decay. There was some evidence of diplacusis in the left ear.

Classification: sensorineural

Diagnosis: Rh incompatibility with kernicterus

not caused by some other factor that might have made the child deaf at birth, such as German measles in the mother's first trimester of pregnancy, anoxia, Rh incompatibility, etc.

Although it is an established fact that deafness can be hereditary, efforts to estimate the probability that a particular child in a given family will be born deaf usually have been unsuccessful—mainly because of the difficulties in accurately diagnosing individual cases of profound nerve deafness and establishing the genetic characteristics of the parents.

The audiogram of a typical case of congenital hereditary deafness with an extraordinary family tree is shown in Figures 138 and 139. Another interesting but disturbing type of hereditary deafness develops at puberty or shortly thereafter. Sometimes this may appear in a person with perfectly normal hearing and without any known background of deafness in his family. Such a person's hearing can deteriorate over a period of several years until practically no useful hearing remains. Occasionally, the hearing loss does not start until the age of 17 or 18.

Usually, the degree of deafness is relatively severe when it is of hereditary origin. However, in many children there is useful residual hearing, and it is particularly important to detect deafness in these children early. Most of them can be prepared effectively in infancy and by preschool training in early childhood so that they are enabled to attend public schools with the help of amplified sound such as a hearing aid and, if necessary, with some supplementary tutoring.

MENASSE TYPE. Falling into this group is the hereditary congenital deafness described many years ago by Menasse and illustrated in Figure 140. The characteristic features of this condition are well defined. The threshold shows a descending curve with a greater loss in the higher frequencies. Similar hearing losses generally are found in other members of the family. A speech defect is present involving particularly the letters *s* and *z*. The hearing loss is bilateral and nonprogressive but also nonreversible.

BASIN-SHAPED CURVE. Another type of hereditary congenital deafness, which produces the basin-shaped curve, is shown in Figure 141.

HEARING AND BEHAVIOR. Children with high tone deafness present a complex and often a deceptive picture. Sometimes they seem to hear and to understand well, particularly when they are looking at the speaker or paying strict attention, but at other times they seem to be inattentive and backward, especially under certain conditions for which the reason often is not apparent to the layman. Most of the adverse effects of early deafness on the child's personality have their origin in the distorted communication caused by the inability to discriminate between high tone sounds.

From this nucleus the development of abnormal behavior and the maladjustment of the child to his immediate social community readily can be predicted. Most such children present behavior problems before the cause of their difficulty is recognized and understood, and the child is properly treated. It is the responsibility of the physician to be aware of the effects of hearing loss, to be able to detect it, and to know what to do for the child. It is also important that he constantly be aware of the considerable difference in the effects of a severe hearing loss, depending on whether its onset was before or after the age of 3, when speech patterns in a child become reasonably well established.

Rh Incompatability. Children who develop cerebral jaundice (kernicterus) and cerebral palsy due to Rh incompatibility in fetal life occasionally evidence a high tone hearing loss such as that shown in Figure 142. The speech defect in such children may be due not only to the muscular incoordination found in cerebral palsy but also to the complications produced by the high tone deafness present, with a resulting loss of the monitoring function on speech development. In these cases deafness is neither progressive nor reversible.

Anoxia. A most impressive amount of clinical experience shows that prolonged periods of anoxia after birth can cause sensorineural high tone deafness. Considerable investigation now is in progress concerning the effect of anoxia on hearing, and the findings reveal a pronounced effect on the auditory nuclei.

ACQUIRED HEARING LOSSES

Hearing losses acquired after infancy or after speech patterns have begun to develop may be conductive or sensorineural and may involve one or both ears to any degree.

MUMPS

Mumps is the most common cause of total sudden unilateral deafness. Histopathologic specimens in such cases show a destruction of the labyrinth with severe damage to the cochlea. Interestingly enough, the labyrinthine mechanism controlling balance rarely is affected in mumps despite its intimate contact with the cochlea. Normal caloric studies in a case of unilateral sudden deafness always should direct suspicion to mumps as the likely diagnosis.

Since many people have subclinical cases of mumps with very few if any symptoms, it is likely that more cases of unilateral total deafness are due to this cause than it is possible to certify from patients' histories. Sometimes physicians find that the patient was exposed to mumps several weeks prior to his deafness but never developed symptoms.

An interesting feature of mumps is that it almost invariably affects only one ear. In rare instances bilateral deafness has been reported, but the incidence is almost negligible. When one considers the likely mechanism by which mumps virus can produce deafness, it is difficult to explain why it should affect only one ear.

The sudden onset of mumps deafness also requires some comment. Patients with total unilateral deafness frequently are unable to describe when and how it started. However, careful investigation reveals that the onset was sudden and due to mumps, occurring sometimes years before the patient was aware of his hearing loss. The deafness in mumps can come so painlessly as to go unrecognized for years, especially if it occurs in childhood and in the right ear (in the case of right-handed people). Since the chief handicap produced by total unilateral deafness is the inability to use that ear on the telephone and reduced ability to localize the source of sound, it is understandable that a patient, particularly a child, can go for many years using his left ear for telephoning, so that he can write with his right hand without being aware that he cannot hear at all in his right ear. It is only when he tries to use the telephone (or, in recent years, a pocket transistor radio) in the right ear that he becomes suddenly aware of his deafness. Under such conditions it is not surprising to encounter some confusion about the onset.

Residual Hearing. Even though mumps deafness is almost always total, patients commonly believe that they have residual hearing, because their audiograms show only a 60- or a 70-db loss, and they may pull a number of audiograms out of their pockets to prove it. At the risk of bearing ill tidings, it is necessary to explain to such patients that when their previous audiograms were taken, the tester simply overlooked the need to mask out the normal ear, and that the tone the patient thought he heard in his bad ear after 60 db was reached, actually was heard in the good ear because of the carry-over. This can be demonstrated readily and conclusively to the patient on the audiometer by turning the masking tone on and off while a tone of 70 db is applied continuously to the bad ear. The masking clearly will blot out the shadow hearing. This conclusive demonstration may be essential to save the patient from seeking unnecessary treatments for his bad ear. All too frequently patients have been treated for years to improve nonexistent "residual hearing" before they are tested properly and told that the "hearing" on their old audiograms was only a shadow curve. As a rule they are grateful when they are given an honest and clear explanation of their handicap.

Irreversibility. According to the best of present-day knowledge, the severe deafness produced by mumps is irreversible. Removal of tonsils and adenoids, submucous resection, eustachian tube inflation, vitamin injections and even exploratory stapes mobilization are contraindicated.

Other Types of Deafness. Mumps can cause also another type of deafness which generally is bilateral. This happens in some cases of encephalitis and is described in Chapter 15. Occasionally, a patient is encountered with partial deafness, presumably due to mumps. In the author's experience cases of this type are rare.

Blows to the Head and Intense Noise

Head trauma and exposure to sudden intense noise such as that from gunfire and cap guns are not uncommon causes of unilateral partial sensorineural deafness. This is accompanied usually by a ringing tinnitus which, when it subsides, leaves some high tone deafness. Direct trauma to the head, such as from falls and head blows, also may produce this kind of hearing loss, but to a greater degree. There may be no visible damage to the eardrum or the middle ear, and there may not be any evidence of a fracture in the temporal bones; yet damage has been shown to occur in the inner ear following such injuries.

Ototoxic Drugs

Another cause of sensorineural deafness is the injudicious systemic use of drugs, such as kanamycin, neomycin and dihydrostreptomycin. When these drugs are injected in daily doses of 1 Gm. or less, they rarely produce any ototoxic effects, unless given in the presence of kidney infection. Reports have shown that children with reduced kidney function may become almost totally deaf by as few as two injections of one of these drugs. They therefore should be withheld from children with kidney malfunction unless they are needed to save life.

Uncommon Cause of Sensorineural Deafness

A relatively uncommon cause of sensorineural deafness beginning between childhood and adolescence and progressing until little useful hearing remains appears to have a hereditary tendency.

Adenoid Hypertrophy

The most common cause of conductive hearing impairment in children is hypertrophied adenoid tissue. The high incidence of hearing loss in children with hypertrophied adenoids, especially with a history of mouth breathing and ear infection, is not fully realized, because routine hearing tests rarely are done in such children, particularly if they are below the age of 6. In a carefully controlled research study, 90 per cent of children referred for conductive hearing losses had adenoid hyperplasia. In some 35 per cent of these cases there had been a previous adenoidectomy, but the symptoms were not controlled because of either adenoid regrowth or ineffective surgery. It was demonstrated further in this study that the vast majority of these hearing losses could be corrected if all hypertrophied adenoid tissue surrounding both eustachian orifices was removed carefully under direct visualization.

Adenoid abnormalities and indications for their removal relate only to cases of conductive deafness and not to other types of hearing loss. Many cases of conductive deafness due to hypertrophied adenoids can be obviated also by early attention with antibiotics, myringotomy, control of allergy, proper humidification and prevention of otitis media following acute upper respiratory infection.

OTITIS MEDIA

One of the monumental achievements in medicine is that it has eliminated in great measure the need for urgent mastoid surgery. Largely this is due to the ability of the practitioner to prevent acute otitis media following upper respiratory infection and his effective management of the disease, if it should develop. The important roles of antibiotics, myringotomy and room humidity should not be overlooked. There is still too high an incidence of otitis media resulting from acute rhinitis and allergies in children. These can be reduced significantly not only by advocating proper room humidification but especially by cautioning children against forceful blowing of their noses. Parents likewise should be made aware that improper nose blowing can force infected mucus into the middle ear and cause infection. In spite of the social stigma attached to the practice, sniffing is far safer than nose blowing unless the latter is done gently and with one nostril left unpinched.

OTHER CAUSES OF CONDUCTIVE HEARING LOSS

There are many other causes of conductive hearing loss. Among these are foreign bodies in the ear, impacted cerumen, secretory otitis media, allergies, external otitis, otosclerosis and ossicular defects in the middle ear. Recently I removed a piece of cotton from the ear of a child who had suffered conductive hearing loss for 3 years. The child had been subjected to two tonsillectomies and adenoidectomies and treated with numerous eardrops to clear up a middle ear infection. Careful examination revealed that the eardrum was not even visible, for a large piece of cotton, possibly from a cotton-tipped applicator, had attached itself to the eardrum and completely shielded it from view. Apparently, the abnormal appearance

of what was supposed to be an eardrum was the motive for all this therapy.

Secretory otitis media seems to be increasing in incidence, and its cause is not yet established. The condition is characterized by the accumulation of fluid in the middle ear, usually straw-colored and sometimes mucoid or gellike in consistency. In many instances this fluid is present even though the eustachian tube is patent, and there is no evidence of adenoid hypertrophy, or the adenoids have been removed. Fluid often accumulates in spite of numerous myringotomies and varied treatments. The hearing loss usually is greater in the higher frequencies, and occasionally there is even reduced bone conduction that may lead to a mistaken diagnosis of sensorineural deafness. The bone conduction is reduced by fluid in the middle ear, but hearing returns to normal when this fluid is removed. For some unexplained reason, secretory otitis generally is self-limiting and may disappear spontaneously, though the credit often is given to the drug used at that particular time. Occasionally, the secretion continues to form and causes a perforation in the eardrum that resists healing and leads to a mistaken diagnosis of chronic otitis media. However, the discharge is free of infectious elements, and no other sign of chronic otitis media is seen.

IN TREATING secretory otitis it is of the utmost importance to avoid unwarranted surgical procedures, particularly an adenoidectomy that is not indicated. It is unwise to perform a tonsillectomy and adenoidectomy on an infant with secretory otitis media without positive evidence that the adenoids are the principal cause of the difficulty.

OBSERVATION OF FLUID. In observing the eardrum in secretory otitis media, one often sees bubbles in a yellowish fluid behind the eardrum. Forcing air up the eustachian tube by politzerization usually shows the tube to be patent, and the fluid level shifts or even disappears while the hearing suddenly improves during this procedure. Only in the performance of myringotomy straw-colored fluid is observed issuing from the hole in the eardrum. Sometimes the appearance of the drum is deceiving: fluid may fill the ear to such an extent that it cannot be seen, and the middle ear may look normal. With air pressure, however, the intact eardrum does not move normally. The physician may miss the fluid level, even when it is present, if he examines the ear while the child is lying on the good ear; in that position the level cannot be seen. Therefore, the patient during examination should be sitting or standing.

HEARING TESTING BY THE OTOLOGIST

It is comparatively simple for the otologist to test the hearing of older children, because they are usually cooperative and give accurate responses to auditory signals. The situation is quite different with infants and young children who have little or no speech, especially if they may have developed some antisocial patterns. The otologist must perform a battery of tests and consider their results in conjunction with the history, particularly the developmental history and the physical examination. Several hearing tests can be performed to insure that the child's responses to auditory signals reliably reflect the level of the child's residual hearing. Such tests include the use of calibrated noisemakers, speech reception tests through calibrated equipment, psychogalvanic skin resistance tests, conditioning tests such as the peep-show technic and other special tests, including an EEG.

NOISEMAKERS

The otologist in most instances will perform the same tests with noisemakers as the referring physician already has done in his office. The otologist's noisemakers will be calibrated in both intensity and frequency, and he will spend a great deal of time repeating tests to insure the reliability of responses.

SPEECH RECEPTION TESTS

Speech tests generally require that the child have some language ability in order to give a response to the test material. In younger children the speech reception tests, that is, the ability of the child to hear speech rather than pure tones, are useful in obtaining thresholds of awareness. The child is placed in a quiet room and spoken to either through earphones, if he will accept them, or through a loudspeaker. The tester may be in an adjoining room, where he can control the loudness of his voice by means of calibrated equipment and watch the reaction of the child through an observation window. The child may put his hand to the earphone in which he hears the voice, he may cease his activity of play, or he may turn his head toward the loudspeaker in free field testing. We must point out again that a lack of response does not mean necessarily that the child does not hear.

PSYCHOGALVANIC SKIN RESISTANCE (PGSR) TEST

Most forms of auditory testing require the cooperation of the child giving subjective responses. In PGSR testing the active participation and cooperation of the child are not essential except that he must accept earphones and remain reasonably quiet. The services of at least two people experienced with children are required; one works directly with the child and tries to keep the examination from becoming an unpleasant experience, and the other examiner operates the equipment. The test is at present a most useful procedure in some children and infants who otherwise cannot be studied. Its reliability in proper hands has been established beyond doubt, but it is not always definitive in all children. It must be viewed as a supplementary test to be correlated with other findings rather than as a single test providing all of the information desired. The testers must be experienced with children and also aware of the electronic and the psychological pitfalls inherent in this technic.

In brief, the child is taught to accept a set of earphones on his head, two small electrodes on his fingers and another pair on his leg. He then is conditioned carefully so that each time sound is introduced into his ear, it is followed a second later by a mild shock to the calf of his leg. The shock must be almost imperceptible to the child and should not cause any obvious discomfort. The shock produces a change in sympathetic nerve activity, causing increased skin perspiration and reduced skin potential. The electrical effect is conducted from the finger electrodes to a recording device. When the child has been adequately conditioned, the shock is stopped except for reinforcement purposes, and the change in skin resistance continues in response to sound alone. In this manner, by reducing the intensity of the sound in the ear until at one level the skin resistance is affected and at a slightly weaker level it is not affected, it is possible to obtain a complete audiogram on most children.

Peep-Show

In this test the child is conditioned to press a button in response to a pure tone. When he does so, a light is turned on which illuminates pictures inside a box or a doll house. If the button or the switch is pressed without the child's having had an auditory stimulus, the light does not appear, and the visual reward is withheld. Other types of conditioning tests require the child to place a ring on a peg, to drop an object in a box, or to press a button on a battery-powered animated toy, all in response to pure tone stimulation. Responses made without auditory stimulation are not rewarded. These and other conditioning tests require that the child be emotionally, physically and intellectually able to cooperate, and the tests may be limited in usefulness for differential diagnosis in a small percentage of children.

Other Objective Tests

Brief mention should be made of two objective tests still in the developmental stage. These are the electroencephalogram and the electrocardiogram for assessing hearing acuity. It is expected that in time these procedures will be standardized and become part of the battery of tests used in evaluating a child's hearing level.

SCHOOL TESTING PROGRAMS

School hearing testing programs are assuming major importance in the early detection of hearing loss in children of school age. Some physicians mistakenly deprecate this work, because often they cannot confirm the presence or the absence of a hearing loss in a child by means of a conversational or a whispered voice test. This is most regrettable. Audiometry as used in these school tests is much more sensitive and exact in detecting early hearing defects than any voice test. Physicians therefore should be the first to understand the valuable preventive possibilities of these routine hearing tests.

The detection of early hearing changes often makes it possible to take corrective action and to prevent further deterioration, with all the serious problems that may follow such neglect.

If the pediatrician or the general practitioner is unable to find the cause of a hearing loss or to suggest proper treatment, it is his obligation to refer the child to an otologist or a hearing clinic that can provide the required services.

The pediatrician or the family doctor can render a valuable service by suspecting hearing losses in school children who are brought to him because they have been inattentive or do poorly at school, or have had repeated ear infections. Sometimes the parents wonder if their child hears normally. In such cases the hearing loss may well have reached a handicapping level. A careful history is of the utmost importance; this should include especially questions regarding the youngster's response to the spoken word.

It is advisable to perform an audiogram on all such children, but even in the absence of an audiometer a physician can obtain a wealth of information by means of simple tests with a 500-cps tuning fork and by speech tests, as by speaking softly into each ear and asking the child to repeat words or phrases that a normal child should be able to hear. If a child hears and repeats softly spoken phrases properly, he obviously hears, but it always must be borne in mind that many times children hear and yet do not respond. If it is assumed that the response is reliable, and the child fails to hear a soft voice, the physician then should use a 500-cycle tuning fork to determine whether the hearing loss is conductive or sensorineural.

THE TREATMENT OF HEARING LOSS

Most patients go to the physician for relief of pain or discomfort or to allay their fears of cancer, deformity or other serious disease. In contrast, a hearing loss is painless and rarely a direct threat to life or health. However, the social and the vocational connotations of impaired hearing are the driving forces that impel the adult patient to go to the physician. In the case of a child, the initiative almost never comes from the patient but usually from a teacher or the parents. When the thought occurs to them that the child may have a hearing handicap, they suddenly realize the serious social and economic implications of deafness and seek the physician's counsel.

It is true that physicians cannot actually cure the hearing loss in all cases. Certainly they are incapable of restoring hearing in cases of sensorineural deafness. However, the physician can tell the patient or his parents whether medicine or surgery will help him and, if not, he can mitigate greatly the social and the emotional consequences of deafness by available rehabilitative measures.

Without a doubt physicians can help to prevent unnecessary deafness by exercising care in the use of ototoxic drugs, particularly dihydrostreptomycin, neomycin and kanamycin. These drugs should be avoided in cases of urinary retention and kidney malfunction.

Families with prominent strains of deafness should be guided in their marriage plans. Pregnant women should be cautioned against vaccination and exposure to certain diseases, particularly rubella, during the early months of pregnancy. Anoxia in the newborn should be avoided meticulously by good obstetric management, and high fevers and convulsions in infants should receive prompt and intensive treatment.

Conductive Deafness

The conductive type of hearing loss is the more suitable for definitive medical treatment, and generally the loss can be cured completely or improved considerably. The following procedures may be indicated: adenoidectomy; eustachian tube inflation; treatment of otitis media, sinusitis or allergies; reconstructive surgery; tympanoplasty or stapes surgery.

In treating infections of the middle ears the physician should keep in mind the importance of intensive and prolonged antibiotic therapy, as well as the surgical principle of incision and drainage in those cases in which there is localized pus, as in an attack of acute otitis media with a bulging eardrum. Frequently, expert handling of such cases will prevent moderate degrees of conductive deafness. Similar emphasis should be placed on a careful adenoidectomy, when it is indicated. Just because a child has had a so-called tonsillectomy and adenoidectomy, it does not follow necessarily that hypertrophied adenoids may not be the cause of persistent ear symptoms and conductive hearing loss. It is essential that the adenoids be removed properly. There may be adenoid tissue left in vital areas behind the eustachian tubes, or a marked regrowth as in allergic children, or even extensive scar tissue and damage to the eustachian tubes from adenoidectomies performed without adequate exposure or without regard for anatomic structure.

Whenever the indications for mastoidectomy are to be evaluated, the hearing status must be given high priority. The type of operation performed should not only clear the infection but also preserve as much hearing as possible.

It is now possible also to close most perforated eardrums by tympanoplastic procedures and to improve hearing in many middle ears. The author has performed a number of these procedures successfully even in children.

The physician can prevent the important complications of hearing loss by forthrightly explaining the problems to the parents and assuming the role of guide and adviser to the parents and the child in their efforts to compensate and to adjust to the hearing handicap.

Sensorineural Deafness

In sensorineural deafness the pathologic process generally is irreversible. As yet there is no incontrovertible proof that any available therapy can restore the function of damaged sensorineural elements in the ear. Nevertheless, a great deal can be done to help children with handicapping deafness of this type, and in such cases the physician must assume a greater responsibility. It is essential to explain to the parents why medical or surgical treatment is presently ineffective, and why all efforts should be directed toward rehabilitation rather than toward a nonexistent cure that thus exposes the child to needless medical and surgical treatments.

First, the primary interest of the physician is not in how much hearing is lost. He is interested in how much hearing is left, and what can be done to help the child to use most efficiently the hearing that he has. We have found it unwise to tell a parent that her child has lost a certain percentage of his hearing. It is far more helpful to say that the child has lost some hearing, but that a certain quantity of hearing remains that can either be corrected medically or surgically or made much more useful with a hearing aid and special training procedures. The atmosphere that the physician creates should be positive rather than negative. The standard audiogram chart unfortunately records in decibels of hearing loss, but it is not advisable to explain it in such a negative manner to the patient and his family. The real purpose of all hearing tests is to determine how much hearing is present.

AUDITORY REHABILITATION

All youngsters with hearing loss severe enough to interfere with their ordinary communication should receive in addition to medical treatment some form of auditory rehabilitation if their auditory deficit cannot be corrected. Usually a 30- or 35-db hearing loss in the speech frequencies in the better ear or a marked high tone loss is considered to be sufficiently handicapping to interfere with communication. Such children must be taught to listen actively and to pay strict attention to all sounds. They must be instructed carefully in how to get the most out of their residual hearing. The early application of a hearing aid and training in its use often will demonstrate to hesitant parents the realistic value of this type of approach and prompt their wholehearted support and cooperation.

Hearing Aids. The hearing aid should be used with an individually molded earpiece placed in the ear that will give the child the most effective hearing. This may be in the worse- or the better-hearing ear, depending on the degrees and the types of hearing loss present. Bone conduction hearing aids have limited use and are suitable primarily for use in the presence of complete atresia of the ear canals or for chronically discharging ears.

When a diagnosis of deafness is established in an infant or a young child, the deafness usually will be of the sensorineural type, and amplification generally will be necessary.

The least possible delay should be permitted in making maximum use of the residual hearing. The author has used amplification in infants. Some children 2 years old have managed extraordinarily well with their own hearing aids. There is convincing evidence that even infants whose deafness is definitely irreversible will benefit from auditory amplification. This can be accomplished by the use of a loudspeaker system or by placing on the infant's head, when the mother speaks to him for any length of time, a helmet such as a pilot might use, with a built-in set of earphones. Exposure to the rhythm of music and the constant background of speech are important experiences for the infant and young child with a marked hearing loss. When an aid is fitted on the child, the parent should be encouraged to report the child's reactions and progress with amplification. In order to obtain maximum use of the aid, the parent should be constantly alert for any changes in the operation of the aid (the need for a new battery or adjustment, etc.).

Speech Reading and Auditory Training

In conductive hearing losses adequate compensation can be secured for the most part by amplification. However, in sensorineural losses amplification does not solve the problem of distortion, and the use of speech reading and auditory training should be added to amplification.

In speech reading training the basic goal is the strengthening of the powers of visual observation. This includes the coordination of lipreading with the interpretation of facial expressions, and an intuitive grasp of the conversational trend.

The child's responses to speech tests will determine largely the type of auditory training that he will need. In many cases the child will need auditory training before he is fitted with an individual hearing aid. He may need this training because he has developed poor listening habits. In any case, the object of this training is to teach him that sounds have meaning, and that sounds can be differentiated and identified. The specific goal is the development of fine discrimination for the sounds of speech.

National Organizations

There are at present too few facilities that can aid the infant or the pre-school child and his parents with the problems of deafness and speech development. Many more are needed. A number of national organizations can be of service in such cases, and the parents should be invited to write to them. Among the foremost are the John Tracy Clinic Correspondence Course, 806 West Adams Blvd., Los Angeles 7, Calif.; The American Hearing Society, 817 14th Street, N.W., Washington 5, D.C.; The Volta Bureau, 1537 35th Street, N.W., Washington 7, D.C., which also publishes an up-to-date list (reprint No. 788) of schools and classes for deaf children under 6. This list covers all 50 states and the provinces of Canada. The National Society for Crippled Children and Adults, 2023 West Ogden Ave., Chicago 10, Ill., can provide lists of literature on speech and hearing rehabilitation, as can The American Annals of the Deaf, Gallaudet College, Washington, D.C.

The American Academy of Ophthalmology and Otolaryngology, through its committee on Conservation of Hearing, has been endeavoring to educate both the public and the medical profession in the importance of early recognition and adequate treatment of the hard-of-hearing child. As an essential component of its program, it has urged the establishment of clinics throughout the country in which these cases could be cared for properly. In some states a really comprehensive program has been developed.

Regional Clinics

Though otologic services may be obtainable in the larger urban centers, the reverse is true for the predominantly rural areas. This emphasizes the need for regional clinics to which cases in these areas may be referred. Each clinic should provide a comprehensive service, including both medical and rehabilitative therapy. Detection clinics are helpful in screening cases found defective in group testing, but practical results come only from a program that actually provides the indicated treatment.

The Coordinator

More than in most handicaps, the hard-of-hearing child requires the integrated attention of **a team of specialists**. One person cannot possibly diagnose, treat, rehabilitate and guide the parents and the child in their efforts to overcome the communicative handicap imposed by deafness. It is the responsibility of the pediatrician to act as the coordinator of the team, which frequently includes the otologist, the audiologist, the speech therapist, the psychologist and even the psychiatrist, as well as social workers and others.

In brief, the physician who suspects the presence of hearing loss in a child should first refer the child for quantitative hearing tests and an accurate diagnosis of the cause of the deafness. He must then determine whether the hearing loss is curable and what measures are necessary to cure it as soon as possible. If the loss is irreversible, and a hearing aid can help, a suitable one and training in its use by an audiologist should be advised. Speech therapy should be given by a teacher who is well aware of the problems of deafness and knows how to use amplified sound. If there is a psychological problem, a trained psychologist should be asked for an evaluation.

Adjustment. The physician must always be available to guide and to support the parents and the child during the trying months of adjustment. He can and should make every effort to relieve the parents of any guilt they may feel in having produced a deaf or hard-of-hearing child. Instead, he can guide their emotional involvement into constructive channels by encouraging them to start auditory training early and to bring up the child in as normal an environment as possible, making the best use of all available methods of communication and utilizing most effectively the residual hearing of the child. The emotional stability of the child and his parents, and not merely the hearing problem, must receive farsighted attention.

Hearing defects in children and the problems of the hard-of-hearing child are basically problems in preventive pediatrics. Their solutions are within practical reach and depend to a great extent on the physician.

Recommended Reading

BOOKS

OTOLARYNGOLOGY

Ballenger, H. C.: Diseases of the Nose, Throat, and Ear, ed. 10, Philadelphia, Lea & Febiger, 1954.

Birrell, J. F.: The Ear, Nose, and Throat Diseases of Children, Philadelphia, Davis, 1960.

Boies, L. R., Hilger, J. A., and Priest, R. E.: Fundamentals of Otolaryngology, ed. 4, Philadelphia, Saunders, 1964.

Coates, G. M., *et al.*: Otolaryngology, Hagerstown, Md. (now Springfield, Ill.), Thomas, 1955.

DeWeese, D. D., and Saunders, W. H.: Textbook of Otolaryngology, St. Louis, Mosby, 1964.

Dolowitz, D. A.: Basic Otolaryngology, New York, McGraw-Hill, 1964.

Eggston, A. A., and Wolff, D.: Histopathology of the Ear, Nose, and Throat, Baltimore, Williams & Wilkins, 1947.

Goodhill, V.: Stapes Surgery for Otosclerosis, New York, Harper, 1961.

Hollender, A. R.: Office Practice of Otolaryngology, Philadelphia, Davis, 1965.

Jackson, C., and Jackson, C. L. (eds.): Diseases of the Nose, Throat, and Ear, Philadelphia, Saunders, 1959.

Korkis, F. B.: Recent Advances in Oto-Laryngology, Boston, Little, Brown, 1958.

Lederer, F. L., and Hollender, A. R.: Textbook of the Ear, Nose and Throat, Philadelphia, Davis, 1947.

Levin, N. M. (ed.): Voice and Speech Disorders: Medical Aspects, Springfield, Ill., Thomas, 1962.

Mawson, S. R.: Diseases of the Ear, Baltimore, Williams & Wilkins, 1963.

Morrison, W. W.: Diseases of the Ear, Nose, and Throat, New York, Appleton, 1948.

Portmann, G.: Diseases of the Ear, Nose, and Throat, Baltimore, Williams & Wilkins, 1961.

Reading, P. V.: Common Diseases of the Ear, Nose, and Throat, ed. 3, Boston, Little, Brown, 1961.

Ryan, R. E.: Synopsis of Ear, Nose, and Throat Diseases, ed. 2, St. Louis, Mosby, 1963.

Schuknecht, H. F. (ed.): Otosclerosis, Boston, Little, Brown, 1962.

Seltzer, A. P.: Ear, Nose and Throat for the General Practitioner, Springfield, Ill., Thomas, 1964.

Shambaugh, G. E., Jr.: Surgery of the Ear, Philadelphia, Saunders, 1959.

Williams, H. L.: Ménière's Disease, Springfield, Ill., Thomas, 1952.

Wilson, T. G.: Diseases of the Ear, Nose, and Throat in Children, ed. 2, New York, Grune & Stratton, 1962.

HEARING

American Industrial Hygiene Association: Industrial Noise Manual, ed. 2, Detroit, American Industrial Hygiene Association, 1966.

Audiometers for General Diagnostic Purposes, American Standards Association Bulletin (Z 24.5-19.51) New York, American Standards Association.

von Békésy, Georg: Experiments in Hearing, New York, McGraw-Hill, 1960.

Bunch, C. C.: Clinical Audiometry, St. Louis, Mosby, 1943.

Canfield, N.: Hearing, New York, Doubleday, 1959.

Davis, H., and Silverman, S. R. (eds.): Hearing and Deafness, rev. ed., New York, Holt, 1960.

Ewing, I. R., and Ewing, A. W. G.: New Opportunities for Deaf Children, London, University of London Press, 1958.

Fletcher, Harvey: Speech and Hearing in Communication, New York, Van Nostrand, 1953.

Glorig, A.: Audiometry—Principles and Practices, Baltimore, Williams & Wilkins, 1965.

Glorig, Aram, Jr.: Noise and Your Ear, New York, Grune & Stratton, 1958.

Hirsh, I. J.: The Measurement of Hearing, New York, McGraw-Hill, 1952.

Jerger, J. F. (ed.): Modern Developments in Audiology, New York, Academic Press, 1963.

Levine, E. S.: The Psychology of Deafness, New York, Columbia University Press, 1960.

Myklebust, H. R.: Auditory Disorders in Children, New York, Grune & Stratton, 1954.

———: The Psychology of Deafness, New York, Grune & Stratton, 1965.

Newby, H. A.: Audiology, ed. 2, New York, Appleton, 1964.

Rosenblith, W. A. (ed.): Sensory Communication, New York, Wiley and the M.I.T. Press, 1961.

Sataloff, Joseph: Industrial Deafness, New York, McGraw-Hill, 1957.

Stevens, S. S. (ed.): Handbook of Experimental Psychology, New York, Wiley, 1951.

Van Itallie, P. H.: How to Live With a Hearing Handicap, New York, Paul S. Eriksson, Inc., 1963.

Watson, L. A., and Tolan, T.: Hearing Tests and Hearing Instruments, Baltimore, Williams & Wilkins, 1949.

Wever, E. G., and Lawrence, Merle: Physiological Acoustics, Princeton, N. J., Princeton University Press, 1954.

PERIODICALS

Acta Oto-Laryngologica, Stockholm, Sweden

Annals of Otology, Rhinology and Laryngology

Archives of Otolaryngology

Eye, Ear, Nose and Throat Monthly

International Audiology, Leiden, Holland

Journal of the Acoustical Society of America

Journal of Auditory Research

Journal of Laryngology and Otology

Journal of Speech and Hearing Disorders

Journal of Speech and Hearing Research

Laryngoscope

Transactions of the American Academy of Ophthalmology and Otolaryngology

MONOGRAPHS AND SUPPLEMENTS

Guide for Conservation of Hearing in Noise, rev. ed., Los Angeles, Subcommittee on Noise of the Committee on Conservation of Hearing, and Research Center, Subcommittee on Noise, 1964; supplement to The Transactions of the American Academy of Ophthalmology and Otolaryngology.

House, W. F. (ed.): Transtemporal Bone Microsurgical Removal of Acoustic Neuromas, monograph, Arch. Otolaryng. *80*:6, 1964.

Index